Kinesiology for the Occupational Therapy Assistant

Essential Components of Function and Movement

THIRD EDITION

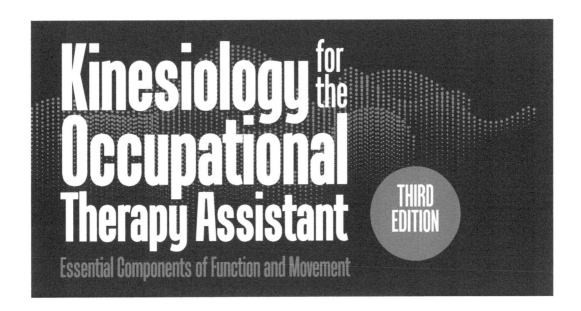

Kinesiology for the Occupational Therapy Assistant

Essential Components of Function and Movement

THIRD EDITION

Susan J. Sain, MS, OTR/L, FAOTA
Independent Contractor
Clinton, Tennessee

Carolyn L. Roller, OTR/L
Staff Occupational Therapist
OrthoTennessee
Knoxville, Tennessee

Jeremy L. Keough, MSOT, OTR/L, FAOTA
Staff Occupational Therapist
Blount Memorial Hospital
Maryville, Tennessee
(Lead Co-Author of the First and Second Editions)

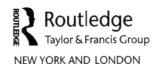
Routledge
Taylor & Francis Group

NEW YORK AND LONDON

Instructors: *Kinesiology for the Occupational Therapy Assistant: Essential Components of Function and Movement, Third Edition* includes ancillary materials specifically available for faculty use. Included are PowerPoints, chapter tests, and student study guides. Please visit www.routledge.com/9781638220336 to obtain access.

Jeremy L. Keough was the lead co-author of the First and Second Editions.

Cover photos taken by and reproduced with permission from Michelle Carr.

First published in 2024 by SLACK Incorporated

Published 2024 by Routledge
605 Third Avenue, New York, NY 10017
4 Park Square, Milton Park, Abingdon, Oxon OX14 4RN

Routledge is an imprint of the Taylor & Francis Group, an informa business

© 2024 Taylor & Francis Group

Library of Congress Cataloging-in-Publication Data
Names: Sain, Susan J., author. | Roller, Carolyn L., author. | Keough,
  Jeremy L. Kinesiology for the occupational therapy assistant.
Title: Kinesiology for the occupational therapy assistant : essential
  components of function and movement / Susan J. Sain, Carolyn L. Roller ;
  lead author of previous edition, Jeremy L. Keough.
Description: Third edition. | Thorofare, NJ : SLACK Incorporated, [2024] |
  "Lead author of previous edition, Jeremy L. Keough." | Includes
  bibliographical references and index.
Identifiers: LCCN 2023045821 (print) | ISBN 9781638220336 (paperback) |
Subjects: MESH: Occupational Therapy | Kinesiology, Applied--methods |
  Musculoskeletal Physiological Phenomena
Classification: LCC RM735.3 (print) | NLM WB 555 |
  DDC 615.8/515--dc23/eng/20231030
LC record available at https://lccn.loc.gov/2023045821

ISBN: 9781638220336 (pbk)
ISBN: 9781003524748 (ebk)

DOI:10.4324/9781003524748

Contents

Acknowledgments

We would all like to express sincere gratitude to the following for their invaluable assistance with preparing this text:

- All of our patients, past and present, for helping us to become better therapists.
- All of our students over the years, in the clinic and in the classroom, who have taught us so much.
- Our families for their love, support, patience, inspiration, and advice.

About the Authors

Susan J. Sain, MS, OTR/L, FAOTA, earned her undergraduate degree in Occupational Therapy from the University of Wisconsin at Madison, along with a degree in Spanish. She later earned a master's degree in Health Promotion/Health Education from the University of Tennessee at Knoxville. Her professional experiences include adult and child psychology, skilled nursing, pediatrics in a variety of settings, early intervention, and academia. Susan has instructed kinesiology for more than 20 years. She has served in a variety of volunteer positions for various state associations, the American Occupational Therapy Association, and the National Board for Certification in Occupational Therapy. Her current interests include aging in place, environmental psychology, and universal design.

Carolyn L. Roller, OTR/L, was an adjunct faculty member in the Occupational Therapy Assistant program at both Roane State Community College and South College, Tennessee, teaching kinesiology and physical dysfunction. She works pro re nata as a hand therapist for OrthoTennessee in Knoxville, Tennessee. Carolyn earned her undergraduate degree in Occupational Therapy from the University of Wisconsin at Milwaukee. Her professional experiences include outpatient rehabilitation, home and job site analysis, ergonomic considerations, and prevention of hand injuries in the wellness community.

Contributing Authors

Dana M. Howell, PhD, OTD, OTR/L, FAOTA (Chapter 12)
Department Chair and Foundation Professor
Eastern Kentucky University
Richmond, Kentucky

Matthew J. Sabin, PhD, LAT, ATC, SMTC, CIDN (Chapter 11)
Associate Chair
Department of PRESS
AT Program Director
Professor
Eastern Kentucky University
Richmond, Kentucky

Maribeth P. Vowell, PT, MPH, EdD (Chapters 5 and 6)
Professor of Physical Therapist Assistant Technology
Roane State Community College
Oak Ridge, Tennessee

Introduction

This text uses a top-down approach to encourage the reader to visualize how all the components of movement fit together and affect each other. This approach allows the student to see the big picture while helping them determine what underlying issues may be causing limitations. The top-down approach maximizes learning vs. memorizing detailed bits of information that later prove difficult to remember and apply in practice. In addition to identifying the underlying components that make movement possible, this text illustrates how kinesiology applies to functional movement and the client. The reader will gain insight into the practice of occupational therapy through solving problems and developing questions needed to assist the client to achieve movement-related goals in tasks, activities, and occupations. Gross range of motion and manual muscle testing are also introduced to further enable individual skill development. This text will refer to those who receive occupational therapy services as clients, following the terminology of the *Occupational Therapy Practice Framework: Domain and Process, Fourth Edition*.

We hope the reader will gain an understanding that movement is a complex symphony of body systems working in harmony. More importantly, we hope the reader is able to perceive how movement enables or hinders function and participation in daily activities and occupations. Information is provided at the occupational therapy assistant level.

This text is divided into 12 chapters to enhance learning of the study of movement.

Chapter 1, "Kinesiology: A Foundation in Occupational Therapy," summarizes kinesiology and how the study of movement applies in occupational therapy. Historical applications are referenced, as well as current influences of kinesiology within the profession. The *Occupational Therapy Practice Framework: Domain and Process, Fourth Edition* is also introduced to help unify chapter organization throughout the text. Client factors and activity demands are also discussed to build on the knowledge needed to identify movement in context.

Chapter 2, "Human Body Functions and Structures Influencing Movement," identifies anatomical features that impact movement. Body functions include skeletal, muscular, and neuromuscular functions. Body structures include specific topics regarding muscles, ligaments, and joints. Body functions are presented prior to body structures in each chapter to build on the top-down approach used in this text. This also helps to maintain the focus on function.

Chapter 3, "Factors Influencing Movement," and Chapter 4, "Introducing Body Movement," provide the basis for understanding movement. Information is presented to better explain how and why abnormal and normal movements occur. Factors are also identified that assist the reader in observing movement of interest to the occupational therapy assistant during engagement in activities, tasks, or occupations by the client.

Chapters 5 through 10 focus on the essential functions and movement of the trunk and neck, lower extremity, and upper extremity. Information is focused on specific areas relevant to the occupational therapy assistant with an overview of peripheral topics. Chapters 5 and 6 address the trunk and lower extremity as a basis for support during movement to allow the student to develop a system for assimilating information prior to progressing to the upper extremity. Chapters 7 through 10 focus on function of the upper extremity including topics on movement. Again, body functions are identified first followed by information related to body structures.

Chapter 11, "Kinesiology and Therapeutic Exercise," and Chapter 12, "Functional Mobility in the Home and Community," are additional chapters that highlight movement and function in daily life. Chapter 11 helps to identify therapeutic exercise implications within the healthy population as well as those in recovery. Chapter 12 helps to identify functional mobility in the home and community identifying considerations and adaptations that enable function.

Unique Features of This Kinesiology Text

Many unique features of this kinesiology text combine to provide an enhanced learning experience for the student and health care professional.

- Incorporates the *Occupational Therapy Practice Framework: Domain and Process, Fourth Edition.*

- Occupation- and life-based activities and questions at the end of each chapter.

- Boxes with additional key information.

- Occupational profiles to present applications to occupational therapy and epilogues that inform the reader of the outcome of each occupational profile.

- Implications of function across the lifespan.

- Written for the occupational therapy assistant student at the occupational therapy assistant level.

- Written by occupational therapy practitioners with more than 30 years of combined experience teaching kinesiology to occupational therapy assistant students.

- Addresses the American Occupational Therapy Association's *Blueprint for Entry-Level Education.*

- Helps meet Accreditation Council for Occupational Therapy Education Standards for occupational therapy assistant education.

- Changes and improves sequence of topics to enhance occupational therapy assistant learning.

- Enables range of motion and manual muscle testing to be incorporated in the course with the use of one book.

- Provides a top-down approach to learning with a focus on application of information vs. rote memorization.

- Allows for occupational therapy assistant program variability in teaching approach to meet the needs of biomechanical- to occupation-based programs and preferences of the instructor.

CHAPTER 1

Kinesiology
A Foundation in Occupational Therapy

Susan J. Sain, MS, OTR/L, FAOTA

Key Terms

activities

activities of daily living

activity limitation

areas of occupation

beliefs

biomechanical model

body functions

body structures

client factors

context

environmental factors

impairment

instrumental activities of daily living

kinesiology

kinetic model

locus of control

motivation

occupation

occupation and activity demands

orthopedic model

participation

participation restriction

performance patterns

performance skills

qualitative

quantitative

spirituality

values

Chapter Outline

Introduction

Foundations in Occupational Therapy

Educational Requirements Related to Kinesiology

National Board for Certification in Occupational Therapy

Historical Influences in Occupational Therapy

Engagement in Human Occupation

International Classification of Functioning, Disability and Health

Occupational Therapy Practice Framework: Domain and Process, Fourth Edition

Summary

References

Applications

Sain, S. J., & Roller, C. L. *Kinesiology for the Occupational Therapy Assistant: Essential Components of Function and Movement, Third Edition* (pp. 1-23).
© 2024 Taylor & Francis Group.

Chapter Objectives

After completion of this chapter, students should be able to:

1. Define key terminology.
2. Identify how kinesiology has influenced occupational therapy practice over time.
3. Understand how kinesiology relates to accreditation standards and initial certification expectations.
4. Organize influences that affect functional movement.
5. Analyze how functional movement is reflected in the *Occupational Therapy Practice Framework: Domain and Process, Fourth Edition*.
6. Compare and contrast the *Occupational Therapy Practice Framework: Domain and Process, Fourth Edition* with the *International Classification of Functioning, Disability and Health*.

BOX 1-1

KINESIOLOGY

"The study of the principles of mechanics and anatomy in relation to human movement."

(Merriam-Webster, n.d.)

Introduction

Kinesiology provides a foundation for studying human movement, but kinesiology alone is not enough to predict outcomes or engagement in **occupation**. Unfortunately, one area of study cannot fully and adequately describe how or why human **activities** occur. In order to better understand human movement and what motivates clients to engage in occupations, one must incorporate the study of many different interrelated constructs. Occupational therapy practitioners use information from various realms, such as physical, social, psychological, biomechanical, or motivational, and then apply this information to individuals and their unique situations to effect change. The multitude of variables to consider is endless; however, the *Occupational Therapy Practice Framework: Domain and Process, Fourth Edition* (OTPF-4) provides a method to identify and apply some of these important variables. To begin with, this chapter will review kinesiology's historical influences in occupational therapy education, including information from the Accreditation Council of Occupational Therapy Education (ACOTE). This will be followed by concepts from the World Health Organization's (WHO) *International Classification of Functioning, Disability and Health* (ICF). The correlation of these concepts to the OTPF-4 domains will be discussed. Next, an overview of how **motivation** impacts human movement will be presented, and, finally, the chapter will mention **occupation and activity demands** considered within the practice of occupational therapy.

Kinesiology incorporates the study of many different subjects in order to provide an understanding of movement. Anatomy, physiology, physics, calculus, and biomechanics all provide information to define or describe how movement occurs. Anatomy provides information on the body components that produce movement, which may include muscles, bones, and joints. Physiology describes the body systems and **body functions** that influence movement. Physics is the study of natural phenomena, such as matter and energy, and, accordingly, provides information to help understand how force, motion, and energy apply to movement. Calculus can be applied to general physics to explain how change occurs and, thus, quantify how movement occurs. Lastly, *biomechanics* refers to the application of mechanical principles to the human body making it directly relevant to kinesiology. A formal definition of kinesiology is provided in Box 1-1.

In addition to considering all of the areas mentioned previously, the therapy practitioner needs to determine the kind of information that would be most helpful. There are two primary types of information or data, **qualitative** and **quantitative**. Qualitative information includes information on movement that may come from observation or interview. Examples of qualitative information include movement analysis through observation, gross range of motion (ROM), gross manual muscle testing (MMT), or an interview of a client's perceived performance and desire to re-engage in occupations. A client's perceived quality of movement or amount of movement are also examples. Several factors may lead the therapist to choose a qualitative approach. A client may be observed performing **activities of daily living** (ADLs) or may be asked to move a certain way to identify preferred movement patterns and movements available to the client. A practitioner can also look for typical patterns of movement as well as deviations in movement patterns. Formal ROM evaluations may not be indicated, or a lack of time may necessitate a gross ROM or MMT observation. Another consideration may be impaired cognition that can hamper a client's ability to follow directions and complete a standardized assessment.

Quantitative information, on the other hand, identifies numerical data under standardized situations to gather information. Examples include obtaining formal ROM measurements with a goniometer, assessing formal MMT grade, standardized fine/gross motor assessments, or using a computer or video to analyze movement. Each method requires the practitioner to use a standardized procedure to gather data about the client. This provides objective information, often numerical, that can be assessed at a later date to identify change or progress toward occupational therapy goals. Standardized assessments often provide client-specific information that can be compared to a population. The complexity of deciding what is important to include in the analysis of movement and how to obtain this information is one reason why kinesiology can be considered one of the hardest courses of study.

As the profession of occupational therapy and the application of kinesiology have changed over time, both have become more holistic, returning interest to the qualitative characteristics of movement and occupation. Descriptions on qualitative and quantitative approaches can be expressed in much more detail than this text allows; however, important information will be identified that is needed for entry-level practice as an occupational therapy assistant. A review of the historical connections between occupational therapy and kinesiology will provide a link to understanding current occupational therapy practice characteristics.

Foundations in Occupational Therapy

Educational Requirements Related to Kinesiology

Occupational therapy practitioners have used kinesiology as a tool for change since the inception of the profession. While the emphasis on kinesiology has changed over the years, the importance of understanding movement and its influence in therapy has remained constant. Kinesiology has always been one of the basic sciences included in occupational therapy training programs. One way to examine

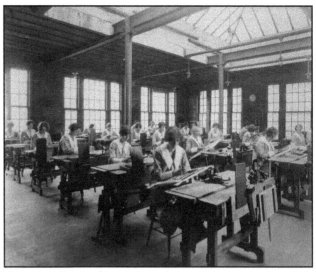

Figure 1-1. Picture of BSOT. (Reproduced with permission from Tufts University, Digital Collections and Archives, Medford, MA.)

the emphasis on kinesiology can be found by looking at the training requirements over time for occupational therapy practitioners.

At the start of the profession, during World War I, reconstruction aides were established to meet the rehabilitative needs of returning injured soldiers. Reconstruction aides could specialize in either physical therapy or occupational therapy. Kinesiology was one of the lectures provided during the training programs for reconstruction aides specializing in occupational therapy (United States Federal Board for Vocational Education [USFBVE],1918). Following World War I, the American Occupational Therapy Association (AOTA) adopted standards for occupational therapy courses in 1923. These standards are reflected in an April 15, 1929 flier describing the Boston School of Occupational Therapy (BSOT; 1929). Figure 1-1 shows students in the classroom at the BSOT in 1925. Courses covering medical, social services, and craft study were provided by the school. Medical study involved subjects such as anatomy, kinesiology, hygiene, and physiology.

In 1935, the essentials of an accredited school in occupational therapy were established by the Council on Medical Education and Hospitals of the American Medical Association in collaboration with AOTA. Again, kinesiology was identified as a required subject listed under the biological sciences (Willard & Spackman, 1947). Kinesiology remained a requirement when the essentials were revised in 1949. Interestingly, kinesiology was viewed as important enough to be included in the first occupational therapy master's degree program at the University of Southern California in 1947 (*American Journal of Occupational Therapy*, 1947). A course listed as advanced kinesiology was included for 2 of the 31 credit hours required to graduate.

The essentials remained consistent until the next major revisions were adopted in 1973. One of the changes that was incorporated in this revision was that course content and

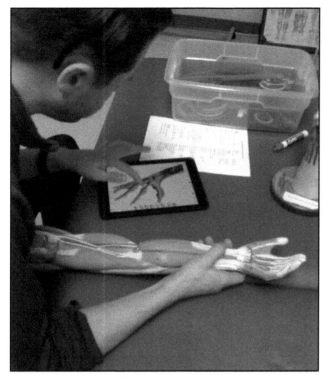

Figure 1-2. Occupational therapy assistant student.

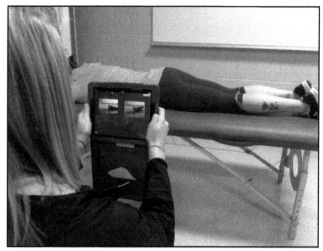

Figure 1-3. Future occupational therapy assistants.

practice as identified by the National Board for Certification in Occupational Therapy (NBCOT) also reflects the role of kinesiology in occupational therapy.

National Board for Certification in Occupational Therapy

The ACOTE educational standards clarified in the "2018 ACOTE Standards and Interpretive Guide" can be compared to the picture of entry-level practice identified by NBCOT. NBCOT provides the national certification examination that identifies whether minimum standards of knowledge and competency are achieved as an entry-level occupational therapy assistant. Entry-level practice, as related to NBCOT exam creation, is described as an occupational therapy assistant up to the third year of practice. To identify entry-level competencies, NBCOT collects information on current practice through a practice analysis. The most recent analysis and competencies were established in 2017 (NBCOT, 2018).

Entry-level practice presented by NBCOT is described by hierarchical components that include domain areas, task statements, and knowledge statements (NBCOT, 2018). Domain areas identify the major performance components of the profession. Task statements indicate activities performed in the domain area. Knowledge statements describe the minimum knowledge required to perform each task. The components of entry-level practice relevant to knowledge of kinesiology that correspond with the ACOTE accreditation standards and NBCOT domains are presented in Table 1-2. ACOTE standards that are relevant to kinesiology are identified in the column on the right while their corresponding NBCOT domains are identified in the left column.

The ACOTE accreditation standards and the NBCOT practice analysis highlight necessary components of the current practice of occupational therapy. The use of kinesiology

hourly requirements were replaced with terminal behavioral objectives (Huss, 1981). There have been many additional revisions to the essentials or standards since 1973. The most recent accreditation standards for occupational therapy assistant programs continue to present requirements stated through terminal behavioral objectives. These standards were established by ACOTE of AOTA in 2018 and were clarified in the "2018 ACOTE Standards and Interpretive Guide" (AOTA, 2018). Figures 1-2 and 1-3 present images of students studying kinesiology in the occupational therapy assistant program at Roane State Community College in contrast to the 1925 picture at the BSOT.

Terminal behavioral objectives reflect what the occupational therapy assistant student should be able to demonstrate upon completion of an occupational therapy assistant program in preparation for becoming an occupational therapy assistant. Some terminal behavioral objectives from the "2018 Accreditation Standards for Educational Programs" for the occupational therapy assistant are identified in Table 1-1. As seen in the table, these terminal behaviors apply to education and learning provided by a course in kinesiology.

While educational standards for occupational therapy have changed over time, the basic science of kinesiology has remained a constant foundation in the educational preparation of the occupational therapy assistant. Understanding the terminal behavioral objectives that apply to a kinesiology course will enhance learning and aid in comprehending how kinesiology fits within occupational therapy. Entry-level

TABLE 1-1

Terminal Behavior Objectives Relevant to Occupational Therapy Assistant Education of Kinesiology

STANDARD	DESCRIPTION	APPLICATION TO KINESIOLOGY COURSE
B.1.1	Demonstrate knowledge of the structure and function of the human body to include the biological and physical sciences, neurosciences, kinesiology, and biomechanics.	Entire course
B.4.4	Contribute to the evaluation process of clients' occupational performance, including an occupational profile, by administering standardized and nonstandardized screenings and assessment tools and collaborating in the development of occupation-based intervention plans and strategies. Explain the importance of using psychometrically sound assessment tools when considering client needs, and cultural and contextual factors to deliver evidence-based intervention plans and strategies. Intervention plans and strategies must be client centered, culturally relevant, reflective of current occupational therapy practice, and based on available evidence.	Ability to administer assessments such as ROM, MMT, and client interview
B.4.24	Demonstrate effective intraprofessional occupational therapist/ occupational therapy assistant collaboration to explain the role of the occupational therapy assistant and occupational therapist in the screening and evaluation process.	Ability to relay assessment parameters and information to the client

Adapted from American Occupational Therapy Association. (2018). 2018 Accreditation Council for Occupational Therapy Education (ACOTE®) standards and interpretive guide. *American Journal of Occupational Therapy, 72*(Suppl. 2), 7212410005p1–7212410005p83. https://doi.org/10.5014/ajot.2018.72S217

TABLE 1-2

Corresponding Entry-Level Practice Descriptions Relevant to Kinesiology Between NBCOT and ACOTE

NBCOT CLASSIFICATION CODE	NBCOT DOMAIN COVERING TASK, KNOWLEDGE, AND SKILL STATEMENTS	CORRESPONDING ACOTE STANDARD *(Not all inclusive)*
Domain 1	Assist the registered occupational therapist to acquire information regarding factors that influence occupational performance on an ongoing basis throughout the occupational therapy process.	B.1.1, B.1.4, B.2.1, B.3.2, B.3.5, B.3.6, B.4.0, B.4.5, B.4.6, B.4.9,
Domain 2	Implement interventions under the supervision of the registered occupational therapist in accordance with the intervention plan and level of service competence to support client participation in areas of occupation throughout the occupational therapy process.	B.1.1, B.2.1, B.3.2, B.3.5, B.3.6, B.4.0, B.4.4, B.4.6, B.4.9, B.4.10, B.4.11, B.4.12, B.4.13, B.4.14
Domain 3	Uphold professional standards and responsibilities by achieving service competence and applying evidence-based interventions to promote quality in practice.	B.1.4, B.2.1, B.3.7, B.4.4, B.4.5, B.4.6

Adapted from National Board for Certification in Occupational Therapy. (2018) Content outline for the COTA exam (based on the results of the 2017 practice analysis). https://www.nbcot.org/-/media/PDFs/2017_COTA_Outline.pdf

TABLE 1-3
Kinesiological Influences During Various Eras of Occupational Therapy

ERA	INFLUENCE
1900s to 1920s	Reconstruction and curative era
1930s to 1950s	Reductionistic era and orthopedic model
1950s to 1970s	Medical era and kinetic model
1970s to present	Occupation era and biomechanical model

in the profession of occupational therapy can be identified as one of these components; however, this does not provide a more in-depth description of how occupational therapy assistants apply the knowledge of kinesiology to daily practice. The OTPF-4 does describe in greater detail how kinesiology is applied in occupational therapy, but, first, a look at the history of the profession may help to provide greater insight into current practice trends.

Historical Influences in Occupational Therapy

The current applications of kinesiology in occupational therapy can be identified over the past century by looking at prior trends in practice. While historical practice of occupational therapy may not be reflective of present practice settings, core components can be identified that remain true today as well as in the past. Trends can be grouped together based on consistent variables, such as the influence of kinesiology in the profession of occupational therapy. The particular trends involving kinesiology in the practice of occupational therapy (Table 1-3) can be broken down into eras ranging from the 1900s to 1920s, 1930s to 1950s, 1950s to 1970s, and 1970s to present. Although various authors subdivide the years from the 1970s until present into different eras of occupational therapy (i.e., evolution of the profession, evidence-based practice, occupational science, and the new millennium), the influence of kinesiology during those eras did not change significantly, thus they will not be presented separately here.

The profession of occupational therapy emerged at the start of the 20th century during the reconstruction and curative era. The moral treatment movement in the 1800s identified a need to provide a higher quality of life for individuals in institutions. As a result, occupational therapy emerged in mental health institutions to enhance individual engagement through craftwork and therapeutic activities. While aspects of kinesiology were not specifically addressed, movement considerations were identified as aspects to consider

in craftwork. Specifically, strength was mentioned 10 times, coordination 3 times, and endurance 1 time throughout the first textbook in the study of occupational therapy, *Studies in Invalid Occupations: A Manual for Nurses and Attendants*, written by Susan Tracy (1910).

With the start of World War I, the professions of occupational therapy and physical therapy emerged as reconstruction aides to provide interventions for injured soldiers. Interventions by reconstruction aides in occupational therapy not only targeted psychological disorders but also the physical disabilities of returning injured soldiers. General exercise, exercises of certain parts of the body, and kinesiology were identified as techniques of occupational therapy in the book *Training for Teachers for Occupational Therapy for the Rehabilitation of Disabled Soldiers and Sailors* (USFBVE, 1918). Reconstruction aides began to consider the available ROM for specific limbs. Surgeons prescribing "work" in occupational therapy also considered specific joints or muscles (Greene & Roberts, 2005; USFBVE, 1918). Occupational therapy became more and more accepted as beneficial for individuals with mental and physical disabilities through the provision of curative occupations.

Throughout the 1920s, the importance of curative occupations continued to grow in occupational therapy. Emphasis was placed on finding specifically chosen, purposeful activities for intervention instead of random activities or "busy work." Sands (1928) was able to express this newfound emphasis in her article, "When is Occupation Curative?" She suggested that if work was to be called occupational therapy, then it should be curative, and that the physical objective of curative work was to strengthen weak muscles. She also recommended that joint measurements should be taken, record keeping should be improved, and the use of haphazard occupations should be discouraged. By the end of the 1920s, the art of craftwork and activities most commonly applied at the start of the century were enhanced with the considerations of anatomy and kinesiology. Clearly, a broader influence of the medical field was beginning to take root in occupational therapy.

Occupational therapy gained further acceptance within the medical community over the next several decades from the 1930s to 1950s. Occupational therapy adopted rational inquiry, as did the medical field, which encouraged a reductionistic approach to treatment (Kielhofner & Burke, 1977). This approach encouraged scientific efforts and attempted to identify all therapeutic components that were the most beneficial in treatment, even to the smallest element. Occupational therapy strengthened ties within the medical community, and the medical community encouraged occupational therapy to further address the motor deficits accompanying physical disabilities (Kielhofner & Burke, 1977). Occupational therapy responded with the development of the **orthopedic model**, among other models, to address motor impairments (Greene & Roberts, 2005; Haworth & Macdonald, 1940).

The orthopedic model took into consideration anatomy, physiology, pathology, and kinesiology in addressing client **impairments** and disabilities. Activities, or occupations,

BOX 1-2

ORTHOPEDIC MODEL

"If the occupational therapist intends to re-educate joints and muscles to perform certain movements it is obvious that she must know something of the structure of joints and the way in which movements are normally produced. A knowledge therefore of anatomy and physiology, of the structure of, and movements performed by, each joint and of the muscles and groups of muscles used in each movement is essential."

(Haworth & Macdonald, 1940, p. 68)

BOX 1-3

KINETIC MODEL

"The aim of Occupational Therapy in the treatment of physical injuries is threefold (1) improve the motion of joints and the strength of muscles, (2) develop coordination, motor skills and work tolerance, (3) prevent building up of unwholesome psychological reactions."

(Willard & Spackman, 1947, p. 168)

were selected depending on the desired movements. Greater care was also undertaken to record client information, number of treatments, results, and remarks. Haworth and Macdonald (1940) provided information on how to apply the orthopedic model, part of which is displayed in Box 1-2. Unfortunately, at the time, few texts and journals were available to further refine this approach, which slowed the development and sharing of professional information.

Following World War II, occupational therapy continued its development within the medical era, and the profession further refined an approach to treating physical disabilities with the **kinetic model** (Greene & Roberts, 2005; Licht, 1950; Willard & Spackman, 1947). This era lasted roughly from 1950 to 1970. The kinetic model provided the basis for future kinesiological approaches to treatment. The first edition of *Willard and Spackman's Principles of Occupational Therapy*, published in 1947, provided three aims of treatment for physical disabilities, which are presented in Box 1-3. Kinesiology was mentioned six times in the text and significant space was provided to address ROM limitations.

Increased availability of texts and literature in occupational therapy supported the use of kinesiology in treating physical disabilities. The *American Journal of Occupational Therapy* printed several articles on joint measurement in 1947 and 1948. Licht (1950) also provided significant information on how to apply the kinetic model. He identified influential variables of the kinetic model to be cycle of motion, types of muscle contractions, joint range, starting position, realism, and tool variants. Increased scientific efforts and reductionism in the 1950s and 1960s further refined the use of

kinesiology in occupational therapy. By the third edition of *Willard and Spackman's Occupational Therapy*, 72 pages were provided to describe the restoration of physical function in further depth and clarity (Spackman, 1963).

Renewed interest in occupation re-emerged in the 1970s, and the **biomechanical model** emerged as a popular model for addressing **activity limitations** due to impairments in **body structure** and body functions. The biomechanical model is a restorative approach that attempts to isolate and remediate impairments in body structure and function with the end result of improving occupational performance (James, 2003). Kinesiology is important to help understand and apply this model. This model is commonly used in occupational therapy as it fits well in today's medical clinics and medical model to effect quick change in therapy for physical disabilities. The biomechanical model is not a holistic approach; however, it can be used effectively and efficiently in conjunction with other treatment approaches. It is important to remember that reducing the client's problems to the smallest component does not always efficiently or effectively address the complexity of human impairments and disabilities.

Kinesiology is one of the basic medical sciences important to occupational therapy practitioners working in the medical model. It is also a common technique used by occupational therapy practitioners to address client limitations and disabilities.

Kinesiology provides a structured method of observation to understand human movement. The OTPF-4 can provide a better grasp of how kinesiology is used in the current practice of occupational therapy.

Engagement in Human Occupation

Describing human nature and behavior can be a daunting task. Perhaps the first thing to reflect on is, "What comprises human occupation?" **Occupation** has individual and unique meanings for each person. In its basic form, occupation can be considered what people do to occupy their time. An occupation can be defined as anything from rest to sleep to work, incorporating everything that occurs throughout the day. Many people define themselves by their occupations or individual daily activities. These chosen pursuits reflect who we are. The anthropologist Bateson (1996) wrote, "The capacity to do something useful for yourself or others is key to personhood" (p. 11). Given its importance, occupation cannot simply be reduced to its mechanics or kinesiology alone. Sociological, cultural, emotional, and psychological domains all play important roles in what we engage in and how we perform the occupations of our choosing.

The OTPF-4 gives occupational therapy practitioners a structure to identify the mechanics of movement while still considering other aspects of occupation. The OTPF is published by AOTA and provides guidelines for the practice of occupational therapy. The most recent revision of the OTPF was adopted in 2020. The format and language of this kinesiology text are based on the 2020 official OTPF-4 document.

International Classification of Functioning, Disability and Health

The OTPF-4 is derived from the ICF, endorsed May 22, 2001 (WHO, 2008). WHO is a global health organization within the United Nations that promotes the health of all people as a basic and fundamental human right. WHO (2020) adopts a broad definition of health as, "a state of complete physical, mental and social well-being and not merely the absence of disease or infirmity." The practice of occupational therapy as reflected in the OTPF-4 embraces this definition of health. The ICF is an international standard used to define and assess health and disability. The most recent comprehensive revision of this document, accepted in 2001, demonstrates a radically different view of disability that moves focus away from a purely medical or biological perspective. All aspects that may contribute to disability, such as societal attitudes, **context**, and environment, are recognized. This holistic perspective is also a hallmark of occupational therapy.

The attitude presented in the ICF suggests that having a disease or diagnosis does not necessarily indicate a disability or a decrease in function. A person may have a diagnosis yet function perfectly well. Conversely, a person may not have any diagnosis or medical condition yet fail to function adequately. Contextual factors, such as societal views on illness or disability, and **environmental factors** may impact, positively or negatively, a person's level of functioning. Disability now becomes viewed as a universal human experience affecting all people. This paradigm shift moves the responsibility from the individual alone to society as a whole. Society becomes responsible for allowing an individual's condition to become a disabling factor or not. In an article describing the meaning of therapy and the virtues of occupation, Englehardt (1977) stated, "people are healthy or diseased in terms of the activities open to them or denied them" (p. 672). In other words, societal attitude, context, and environment can enable or disable a person.

The ICF is divided into three sections: body, activities and **participation**, and environmental factors. The section on body includes body functions and body structures organized according to major anatomical divisions, such as cardiovascular, neuromuscular, skin, sensory, mental, speech, digestive, and genitourinary. Activities and participation includes broader categories that involve actions a person is capable of performing based on body functions and structures. Examples include learning and applying knowledge, communication, mobility, self-care, community, social, and civic life. Environmental factors span a wide range from the natural and human-made environment to things such as attitudes of people, services, systems, policies, and technology (WHO, 2002). The OTPF-4 also reflects these categories.

Body functions and body structures have historically been addressed by medical or rehabilitative models using the principles of kinesiology. The reductionistic approach in the medical model proposes that if the impairments are corrected or improved, function will also improve. This approach, however, does not address the multitude of contextual and environmental factors and furthermore places too much emphasis on the individual.

Contextual and environmental factors are addressed by social models. The social model looks at disability as a socially or environmentally created problem, wherein the physical environment and social or cultural attitudes create the disability by lack of access or acceptance. In the social model, the responsibility for, or cause of, the disability is taken off of the individual and placed on society. This model pays little attention to the disease or disability that may exist. Refer to Table 1-4 for a comparison of these models.

As neither the medical nor social model fully captures the nature of disability or functioning, a third model is used in the ICF. This model, known as the *biopsychosocial model*, attempts to merge the medical and social models, incorporating the strengths of each model. The biopsychosocial model was introduced by George Engel in 1977. His model interconnects biological, psychological, and sociological fields and applies them to health and illness. The shift in focus is toward health and functioning, incorporating all domains, rather than using diagnosis alone as a predictor of success or engagement in occupation. The philosophy reflected in the OTPF-4 is aligned with this holistic approach to health and functioning.

TABLE 1-4
Comparison of the Medical Model and Social Model

	MEDICAL MODEL	SOCIAL MODEL
Cause of disability	Diagnosis or disease	Environmental barriers, social stigma, lack of support system
Responsible party	Individual	Society
Treatment, care given to address disability	Surgery, medication, individual therapy	Environmental modifications, policy change, legislation, change of societal perceptions
Disability primarily affects	Individual, family	Community, social system or groups, society as a whole

BOX 1-4

Impairments are defined as "problems in body function or structure such as a significant deviation or loss."
Activity is defined as "the execution of a task or action by an individual."
Activity limitations are defined as "difficulties an individual may have in executing activities."
Participation is defined as "involvement in a life situation."
Participation restrictions are defined as "problems an individual may have in executing activities."

(WHO, 2002)

The ICF identifies three levels of human functioning: body or body part, the whole person, and the person in context of the society in which they live. These levels coincide with levels of dysfunction labeled impairment (body part, function or structure), activity limitation (individual level or whole person, difficulty carrying out activities), and **participation restriction** (societal, difficulty engaging in life activities). Refer to the definitions in Box 1-4.

A person may have impairments in a body part, but this may or may not translate into an activity limitation or restriction in social participation. An impairment example at the body part level would be scarring from a severe burn, which may cause limitations in activity or social participation. The person may be physically able to engage in any occupation of their choice, therefore demonstrating no activity limitation; however, actual participation may be reduced or denied due to societal stigma and unacceptance of someone who looks different. This would result in participation impairments at the societal level. Conversely, a child with a lower extremity amputation, which is a body part impairment, may be provided with a prosthesis and encouraged to interact as any other child. In this case, there are no activity or participation limitations. Additionally, it is possible to have activity or participation restrictions without having an impairment of the body or a body part. A person may be diagnosed with HIV, but not currently have any symptoms or impairments affecting the body level. The person, however, may be limited in activity or denied social participation because of social or cultural stereotyping or stigmatization. This situation creates a restriction at the societal/participation level in the absence of body level impairment. Table 1-5 depicts how impairments, activity limitations, and participation restrictions relate to certain conditions.

Although the focus of this kinesiology text will be on the categories of body function and body structure, as well as the study of movement as it relates to the practice of occupational therapy, one cannot ignore the other factors that contribute to health and functioning. As occupational therapy practitioners, we are called to use a holistic approach, addressing all domains while treating the total person. The OTPF-4 helps to identify the other factors contributing to health and functioning.

TABLE 1-5
Levels of Dysfunction to Body Level Impairments

CONDITION	IMPAIRMENT (Body/Body Part)	ACTIVITY LIMITATION (Individual)	PARTICIPATION RESTRICTION (Societal)
Severe facial burn	Yes	None	Yes—due to society not accepting how person looks
Lower extremity amputation	Yes	Maybe—gait, sports	No—school, playground, community activities all accessible
HIV positive	No	Maybe	Yes—denied insurance or services, denied access to certain community activities due to fear and stereotypes

Occupational Therapy Practice Framework: Domain and Process, Fourth Edition

The original *Occupational Therapy Practice Framework: Domain and Process* was developed to define occupational therapy's perspectives and contributions to health and participation. This document is reviewed every 5 years to determine if it is still relevant and current to the practice of occupational therapy. The second edition (OTPF-2) evolved to serve as a guide to the practice of occupational therapy and was designed to help organize and delineate occupational therapy services in a uniform manner that is understood by all practitioners. The OTPF-3 was created to further define the vision of the profession of occupational therapy as "occupation based, client centered, contextual, and evidence based" (AOTA, 2014, p. S3). As with the other revisions, the OTPF-4 delineates emerging concepts and changes within the profession of occupational therapy along with modifying language to better reflect WHO taxonomy. Additionally, OTPF-4 identifies the cornerstones of occupational therapy practice (core values rooted in occupation, therapeutic use of occupation, professional behaviors, and therapeutic use of self) as well as increasing the focus on the transactional relationship between client, occupation, and context in intervention. Occupational therapy's focus on function aligns with the WHO's view of health. The classifications and language of the ICF, recognized by health care professionals worldwide, were originally adopted for use in the OTPF-2 and remain in use in the OTPF-4. Table 1-6 demonstrates the parallels between the OTPF-4 and the ICF.

The OTPF-4 identifies those who receive occupational therapy services as *clients*. Clients are defined as persons, groups, or populations. The category labeled *persons* refers not only to an individual receiving occupational therapy services but to their family and caregivers as well. Individuals involved with the client, such as teachers, employers, or any other relevant person are also included at the person level. *Groups* refers to a collection of individuals, such as families or students. The largest category for clients is populations. *Populations* include various people either living in or sharing similar situations (e.g., residents of the same city, refugees, people with chronic health conditions, or older adults; AOTA, 2020). For the purposes of this kinesiology textbook, emphasis will be on the persons or individual level. Additionally, this text will refer to anyone receiving occupational therapy services as *client* in accordance with the language of the OTPF-4.

The OTPF-4 is divided into two sections: domain and process. The *domain* section outlines areas of knowledge and expertise that pertain to occupational therapy. All aspects of the domain are interrelated and are of equal importance. The areas of the domain encompass building blocks that come together so that a client can engage in an activity or occupation of choice. As delineated in the OTPF-4, the domain of occupational therapy includes occupations, contexts, **performance patterns**, **performance skills**, and **client factors**. Table 1-7 delineates these in a visual format. The OTPF-4 section labeled *process* describes the steps involved in providing services to the client. The process of occupational therapy includes evaluation, intervention, and targeted outcomes. Table 1-8 outlines features of the process of intervention that are more directly related to kinesiology and its applications. The two sections, domain and process, are designed to be used together to guide therapy and enhance client engagement in occupation. Information gathered regarding the client from all components of the domain is used purposely to plan the therapy process, including interventions. During the intervention process, the occupational therapy practitioner's expertise in activity and occupational analysis comes into play. As part of this skill set, the practitioner analyzes demands for client-valued activities and occupations.

TABLE 1-6

Similarities of the OTPF-4 and the ICF

OTPF-4 DOMAIN (D) AND PROCESS (P)	ICF BODY FUNCTIONS AND STRUCTURES	ICF ACTIVITY	ICF PARTICIPATION	ICF CONTEXTUAL FACTORS
Occupations (D)		X	X	X
Contexts (D)		X	X	X
Performance patterns (D)	X	X	X	X
Performance skills (D)	X	X	X	X
Client factors (D)	X	X	X	X
Occupation and activity demands (P)	X	X	X	X

TABLE 1-7

Aspects of Occupational Therapy's Domain

OCCUPATIONS	CONTEXTS	PERFORMANCE PATTERNS	PERFORMANCE SKILLS	CLIENT FACTORS
• ADLs* (includes sexual activity) • IADLs • Health management (new category) • Rest and sleep • Education • Work • Play • Leisure • Social participation (includes intimate partner relationships)	• Environmental factors • Personal factors	• Habits • Routines • Roles • Rituals	• Motor skills • Process skills • Social interaction skills	• Values, beliefs, and spirituality • Body functions • Body structures

*Also referred to as basic activities of daily living (BADLs) or personal activities of daily living (PADLs).

Adapted from the American Occupational Therapy Association. (2020). Occupational therapy practice framework: Domain and process (4th ed.). *American Journal of Occupational Therapy, 74*(Suppl. 2), Article 7412410010. https://doi.org/10.5014/ajot.2020.74S2001

The domain labeled occupations includes a broad spectrum of activities. These range from getting up and performing morning routines to attending school or contributing at work. Occupations can also include what one chooses to do during free time. General categories in the domain of occupations include ADLs, **instrumental activities of daily living** (IADLs), health management, rest and sleep, education, work, play, leisure, and social participation (AOTA, 2020). A specific activity may fit under a variety of occupational areas. How the individual categorizes an activity is based on personal values that may change over time. Not all people will categorize activities similarly. Some people will put an activity in one **area of occupation**, while others will place the same activity in a different occupational area. This is understandable because different activities mean different things to different people. One person might view cooking as the area of occupation labeled work while another might place cooking in the category of leisure activity or social participation. Likewise, one individual might consider cleaning an IADL while another may consider it relaxation or leisure. Box 1-5 defines key terms related to activity and occupational analysis as well as some areas of occupation.

TABLE 1-8

Aspects of Occupational Therapy's Process: Selected Types of Occupational Therapy Interventions

OCCUPATIONS AND ACTIVITIES— ACTIVITY DEMANDS	INTERVENTIONS TO SUPPORT OCCUPATIONS
• Relevance and importance to the client • Objects used and their properties • Space demands • Social demands • Sequencing and timing • Required actions and performance skills • Required body functions • Required body structures	• Preparatory methods • Splints • Preparatory tasks • Physical agent and mechanical modalities • Orthotics and prosthetics • Assistive technology and environmental modifications • Wheeled mobility • Self-regulation

Adapted from the American Occupational Therapy Association. (2020). Occupational therapy practice framework: Domain and process (4th ed.). *American Journal of Occupational Therapy, 74*(Suppl. 2), Article 7412410010. https://doi.org/10.5014/ajot.2020.74S2001

BOX 1-5

Activity analysis: Generic analysis to help understand the typical requirements of specific components of activities. An **activity** is objective and not related to a specific client, but does support the development of performance skills and patterns leading to engagement in occupations.

Occupational analysis: More specific than activity analysis, considers the specific client as well as the client's chosen occupations and the contexts surrounding the occupation. Occupations are personalized activities that are meaningful to the individual's life.

Activities of daily living (ADLs): Self-care tasks performed to take care of one's body, such as bathing, brushing teeth, dressing, eating, bowel and bladder functions, and mobility, and are completed on a daily basis.

Instrumental activities of daily living (IADLs): More complex tasks than ADLs, IADLs support daily life and may occur in the community as well as the home. Examples include caring for pets or other people, financial management, meal preparation, shopping, and home management.

Health management: Occupations focused on creating and practicing routines for health and wellness that support participation in other occupations.

(AOTA, 2020)

Participation in occupations is influenced by the various facets of the domain titled contexts. Contexts describe environmental and personal factors impacting function. Human activities do not take place in a vacuum, and all actions are modified and molded by the surroundings in which they occur. Contexts impact the occupations available to an individual and whether or not they will become engaged. Environmental factors, which tend to be external to the person, are traditionally used to depict the physical or external atmosphere of nonhuman objects as well as the presence and attitudes of other people within the environment. The attribute of human presence is termed the *social environment*. Specific categories within environmental factors include natural and human-made environments, products and technology, support and relationships, attitudes and

services, systems, and policies. Personal factors also fall within the domain of contexts. Personal factors are the unique characteristics of each individual and tend to be internal. Customs, beliefs, activity patterns, age, gender identity, and cultural expectations are some examples of personal factors. Performance can be affected either positively or negatively by any of these contexts.

The domain of performance patterns includes habits, routines, roles, and rituals (AOTA, 2020). Performance patterns attempt to describe the manner in which the person uses performance skills to provide structure for daily life. A person may have the ability to perform a skill but, if the skill is not embedded into a pattern, it may not be used enough to be of value. One example is a child who knows how to, and can independently, brush their teeth but does not do so unless reminded. The performance of this skill has not developed into a pattern that is used consistently. In another case, a college student who has the performance skills to succeed but has not fully identified with the role of student, has not developed the routine of daily study, and is in the habit of arriving late or missing classes is, therefore, not utilizing their abilities and skills. The result is that the student will most likely do poorly.

Performance skills, another domain, are defined in the OTPF-4 as "observable, goal directed actions that result in a client's quality of performing desired occupations" (AOTA, 2020, p. 80). Included in this domain are the interrelated skills of motor, process, and social interaction. Motor skills include movements such as positioning, obtaining and holding objects, moving self, and sustaining performance. Process skills include applying knowledge, organizing, and adapting performance. Social interaction skills include things like initiating and terminating social interactions, with subskills such as speech, eye contact, expressing emotions, and empathizing. These skills are learned and developed over time and require that the individual recruit and apply various body functions and structures in specific ways to successfully complete the action. Often, many performance skills are used simultaneously to engage in an occupation. For example, if a person wants to complete a crossword puzzle, they must use process skills to see and interpret the words and spaces on the paper. This must be accompanied by the motor skills needed to write. Social interaction skills may be required as well if the person seeks assistance from someone else to solve one of the clues.

The last domain area is client factors, which includes personal belief systems, body functions, and body structures. Personal belief systems incorporate spirituality, a person's sense of right and wrong, and other thought processes and patterns that influence an individual's life decisions. The subdomain of client factors, personal belief systems, will be discussed more thoroughly in this chapter. Body functions and body structures are based on human anatomy and physiology and will be discussed throughout this book.

As stated earlier, the process section of the OTPF-4 focuses on treatment planning and consists of evaluation, intervention, and targeting of outcomes. The intervention process of occupations and activities considers client factors, activity demands, and occupational demands. **Activity demands** include all aspects typically required to carry out the activity. **Occupational demands** are those requirements specific to an individual person attempting to engage in an occupation, including importance to the client. Both activity and occupational demands may include the objects used, space demands, social demands, sequencing and timing, required actions, and performance skills. Additionally, the underlying required actions, body functions, and body structures are taken into consideration when determining whether or not a client can engage in a certain activity or occupation.

Client Factors

The domain of client factors is described as things that are mostly internal to the client that may positively or negatively affect performance. Client factors are divided into three sections. The first section includes **values**, **beliefs**, and **spirituality**. This is followed by body functions in the second section, and body structures in the third section. The client factors of values, beliefs, and spirituality are formed over a lifetime of learning and through life experiences. Values, beliefs, and spirituality influence motivation. Body functions and structures relate to the actual physiologic and anatomic make-up of each person. These client factors are evident at birth for the most part. Body functions focus on the physiologic functions of body systems, such as specific and global mental functions, sensory, neuromuscular, cardiovascular, respiratory, and skin functions. Physiologic function can support or hamper engagement in occupations. Anatomy and specific body parts are discussed in the body structures section of client factors. Organs, skin, muscles, bones, limbs, structures of the nervous system, and other anatomical features are grouped under body structures. A basic understanding of anatomical features is necessary in order to understand kinesiology, biomechanics, and human movement; however, the presence, absence, or alteration of a specific body function or structure does not dictate a person's engagement in occupations. The OTPF-4 uses the classifications and definitions found in the ICF to categorize and define body functions and structures. Subsequent chapters in this text will focus in greater detail on body functions and body structures as they relate to kinesiology (AOTA, 2020).

An early kinesiologist and scholar of the symbolic nature of movement, Eleanor Metheny (1954), eloquently incorporated all of the client factors inherent in movement and how they interrelate with one another. Her reflective statement is presented in Box 1-6.

Values, Beliefs, and Spirituality

A person's belief system influences all that they do. Each individual's personal set of values and beliefs gives unique meaning to their life and guides the manner in which they live each day. Values may be defined as culturally acquired principles and standards that an individual considers to be essential to follow in order to lead a good life. A person might value honesty, integrity, hard work, or family relationships, to name a few. What the person understands as truth and fact make up their beliefs. A person's beliefs are true to them regardless of what another person might say, think, or believe. Some people might believe that a certain president was the best ever, even though not everyone would agree with this. Personal beliefs may not always be accurate. Consider the past when it was a commonly held belief that the world was flat. Spirituality is defined as the search for meaning in all that one does, which includes values and beliefs. Spirituality is considered to be dynamic and evolving. It

---

BOX 1-6

"The body is the physical manifestation of the person, his mind, his emotions, his thoughts, his feelings…Through its movements he expresses and externalizes the thinking and feeling which makes him a unique person. And as he moves, the very act of movement modifies and affects his thinking and feeling and being."

(Metheny, 1954, p. 27)

---

is an overarching principle. As implied with the example on beliefs, any of these client factors (values, beliefs, or spirituality) can change over time as a result of life experiences.

Illness or change in personal health status or that of a significant other can alter the way that values, beliefs, and spirituality are interpreted and used. For example, following a heart attack, a client may not immediately have the abilities they had previously; therefore, life activities are impacted. Likewise, even after physical improvement, the person's outlook on life may have changed. What was once important (e.g., climbing the corporate ladder) may be replaced with other beliefs or values, such as spending more time with family. Another consideration is that a client may not engage in an activity because of associations or beliefs formed by previous experiences. In this example, the person who had the heart attack experienced it while golfing and may never want to golf again. In the same example, the client, following their personal religion, may choose not to include certain medical options available because of their beliefs.

Motivation

Client motivation is derived from and affected by individual factors, such as personality, values, beliefs, and spirituality; however, motivation may also be affected by external factors. A literature review dealing with physical rehabilitation of individuals who had a recent medical diagnosis identified three major groups or theories addressing motivation (Maclean & Pound, 2000). These groups included internal or personality-based theories, external or social theories, and a combination of internal and external factors. One assertion found in the literature review is that the combination of internal and external factors enhances motivation more than using only one or the other. The review also acknowledged the difficulty of studying motivation as there is no consensus on the definition of motivation per se (Maclean & Pound, 2000). An internal factor for the kinesiology student might be feeling good about oneself for reaching a goal. External motivators might include a high grade, parental approval, or retention of scholarship monies. As seen, motivation can be intrinsic, coming from internal sources, or extrinsic, reinforced by external factors.

As stated, some experts propose a combination of internal and external motivators. One such model is termed *self-determined extrinsic motivation*. This is defined as when

the person will attempt an activity for external reasons, but these external reasons hold value for the person; they have been chosen by the individual because they are important to that person (Dacey et al., 2008). External factors need to have significance to the person or have some type of internalized personal value or they will not be motivating. An example of a personally valued or endorsed extrinsic motivator may be appearance.

Self-determined extrinsic motivation grew out of the self-determination theory, which recognizes the importance of autonomy and competence on motivation. Both intrinsic and extrinsic motivators are viewed as important (Dacey et al., 2008). This is a dynamic theory acknowledging that levels of motivation as well as what actually motivates a person are individual and can change throughout the lifespan. For example, exercise may be important to a young individual because it enhances appearance. As this person ages, exercise may become important for health reasons. The person's motivation for exercise has changed. Related to the importance of autonomy and competence on motivation, research by Laliberte-Rudman (2002) has shown that when goals are selected by the client, performance increases. Another study by Saebu et al. (2013), demonstrates that increased autonomic motivation leads to increased levels of physical activity during rehabilitation with carryover after therapy ends.

Another theory describing motivation is named **locus of control** (Rotter, 1966). Locus of control theory has similarities to self-determination theory, as it also addresses internal and external beliefs. Rotter's theory further postulates that control and motivation are based on personal experience and can be modified by learning, culture, and family. The term locus of control refers to who or what has impact over outcomes. An internal locus of control indicates that a person believes they have control over what will happen to themselves. The person believes that their actions will make a difference. On the other hand, someone with an external locus of control believes that what happens to them is a result of outside influences and that the outcome is not under personal control. The person believes that their efforts will not make a difference in the situation. Locus of control theory also acknowledges that an individual's perspective can change over time. Other research has found that the desire to control one's environment is fundamental to motivation

(Heckhausen, 2000). This research states that behavior directed at controlling one's environment is broad reaching and can impact any number of functional domains and activities.

Research indicates that several factors impact client motivation to engage in occupation. These factors include internal characteristics inherent in personality, personal values and beliefs, external factors that the client views as important, locus of control (the belief that one's actions have an impact on the outcome), autonomy in decision making, and the desire to control one's environment. Additionally, research indicates that motivational factors are dynamic and can change over the lifespan.

All people begin life with an innate drive for movement and mastery over their environment. In infancy, children have the intrinsic desire to explore and learn about their environment through reaching, grabbing, and mouthing items. This desire to explore continues as the infant's world expands with crawling and, later, walking. As the child masters basic motor skills with physical maturation, motivation becomes somewhat more extrinsic. Factors such as competition and a desire to prove oneself emerge. In adulthood, motivators commonly include health, appearance, being fit, stress reduction, emotional benefits, and weight reduction. As people age, intrinsic and extrinsic motivation toward physical activity decreases, and motivators such as appearance and weight management are no longer as important. In research studies, the motivator found to have the greatest positive impact on older individuals remaining physically active is an internal motivator called *enjoyment* (Dacey et al., 2008).

As occupational therapy practitioners, we need to remain mindful of our client's motivational level. We need to pay attention to what is specifically motivating for the client at any given point in time. It is important to remember that motivation can and does change and that motivation may come from internal or external sources.

Activity Demands

When working with a client and establishing an intervention plan, it is crucial to analyze the activities and occupations that one uses to address goals. To enable participation by the client, occupational therapy practitioners analyze activities to determine which demands are essential, which can be modified, and how to modify them. Activity demands describe the unique qualities of an activity, regardless of client or context. In comparison, occupation demands are specific to the client. Both activity and occupation demands determine the type and amount of effort needed to engage in the activity (AOTA, 2020). Occupational therapy practitioners can manipulate various activity and occupation demands in order to enhance or further challenge a client's engagement in the activity. The OTPF-4 breaks activity demands into several types: relevance and importance to the client, objects used and their properties, space demands, social demands, sequencing and timing, required actions and performance skills, required body functions, and required body structures. Changing any one of these areas will impact the other areas as well as the overall activity or occupation.

First and foremost, if an activity or occupation is not relevant or important to the client, it will not be useful as a therapeutic tool. The activity or occupation must support the client's interests, goals, and values. Objects used and their properties include things like tools, supplies, equipment, or resources necessary to carry out the activity or occupation. Space demands relate to the physical environment. This can include the room or outdoor space used as well as any physical characteristics of the environment. Characteristics take into account lighting, sound, temperature, humidity, furniture or equipment, and its placement. The structure itself is part of the physical environment. Component parts of the structure, such as the threshold of a door, are also considered. Any or all of these structures and component parts can be altered to enhance functioning and performance. Space demands often need to be modified to accommodate for mobility or movement issues such as the use of a wheelchair. One such example is to use space-saving hinges or removing a door to add width to the opening so that a wheelchair can pass through.

Social demands have to do with the social and attitudinal aspects of an activity. Social demands may include other people and the need to share, communicate, respect other's viewpoints, or take turns. Social demands also include things like the rules of a game. Attitudinal aspects may relate to the activity itself or to the participants. Attitudinal demands can vary greatly. Attitudinal and social demands may even have an impact on when or how a person gains a skill. For example, many children adopted from other countries are asked to play pat-a-cake when initially assessed by the pediatrician in the United States. This is not a universally practiced activity with children, so the child is unable to do it. After exposure to the activity, the child who is functioning normally quickly learns the game. Social demands, such as rules to a game, can be easily modified. A one-on-one game could become a team effort with one team playing against another. Attitudinal aspects are usually more difficult to modify as they reflect underlying beliefs and practices of the individual and their society. Sequencing and timing of activities are as crucial to successful performance as the physical ability to carry out the activity. A client might have the physical ability to perform an ADL such as bathing, but may not be able to complete this activity independently if unable to plan and sequence each step. When bathing, for example, the water must be turned to the correct temperature to avoid scalding. The person must remember to undress prior to entering the tub or shower. The person must allocate enough time to complete the bathing activity before they need to leave the home. If even one of these activity demands is not met, the task may not be completed successfully. Often, the occupational therapy practitioner initially needs to assist the client in breaking the activity down into manageable steps, then direct the client to perform the steps in the correct sequence.

Required actions, performance skills, and body functions and structures will be covered throughout this text. These activity demands incorporate the anatomy and physiology required to carry out an activity as well as the skill sets that need to be learned in order to perform the activity. These include not only physical abilities but cognitive, sensory, perceptual, and communication skills as well

Summary

Kinesiology is a specific topic that can be traced back through the history of occupational therapy education and practice that continues to be identified in current practice trends of the profession. Knowledge of kinesiology is an expectation of entry-level practitioners and is often used to assist clients in participating or engaging in areas of occupation or purposeful activities. The role of kinesiology in occupational therapy cannot be fully appreciated by using a minimal, reductionistic approach to understanding how or why movement occurs. The OTPF-4 provides the most comprehensive approach to understanding how and why movement occurs within the practice of occupational therapy. The focus of this kinesiology textbook will be primarily on the first section of the OTPF-4, domain, and will highlight client factors including body functions, body structures, and values. These aspects relate most directly to kinesiology, biomechanics, and human movement related to function. Incorporation of the OTPF-4 supports a focus on occupation and the top-down approach to addressing client problems.

In subsequent chapters, additional areas of domain will be attended to, especially within the context of the occupational profiles. A brief discussion of the process of treatment planning to include activity and occupational demands and their impact on intervention will occur. Finally, interventions to support occupations will be referred to. Fully presenting the process section of the OTPF-4, which encompasses the delivery of occupational therapy services, is not within the intended scope of this kinesiology

References

American Journal of Occupational Therapy. (1947). Special notices: Master's curriculum at USC. *American Journal of Occupational Therapy, 1*, 57.

American Occupational Therapy Association. (2014). Occupational therapy practice framework: Domain and process (3rd ed.). *American Journal of Occupational Therapy, 68* (Suppl. 1), s1-s48.

American Occupational Therapy Association. (2018). 2018 Accreditation Council for Occupational Therapy Education (ACOTE®) standards and interpretive guide. *American Journal of Occupational Therapy, 72*(Suppl. 2), 7212410005p1–7212410005p83. https://doi.org/10.5014/ajot.2018.72S217

American Occupational Therapy Association. (2020). Occupational therapy practice framework: Domain and process (4th ed.). *American Journal of Occupational Therapy, 74*(Suppl. 2), Article 7412410010. https://doi.org/10.5014/ajot.2020.74S2001

Bateson, M. C. (1996). Enfolded activity and the concept of occupation. In R. Zemke & F. Clark (Eds.), *Occupational science: The evolving discipline* (pp. 5-12). F. A. Davis Company.

Boston School of Occupational Therapy. (1929). *Training young women for a new profession* [Brochure]. Author.

Dacey, M., Baltzell, A., & Zaichkowsky, L. (2008). Older adults' intrinsic and extrinsic motivation toward physical activity. *American Journal of Health Behavior, 32*(6), 570-582.

Englehardt, T. (1977). Defining occupational therapy: The meaning of therapy and the virtues of occupation. *American Journal of Occupational Therapy, 31*, 666-672.

Greene, D. P., & Roberts, S. L. (2005). *Kinesiology: Movement in the context of activity* (2nd ed.). Elsevier-Mosby.

Haworth, N. A., & Macdonald, E. M. (1940). *The theory of occupational therapy*. Bailliere, Tindall, & Cox.

Heckhausen, J. (2000). Evolutionary perspectives on human motivation. *American Behavioral Scientist, 43*(6), 1015-1029.

Huss, A. J. (1981). From kinesiology to adaptation. *American Journal of Occupational Therapy, 35*(9), 574-580.

James, A. B. (2003). Biomechanical frame of reference. In E. B. Crepeau, E. S. Cohn, & B. A. Boyt-Schell (Eds.), *Willard and Spackman's occupational therapy* (10th ed., pp. 240-242). Lippincott Williams & Wilkins.

Kielhofner, G., & Burke, J. P. (1977). Occupational therapy after 60 years: An account of changing identity and knowledge. *American Journal of Occupational Therapy, 31*(10), 675-689.

Laliberte-Rudman, D. (2002). Linking occupation and identity: Lessons learned through qualitative exploration. *Journal of Occupational Science, 9*(1), 12-19.

Licht, S. (1950). Kinetic occupational therapy. In W. R. Dunton & S. Licht (Eds.), *Occupational therapy principles and practice* (pp. 63-69). Charles C. Thomas Publisher.

Maclean, N., & Pound, P. (2000). A critical review of the concept of patient motivation in the literature on physical rehabilitation. *Social Science and Medicine, 50*, 495-506.

Merriam-Webster. (n.d.). *Merriam-Webster.com dictionary*. http://www.merriam-webster.com/dictionary

Metheny, E. (1954). The third dimension in physical education. *Journal of Health, Physical Education, and Recreation, 25*, 27-28.

National Board for Certification in Occupational Therapy. (2018). Practice analysis of the certified occupational therapy assistant COTA: Executive summary. https://www.nbcot.org/-/media/NBCOT/PDFs/2017-Practice-Analysis-Executive-COTA.ashx?la=en&hash=90406F04B1E58C4F7CD8BF678B57446127BE68E0

Rotter, J. B. (1966). Generalized expectancies for internal versus external control of reinforcement. *Psychological Monographs, 80*(1), 1-28.

Saebu, M., Sørensen, M., & Halvari, H. (2013). Motivation for physical activity in young adults with physical disabilities during a rehabilitation stay: A longitudinal test of self-determination theory. *Journal of Applied Social Psychology, 43*(3), 612-625

Sands, I. F. (1928). When is occupation curative? *Journal of Occupational Therapy and Rehabilitation, 7*, 115-121.

Spackman, C. (1963). Occupational therapy for the restoration of physical function in occupational therapy. In H. Willard & C. Spackman (Eds.), *Willard and Spackman's occupational therapy* (pp. 167-239). J. B. Lippincott Company.

Tracy, S. E. (1910). *Studies in invalid occupations: A manual for nurses and attendants*. Thomas Todd Co.

United States Federal Board for Vocational Education. (1918). *Training for teachers for occupational therapy for the rehabilitation of disabled soldiers and sailors*. GPO.

Willard, H. S., & Spackman, C. S. (1947). *Principles of occupational therapy*. J. B. Lippincott Company.

World Health Organization. (2002). Towards a common language for functioning, disability and health. https://www.who.int/publications/m/item/icf-beginner-s-guide-towards-a-common-language-for-functioning-disability-and-health

World Health Organization (2008). *International classification of functioning, disability and health*. WHO Press.

World Health Organization. (2020). Basic documents (49th ed.), Supplement. https://www.who.int/about/governance/constitution; https://apps.who.int/gb/bd/

Applications

The following activities will help you identify domains of the OTPF-4 that will be highlighted in this text. Activities can be completed individually or in a small group to enhance learning.

1. **Qualitative Versus Quantitative Information**: The purpose of this activity is to help identify what is qualitative information vs. quantitative information. Qualitative information includes information that may come from observation or interview. This may include information that can be different depending on the situation. Quantitative information identifies numerical data under standardized situations to gather information. As long as the information follows the standardized format, it should yield similar information. Through observation of the classroom, identify examples of information that might be qualitative or quantitative. A qualitative example might include the comfort of the seat for students. A quantitative example that is measurable might be the temperature of the room. Individually or within groups, see how many other examples you can find.

2. **Variation of Health Condition Related to Levels of Dysfunction**: The purpose of this activity is to help the student to see how the impact of health conditions may vary depending on the client. This activity supports the view of health and disability put forth in the ICF and OTPF-4 that a diagnosis does not always imply a disability. It is possible that the client may have impairments, activity limitations, and/or participation restrictions. Individually or in groups, identify the possible results of the health condition related to the problem identified in Table 1-9.

TABLE 1-9
Variation of Health Condition Related to Levels of Dysfunction

HEALTH CONDITION	LEVELS OF DYSFUNCTION	RESULT OF HEALTH CONDITION RELATED TO THE PROBLEM
Generalized anxiety disorder	Impairment (body part)	Anxiety
	Activity limitation (individual or whole person)	Extremely uncomfortable in going out, or does not go out alone
	Participation restrictions (societal)	People's reactions lead to social isolation and minimal relationships
Your example here	Impairment (body part)	
	Activity limitation (individual or whole person)	
	Participation restrictions (societal)	

    a. What category was most difficult to identify for the result of the problem?

    b. Were all levels of dysfunction impacted?

    c. Can you provide solutions to each level of dysfunction to alleviate each concern?

3. **OTPF-4 Areas of Occupation**: The purpose of this activity is to help identify the areas of occupation, which are of key interest to the occupational therapy practitioner. Areas of occupation include ADLs, IADLs, health management, rest and sleep, education, work, play, leisure, and social participation (AOTA, 2020). Areas of occupation include those individual daily activities that have meaning and purpose in our lives. Identify those daily activities in Table 1-10 that apply to you at this time in your life. Try to only place the activity in the most applicable column, realizing that an activity can apply to more than one area of occupation.

TABLE 1-10

Occupational Therapy Practice Framework: Domain and Process, Fourth Edition
Domain Aspect: Occupations

AREAS OF OCCUPATION

Activities of Daily Living	Instrumental Activities of Daily Living	Health Management	Rest and Sleep	Education	Work	Play	Leisure	Social Participation
Brushed teeth	Swept floor	Physical activity	Slept 4 hours	Kinesiology occupational therapy assistant class	Sandwich artist	Tennis, video games	Titans football	Student occupational therapy assistant association
Your example here								
Your example here								
Your example here								
Your example here								
Your example here								
Your example here								
Your example here								

a. At other times in your life, would you have checked different domain categories? Can you identify current or past activities for each category of areas of occupation that applied to you?

b. Compare your perspective to that of family or friends for this same activity. How do your friends and family compare to your selections? Were there specific similarities or differences?

c. If you could, what area of occupation would you engage in more to make your life more balanced? Your perspective can have an impact on how you view and categorize your activities or occupations. If you are stressed and categorize everything as work, then you will have little time for play or leisure in your life. You may also procrastinate and put off doing things, resulting in even less time available for required tasks. If you can alter your perspective and consider, for example, the time spent preparing a meal as a relaxing, leisure hobby time (either solitary or social depending on your preference) and enjoy the process rather than dreading it, you will be more satisfied and use your time more efficiently.

4. **OTPF-4 Occupation and Activity Demands**: Occupation and activity demands include all aspects of the actual activity, which also includes relevance and importance, the objects being used and their properties, space and social demands, and sequencing. Underlying required actions, performance skills, body functions, and body structures are also considered. The purpose of this learning application is to be more mindful of the life demands that impact what appears to be a simple occupation or activity. This learning application should raise your awareness of what is really involved in completing an occupation or activity. It is important to realize that you have control over many of these demands and can modify or change them to enhance your overall success in performing the occupation or activity. Identify an activity and area of occupation in Table 1-11 that is relevant in your life and its associated activity demands.

TABLE 1-11
Occupational Therapy Practice Framework: Domain and Process, Fourth Edition Activity Demands

ACTIVITY AND AREAS OF OCCUPATION	RELEVANCE AND IMPORTANCE	OBJECTS USED	SPACE DEMANDS	SOCIAL DEMANDS	SEQUENCING AND TIMING	REQUIRED ACTIONS AND PERFORMANCE SKILLS	REQUIRED BODY FUNCTIONS	REQUIRED BODY STRUCTURES
Studying; area of occupation is education	Life-long desire/goal to become an occupational therapy assistant	Books, notes, paper, pencils, computer, friends	Minimal desk, seating, good lighting	Alone or with others	Work, child care, no big blocks of time, what to do first—prioritizing, how much time	Create schedule, consider lowering work hours, find child care	Cognitive, motor, sensory	Nerves, muscles, eyes, ears
Your example here								
Your example here								
Your example here								
Your example here								
Your example here								
Your example here								

a. Are there activity demands that interfere with the completion of an occupation or activity? Identify them with a negative sign (-), and identify activity demands that promote an activity with a positive sign (+).

b. Is there an example where one student identified a negative activity demand and another student identified that same activity demand as a positive?

c. What activity demands do you feel are out of your ability to control? How can you change any of the activity demands with a negative sign to enable your engagement in the occupation or activity?

5. **OTPF-4 Consideration of Health Condition**: The purpose of this activity is to help the student bring the OTPF-4 all together in considering health conditions. Again, the OTPF-4 was created as a construct to manage all of the necessary information related to client interventions. Having a disease or diagnosis does not necessarily indicate a disability or a decrease in function. Levels of dysfunction identified by the ICF include impairment, which occurs at the body part; activity limitation, which occurs at the individual level; and participation restriction, which occurs at the societal level. Health conditions are identified in Table 1-12. For each health condition, identify which domain aspects are affected and their associated level of dysfunction. Additionally, identify the level of human functioning that is being affected. This would either be the body part, individual, or societal level.

TABLE 1-12
Consideration of Health Condition

HEALTH CONDITION	DOMAINS	DOMAIN ASPECTS	BROKEN ARM		ANXIETY DISORDER	
			Level of Human Functioning	*Level of Dysfunction*	*Level of Human Functioning*	*Level of Dysfunction*
Impact of health condition on domains	Occupations	ADLs				
		IADLs				
		Health management				
		Rest and sleep				
		Education				
		Work				
		Play				
		Leisure				
		Social participation				
	Contexts	Environmental factors				
		Personal factors				
	Performance patterns	Habits				
		Routines				
		Roles				
		Rituals				
	Performance skills	Motor skills				
		Process skills				
		Social interaction skills				

(continued)

TABLE 1-12 (CONTINUED)
Consideration of Health Condition

HEALTH CONDITION	DOMAINS	DOMAIN ASPECTS	BROKEN ARM		ANXIETY DISORDER	
			Level of Human Functioning	*Level of Dysfunction*	*Level of Human Functioning*	*Level of Dysfunction*
Impact of health condition on process	Client factors	Values, beliefs, and spirituality				
		Body functions				
		Body structures				
	Occupation and activity demands	Relevance and importance				
		Objects used				
		Space demands				
		Social demands				
		Sequencing and timing				
		Required actions				
		Required body functions				
		Required body structures				

a. For each health condition, which OTPF-4 domain appears to be the most affected?

b. Were there any domain aspects that could have been answered either yes or no? Why do you think there is this variability?

c. Is it possible to make changes to that domain aspect to eliminate the level of dysfunction? Provide some examples.

d. Was it difficult to identify the level of human functioning and its corresponding level of disability? Explain your reasoning.

CHAPTER 2

Human Body Functions and Structures Influencing Movement

Susan J. Sain, MS, OTR/L, FAOTA

Key Terms

accessory motions

afferent

amphiarthrodial

anatomical position

central nervous system

concentric

dermatome

diarthrodial

eccentric

efferent

extrinsic muscles

flaccid paralysis

hypertonia

hypotonia

intrinsic muscles

isometric

isotonic

lower motor neurons

peripheral nervous system

plexus

reversal of muscle function

spastic paralysis

synarthrodial

synovial joints

upper motor neurons

Chapter Outline

Introduction

Body Functions

    Neuromuscular and Movement-Related Functions

    Cardiovascular and Respiratory System Functions

    Muscular Functions

    Skeletal Functions

Body Structures

    Nervous System

    Muscular System

    Skeletal System

Summary

References

Applications

Sain, S. J., & Roller, C. L. *Kinesiology for the Occupational Therapy Assistant: Essential Components of Function and Movement, Third Edition* (pp. 25-50).
© 2024 Taylor & Francis Group.

Chapter Objectives

After completion of this chapter, students should be able to:

1. Define key terminology.
2. Identify how the nervous system directs movement.
3. Discuss the difference between isometric and isotonic contractions and when they are utilized.
4. Organize and classify the various joints of the body according to function.
5. Analyze how functional movement is impacted by other body systems (e.g., cardiovascular, respiratory).
6. Compare and contrast a variety of factors that impact movement, noting what enhances movement and what impedes it.

Introduction

This chapter discusses anatomical and physiological components of movement. The *Occupational Therapy Practice Framework: Domain and Process, Fourth Edition* (OTPF-4) considers body functions (physiology) and structures (anatomy) as interrelated parts under client factors. The physiology and anatomy of the nervous and musculoskeletal systems will be addressed as they relate to movement. A basic understanding of the **central nervous system** (CNS) and **peripheral nervous systems** (PNS) will be presented, including the functions of a **dermatome** vs. a **plexus**. This section will include definitions of **upper motor neurons** (UMNs) and **lower motor neurons** (LMNs) along with a comparison of outcomes for damage in either system. Differences in the roles of **efferent** and **afferent** neurons will also be presented. A review of muscle types and function will be offered, including explanations of **isometric**, **isotonic**, **eccentric**, and **concentric** contractions. The terms **intrinsic muscle** and **extrinsic muscle** will be defined as will the concept of **reversal of muscle function**. Additionally, various ways to classify joints will be deliberated with an emphasis on how the joint structure impacts movement. Body functions and structures reflect capacities residing within the body. For functional use, or engagement in occupation, these innate capacities need to be converted into performance skills by the client. Many, if not most, of these skills rely on movement to complete the action.

Body Functions

Movement constitutes a basic drive for all people. Even before birth, the fetus has the potential and need to move. Indeed, movement is what enables people to survive, gather or hunt for food, communicate, and, among multiple other things, engage in daily activities or occupations. As noted by Whiting and Rugg (2006), "Movement is a fundamental behavior essential for life itself. Life processes such as blood circulation, respiration, and muscle contraction require motion, as do activities such as walking, bending, and lifting" (p. 6). More energy is used for locomotion and movement than for any other purpose of the body (Alexander, 1992). Consequently, it is important to move in an efficient manner. Fortunately, the body strives to move efficiently on its own. Research by Alexander (1992) indicates that animals, including humans, automatically adjust gait patterns to use the most efficient pattern available for the speed that they are traveling. The most efficient use of energy is near the middle of the speed range for whatever type of gait is used. More energy is consumed at the beginning or end of the speed range for gait. For example, when hiking, it is much easier and less tiring to hike at your own pace, or in your stride, than to speed up or slow down in order to stay in pace with a partner. Additionally, a slower speed of travel requires increased control. This phenomenon is well known by the fly-fisherman who slips and falls less when "rock hopping" vs. trying to carefully put each foot on the next rock.

One might ask what causes us to move and what allows us to move efficiently without apparent thought? Many interrelated systems interact to enable our ability to move. Some of these systems include neuromuscular, muscular, and skeletal structures. Without the muscular system and muscle contractions creating force, we could not move. Perhaps more muscle tissue exists in the body compared to any other kind of tissue because of this (Alexander, 1992). On average, muscle tissue makes up 40% to 50% of the body weight in humans (Thompson & Floyd, 2004). There are three primary types of muscle: skeletal, smooth, and cardiac. This chapter will focus on skeletal muscle and its relationship to movement. Smooth and cardiac muscle allow all other body and organ systems to function.

For muscle tissue to contract, the muscle must be connected to a nervous system. Additionally, if skeletal muscle is going to be able to move the body, it needs to be attached to a bony system. The human bony system, the skeleton, provides support as well as allows movement at the joints.

TABLE 2-1

Nervous System Definitions

TERM	DEFINITION
Autonomic nervous system (ANS)	Part of the PNS; efferent or motor innervation controlling the viscera; innervates smooth and cardiac muscle, as well as glands; supplies information from the internal environment.
Central nervous system (CNS)	The division of the nervous system that includes the brain and spinal cord.
Motor neuron	Also called *efferent*; relays information from the CNS to structures that need to react or respond; carries information away from the CNS.
Peripheral nervous system (PNS)	The division of nervous system that links the CNS with the muscles and glands; provides sensory information to the CNS; further subdivided into autonomic and somatic divisions.
Sensory neuron	Also called *afferent*; transmits signals from receptors to the CNS; carries information toward the CNS.
Somatic division	Subdivision of the PNS; sensory receptors and nerves related to the external environment; nerves linking these to the CNS, and efferent nerves returning to the skeletal muscle.
Viscera	Organs located within body cavities.

Adapted from Kiernan, J. A. (2009). *Barr's the human nervous system: An anatomical viewpoint* (9th ed.). Lippincott Williams & Wilkins and Solomon, E. P. (2009). *Introduction to human anatomy and physiology.* Saunders-Elsevier.

BOX 2-1

"Cranial nerves [are] highly specialized peripheral nerves."
(Angevine & Cotman, 1981, p. 50)

There are 12 pairs of nerves leaving the brain. They include sensory, motor, or mixed input.
(McMillan & Carin-Levy, 2012)

Some of these body systems, such as the respiratory and cardiovascular, both rely on and contribute to the functioning of the musculoskeletal system. Additionally, adequate sensory systems and mental functions, such as cognition, motivation, and perception, are necessary for functional movement. This chapter will identify how these interrelated systems work together to provide us with desired movement.

Neuromuscular and Movement-Related Functions

Muscles cannot be active without nerve innervations; therefore, we will begin our discussion by looking at the nervous system. The nervous system can be broken down into two major parts: the CNS and PNS. The entire nervous system is made up of sensory and motor neurons. Motor neurons are generally regarded as efferent, or exiting the CNS, and terminate on muscle fibers, causing a contraction when activated. Sensory neurons are afferent, or ascending to the CNS, and send sensory information to the cortex for interpretation (Solomon, 2009). Sensory input can be received from any stimulation, internal or external, to the body. Touch is an example of external stimulation, whereas a muscle ache is a source of internal stimulation. Table 2-1 contains definitions related to the nervous system.

The CNS is commonly defined as the brain and spinal cord. It ends at the last synapse where nerve fibers exit the brain or spinal cord. Motor neurons in the CNS are referred to as *upper motor neurons* (UMNs). The cerebral cortex and brainstem house the cell bodies for UMNs. The remainder of the nervous system components, or all nervous tissue that is not part of the CNS, is called the *peripheral nervous system* (PNS). The PNS transmits information between the CNS and the rest of the body; it provides the link between brain and body.

Nerves of the PNS exit either the brain (cranial nerves) or the spinal cord (spinal nerves). Most cell bodies of the cranial nerves are located in the brainstem. Refer to Box 2-1 for a definition of cranial nerves. Spinal nerves are paired

Figure 2-1. As seen in the drawing, UMNs originate in the primary motor cortex. UMNs synapse with LMNs and exit the CNS from either the brainstem or spinal cord. LMNs that exit the CNS in the brainstem are referred to as *cranial nerves*. LMNs exiting from the spinal cord are referred to as *spinal nerves*. (VectorMine/shutterstock.com)

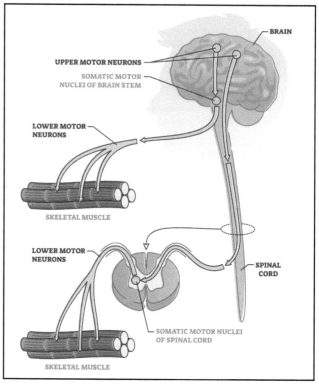

BOX 2-2

Tract is defined as:

"Axonal bundles of UMNs with common origin, function, and termination."
(Houglum & Bertoti, 2012, p. 683)

"A group of nerve fibers that are similar in origin, destination, and function that carry impulses to and from various areas within the nervous system, sometimes travelling on one side (ipsilateral) and sometimes crossing (contralateral)."
(Bertoti, 2004, p. 400)

"…bundles of UMN axons that travel together in the white matter of the brainstem and spinal cord."
(Dvorak & Mansfield, 2013, p. 203)

and exit the spinal cord bilaterally, or to both sides. The motor neurons found in the PNS are called *lower motor neurons* (LMNs). Refer to Figure 2-1 for a depiction of UMNs, LMNs, cranial nerves, and spinal nerves.

Cell bodies of the spinal nerves are located in the anterior horn of the spinal cord and are sometimes referred to as *anterior horn cells*. The anterior horn cells mark the last synapse of the CNS and the beginning of the PNS for spinal motor neurons. The axons of LMNs are found outside of the spinal cord. UMNs send neural messages directly to the LMNs, thus providing the connection between LMNs and the brain. LMNs innervate skeletal muscle. LMNs can be divided into two types: alpha and gamma motor neurons. Alpha motor neurons produce movement whereas gamma help regulate muscle tone (Dvorak, 2013; Kiernan, 2009; McMillan & Carin-Levy, 2012).

UMNs and spinal LMNs are interconnected via tracts. A tract is a bundle of UMN axons that are grouped together within the brainstem and spinal cord. Tracts can be descending (going from the CNS to the PNS) or ascending (going from the PNS to the CNS). See Box 2-2 for other definitions of tracts.

The PNS is further divided into the somatic nervous system and the autonomic nervous system (ANS). The somatic division is primarily responsible for responding to the external environment, or things happening outside of the body. The autonomic division helps maintain an internal balance as it responds to internal stimuli, providing functions such as maintaining body temperature, regulating heart rate, and regulating blood pressure (Solomon, 2009). Interestingly, the ANS has cell bodies in both the CNS and PNS. The ANS regulates the function of our vital organs (Farber, 1982). The

BOX 2-3

Peripheral nerves have the capacity, to a certain degree, for regeneration and repair if the cell body remains intact. In general, peripheral nerves regenerate at about 2 to 4 mm per day.

(Kiernan, 2009)

ANS is split into the sympathetic and parasympathetic systems. The sympathetic system is responsible for the fight or flight reaction experienced during stressful or emergency situations. In contrast, the parasympathetic system maintains and restores energy. Further review of the ANS can be found in anatomy and physiology texts.

Even though both CNS/UMN and PNS/LMN injuries can cause loss of voluntary movement (paralysis), they present quite differently clinically. Injury to an LMN, anywhere from the cell body to the motor end plate, results in **flaccid paralysis**, **hypotonia** (decreased muscle tone), **hyporeflexia** (loss of deep tendon reflexes), and significant atrophy. Examples of LMN injuries include poliomyelitis, radial nerve palsy, or a deep cut on a limb that severs a peripheral nerve (Kiernan, 2009). Box 2-3 includes an interesting fact related to an LMN injury.

Although the outcome is variable, a UMN lesion, such as seen in a cerebral tumor, traumatic head injury, or cerebrovascular accident, often causes **spastic paralysis**, **hypertonia** (increased muscle tone), hyperreflexia (exaggerated deep tendon reflexes), clonus, and little to no atrophy except with prolonged disuse. Unfortunately, it is not always as straightforward as this. There are variations in how a client who has had a UMN lesion presents clinically. Frequently, during the initial phase, a client will present with flaccid paralysis due to a condition analogous to spinal shock. Spinal shock is thought to be caused by the sudden loss of input to the spinal reflex circuits from the motor cortex and brainstem. These reflex circuits involve LMN feedback loops that regulate tone and reflexes. If the brain (UMN) is not exerting any control over the spinal reflexes, they can become hyperactive when they begin to work again. This renewed, unregulated activity in the LMN reflex circuit can result in increased spasticity and an increase in muscle tone. An example of a spinal circuit is the stretch reflex. The stretch reflex is regulated by gamma motor neurons, which, as discussed previously, assist in regulating muscle tone (McMillan, 2012; Purves et al., 2001). Refer to Figure 2-2 for an illustration of the stretch reflex.

Table 2-2 presents a summary of the typical results of a UMN or LMN lesion. Keep in mind that this table represents a typical progression of symptoms, including the initial spinal shock phase for UMN injuries. UMN injury stages may be skipped or may overlap depending on multiple factors,

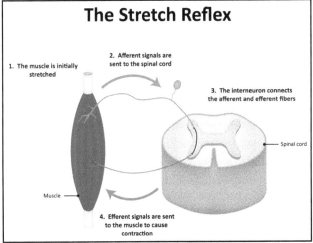

Figure 2-2. Spinal reflex circuit-stretch reflex. Note the feedback loop consists only of LMNs; there is no communication with the primary motor cortex or UMNs. Numbers 1 and 2 indicate a sensory nerve going from a sensory receptor within the muscle to the spinal cord. Number 3 depicts the synapse where the afferent, sensory nerve (in orange) connects or communicates with the efferent, motor nerve (in blue). Number 4 indicates a motor nerve leaving the spinal cord and directing the muscle to contract. (joshya/shutterstock.com)

such as the location of the injury (which area of the brain and, thus, which tracts are damaged) and time since the injury (e.g., acute). An in-depth discussion of the variations in UMN lesions is beyond the scope of this text.

As discussed previously, UMNs oversee voluntary movement; however, human movement incorporates many components in addition to voluntary control of the muscles. UMNs are influenced by many areas of the brain, each having its own responsibilities. Damage to any of these areas will impact the quality and quantity of movement available. Likewise, damage or lesions to these areas can cause movement disorders other than, or in conjunction with, paralysis. Some capabilities necessary for functional movement include coordination, timing, motor learning and retrieval, motor planning, motivation, initiation, and inhibition of movements.

The CNS is often divided into the following five levels of control: the cerebral cortex, basal ganglia, cerebellum, brainstem, and spinal cord. Basically, the cerebral or motor cortex is concerned with voluntary movement. The basal ganglia regulate posture, equilibrium, and planning, initiation, and inhibition of movements. The responsibilities of

TABLE 2-2

Comparison of Typical Outcomes for Lower Motor Neuron and Upper Motor Neuron Lesions

LOWER MOTOR NEURONS	UPPER MOTOR NEURONS
• Flaccid paralysis • Hypotonia • Loss of reflexes • Atrophy • Affects limited or small groups of muscles	• Initial phase (spinal shock; usually short term) ○ Flaccid paralysis ○ Loss of tendon reflexes • Later phases ○ Spastic paralysis ○ Hypertonia ○ Hyperactive reflexes ○ Affects several muscle groups

the cerebellum include timing, intensity, and refinement of smooth, coordinated movements. The cerebellum also incorporates sensory feedback related to actual movements, which allows for comparison between past performance and current ability and want. Integration of all CNS activity occurs in the brainstem, which allows it to regulate things such as muscle tone, respiratory rhythm, and control of posture during movement. The brainstem helps maintain optimum conditions within the body and its various functions. Finally, the spinal cord integrates various reflexes and higher-level activities in order to send neural messages to most of the body and return messages to the brain (Thompson & Floyd, 2004).

As each CNS division has its own specific roles, it makes sense that damage to each area will result in different functional outcomes. Injury to the motor cortex, such as in a cerebrovascular accident, will affect voluntary movement, frequently leading to spastic paralysis. Damage to the basal ganglia will cause dyskinesias, or movement disorders, including chorea. Cerebellar injury will cause errors in rate, range, direction, and force of movements, resulting in ataxia. Injury to the brainstem can cause a great variety of outcomes depending on the extent and location of the lesion. Effects of injury to the brainstem may include vertigo, facial paralysis, and tremor. Injury or disease of the spinal cord can also produce a wide variety of symptoms depending on the level of the CNS, severity of injury, and specific location of the injury (Angevine & Cotman, 1981; Kiernan, 2009).

Sensory systems that provide afferent information to higher levels of the CNS profoundly affect movement. Some sensory input elicits immediate reflex activity, such as in flexor withdrawal, which is an automatic reaction that acts to protect a limb or body part from injury. An example of this is when a person touches a hot object and immediately withdraws their hand without actually thinking about performing the action; it is automatic, or reflex based. Other sensory input is relayed to the cerebral or motor cortex for

interpretation and may be determined irrelevant, so the body ignores it. An example of this might be the buzzing of the overhead lights in your classroom. The majority of sensory input is analyzed by the cortex and then used or discarded to direct movement. Various sensory systems provide us with the ability to use pain, sight, hearing, taste, smell, touch, temperature, and vestibular and proprioceptive feedback to modify movement. Sensory receptors are defined as exteroceptors or interoceptors. A summary of key terminology can be found in Table 2-3.

In summary, the neuromuscular system describes the interdependency of the nervous system's innervations and its communication with the muscular system to enable movement. These two systems relay information back and forth between each other in order to coordinate movement and respond to stimuli. If there is a malfunction in either system, movement will be affected.

Cardiovascular and Respiratory System Functions

On a basic anatomical level, muscles need oxygenation and nutrition via the lungs and blood to thrive. The cardiopulmonary system delivers, among other things, oxygenated blood to all organs, allowing each organ to survive. Adequate cardiopulmonary function also supports endurance. Muscles metabolically generate the energy they need to execute movement via nutrients obtained in vascular and interstitial tissues. Additionally, the cardiovascular and respiratory systems remove carbon dioxide and other waste products to keep the muscles and organs functioning at optimum levels. In other words, the muscular component of movement relies on the cardiovascular and respiratory systems in order to function. Likewise, the cardiovascular and

TABLE 2-3

Definitions of Common Terms

TERM	DEFINITION
Ataxia	Incoordination; inability to execute coordinated voluntary movement; loss of smooth execution of movement; ataxic gait often described as "drunken."
Atrophy	Wasting of tissue, especially in muscle due to lack of use.
Chorea	Irregular, involuntary movements of the limbs or facial muscles, often described as dance-like motions.
Clonus	Caused by hyperactive stretch reflex as a result of a UMN lesion, rapid alteration of muscular contractions between agonist and antagonist muscle groups.
Dyskinesia	Difficulty in performing voluntary movements; "dys" meaning bad or difficult, "kinesia" referring to movement.
Edema	Accumulation of excessive amounts of watery fluid in cells, tissue, or serous cavities.
Exteroceptors	"External receivers"; afferent nerve endings that respond to stimulation by external agents, specialized in receiving information from the external environment, such as the eyes.
Flaccid	Relaxed, without tone.
Flexor withdrawal	Sometimes referred to as *flexor reflex*, protective; the withdrawal of a limb in response to painful stimulation.
Hypertonia	"Above or over tone"; extreme tension of the muscles.
Hypotonia	"Under tone"; having a lesser degree of tension; diminished muscular tone; abnormally low muscle tone.
Interoceptors	"Internal receivers"; afferent nerve endings or receptors that respond to stimulation from within the body, primarily from visceral organs.
Paralysis	Loss of power of voluntary movement in a muscle through injury or disease to its nerve supply.
Proprioceptor	A sensory end organ in muscles, tendons, joint capsules, and inner ear allowing one to know the location of one body part in relation to another; activated by movement or action of the organism itself.
Spasticity	A state of increased muscular contraction in response to sensory stimuli; a sign of UMN damage, velocity-dependent increase in resistance of a muscle to stretch; a unique type of hypertonia in which muscle spasms are increased by movement and often associated with exaggerated reflexes.
Stretch reflex	Slight stretching of a muscle lengthens fibers, causing stimulation of sensory endings, which leads to contraction of the muscle. This is a protective reflex to avoid overstretching. One role of the muscle spindle is to detect stretch and respond to it via the stretch reflex; this phenomenon is in constant use and provides adjustment to muscle tone.
Tone	Also called *muscle tone*; the normal state of tension of muscles caused by partial contraction of some of the muscle fibers.
Vestibular	Related to the vestibule of the ear; a vestibule is a small space or region at the entrance of a canal; vestibular organ, the organ of equilibrium.

Adapted from Angevine, J. B., & Cotman, C. W. (1981). *Principles of neuroanatomy*. Oxford University Press; Bertoti, D. B. (2004). *Functional rehabilitation through the life span*. F. A. Davis Company; Kiernan, J. A. (2009). *Barr's the human nervous system: An anatomical viewpoint* (9th ed.). Lippincott Williams & Wilkins; Solomon, E. P. (2009). *Introduction to human anatomy and physiology*. Saunders-Elsevier; Steadman, T. (1982). *Steadman's medical dictionary* (24th ed.). Williams and Wilkins; and Venes, D. (2013). *Taber's cyclopedic medical dictionary* (22nd ed.). F. A. Davis Company.

respiratory systems rely on the musculoskeletal system to operate properly. This occurs, for example, when there is a contraction of muscles in a limb that aids the return of blood to the heart and decreases the occurrence of edema in the extremities. Regarding the respiratory system, certain skeletal muscles also aid in both the inspiration and expiration phases of respiration.

Disease or limitations in the cardiovascular or respiratory systems can have a negative impact on skeletal muscular function and movement (Cronin & Mandich, 2005). One example of a respiratory system disease that affects skeletal muscle function and movement is chronic obstructive pulmonary disease (COPD). COPD is characterized by degenerative changes of the alveoli, resulting in breathlessness on exertion, even if the exertion is minimal. The oxygen–carbon dioxide gas exchange is lessened, causing less oxygen to travel to other tissues, which results in fatigue, less energy production, and decreased functioning overall (Venes, 2013). A person with COPD may have a difficult time breathing and often will prop themselves on their elbows in a standing position. This position allows the recruitment of additional skeletal muscles to aid in the breathing process. Because breathing is more difficult during movement, the person becomes more sedentary.

Other body functions, such as mental functions, are also involved in the choice to become more sedentary in a person with COPD. In the OTPF-4, mental functions include cognitive areas, such as memory and judgment, as well as affective and perceptual functions that may include temperament and attention span. In the case of the client with COPD, anxiety is associated with the fear that breathing will be further diminished. Increased anxiety puts further strain on breathing and oxygen uptake. In addition, leaving the home often causes increased anxiety and requires more energy expenditure. The person may then decide to remain at home, at rest, to decrease anxiety and enhance breathing. Thus, a negative cycle begins. The decreased ability for efficient breathing leads to decreased movement. Decreased movement leads to an even further decrease in capacity for the lungs to perform their job, and so on. Many such examples of decreased functional performance in respiratory or cardiovascular systems exist, which, in turn, will affect movement. Other texts are dedicated to describing the disease process and can be referred to for detailed information on a specific diagnosis. The goal of this text is that the reader will gain an appreciation of how all body systems are interrelated and affect movement abilities and choices.

Muscular Functions

As your study of human movement progresses, you will find that no two people perform the same movements in the same way. Indeed, one person might perform the same movement in different ways at different times depending on the level of fatigue, pain, motivation, or other factors. Keep in mind that although people often do not use ideal movement patterns in daily activities, they are still able to function at required levels, usually without undue stress on body systems (Fisher & Yakura, 1993). Occupational therapy may become involved when a client's movement patterns stray far enough from what is ideal, causing the client excessive stress. The inefficient movement patterns may increase energy consumption or become ineffective for daily occupations; thus, the client seeks intervention. To move efficiently, people incorporate the laws of physics, biomechanics, and physiology. These concepts and how they affect movement will be discussed in depth in subsequent chapters of this text.

One focus of this chapter is skeletal muscle. Skeletal muscles are a primary feature influencing movement. Skeletal muscles are not only responsible for movement, but also provide a degree of protection, especially for internal organs. In addition, skeletal muscles support posture and produce body heat.

Muscles are able to perform a variety of roles that allow for both mobility and stability against gravity. Muscles must act in cooperation with one another to produce either movement or stability. Muscles are capable of maintaining or

switching these roles instantaneously to meet the demands of the movement required. The various roles a muscle can perform are defined in greater detail in Table 2-4.

When a muscle is activated, it can only develop tension. Muscles produce force or tension by contracting. There are two main types of contractions: isometric and isotonic. Both types of contractions have roles in most movements. Isotonic contractions can be further divided into concentric and eccentric contractions.

The word isometric literally means same measure. The Greek origins of this word tell us its meaning. "Isos" translates as equal, and "metric" is derived from "metron," meaning measure (Venes, 2013). During an isometric contraction, muscle tension develops, but the muscle length does not change. This means that the joint angle or measurement does not change either. Isometric contractions may be thought of as static as they maintain the joint angle in a relatively stationary, nonmoving position. An example of an isometric contraction is when a person is holding the rail on a moving bus or tram while standing. The person's arm muscles produce tension to maintain posture against the forces of acceleration and deceleration, but there is little or no change in joint positions of the arm.

The term *isotonic* is derived from the Greek words "isos," meaning equal, and "tonos," meaning tension (Venes, 2013). Isotonic contractions maintain the muscle at equal tension. This means that the length of the muscle changes, causing joint movement. Isotonic contractions may be thought of as dynamic because the tension produced by the contraction causes movement.

An isotonic contraction is considered concentric when the muscle shortens and the origin and insertion move closer together. This occurs at the elbow when you bring a glass to your mouth. If the muscle contracts with less force than needed to overcome the resistance, an eccentric contraction occurs (Solomon, 2009). Resistance may include gravity, an object, or other muscles. In the case of an eccentric contraction, the muscle is actually lengthening under stress and the attachments move further away from one another. Eccentric contractions work to decelerate the movement, as a brake would do for a car. Consider the movement of placing your glass on the table. Eccentric contractions control the speed and placement of the glass back onto the table. If eccentric contractions of the elbow flexor muscles were not occurring in response to the resistance provided by gravity and the weight of the glass, the glass would crash into the table. Eccentric contractions allow for slow, smooth, controlled movements. Lieber and Bodine-Fowler (1993) believed that muscle injury and soreness are more often associated with eccentric, or lengthening, contractions.

Various muscle properties determine how much a certain muscle can shorten or lengthen. Four properties defined in the literature are contractility, extensibility, elasticity, and irritability. Contractility has been defined as a muscle's ability to shorten in length; however, as discussed previously, not all contractions result in muscle shortening. Perhaps a more

TABLE 2-4	

Muscle Roles

MUSCLE TYPE	ROLE/DESCRIPTION
Agonists	Sometimes referred to as *prime movers*; the agonist can contract concentrically or eccentrically; at most joints, several muscles act together, each as an agonist, causing the movement. In this situation, some texts refer to *primary agonists* and *assistant agonists*.
Antagonists	Muscles with actions opposite those of the agonist, muscles acting against a position or movement, often located on the opposite side of the joint as the agonist; during many movements, the antagonists are passive so as not to impede the movement; however, at times antagonists slow the movement or decelerate to help control the movement.
Coactivation	Sometimes referred to as *cocontraction*; limited to simultaneous action of agonist and antagonist to provide stability, to increase torque at a joint, when learning a new movement.
Neutralizers	Muscles that prevent unwanted accessory actions or substitutions or cancel out multiple actions by the same muscle. When a muscle with multiple actions contracts, it attempts to perform all of its actions, unable to determine which one is necessary for the movement. For example, the biceps brachii both flexes the elbow joint and supinates the forearm. If elbow flexion is the desired goal, neutralizers will cancel out the supination action of the biceps muscle.
Stabilizers	Sometimes referred to as *fixators*; muscles that surround a joint or body part to stabilize the joint against unwanted movement. When muscles contract, the insertion can move toward the origin, or vice versa. Stabilizers prevent motion at one of these locations in order to allow controlled movement at the other location; during normal muscle use, these muscles stabilize the origin of the agonist; muscles that stabilize a portion of the body against a particular force, which may be internal from other muscles or external, such as gravity or a weight being lifted.
Synergists	Muscles that are not prime movers but assist the agonist in the motion and also help to cancel out undesired motions.

Adapted from Hall, S. (1999). *Basic biomechanics* (3rd ed.). WCB/McGraw-Hill; Solomon, E. P. (2009). *Introduction to human anatomy and physiology.* Saunders-Elsevier; Thompson, C. W., & Floyd, R. T. (2004). *Manual of structural kinesiology* (15th ed.). McGraw-Hill; and Whiting, W. C., & Rugg, S. (2006). *Dynatomy: Dynamic human anatomy.* Human Kinetics.

accurate description of *contractility* refers to a muscle's ability to develop tension against resistance. The extensibility of a muscle depicts its capacity to be stretched or lengthened. Conversely, elasticity describes the muscle's ability to return to its original length after it has been stretched. *Irritability* is the term used to describe the capacity of the muscle to receive and respond to a stimulus, whether the stimulus is chemical, electrical, or mechanical (Hall, 1999; Thompson & Floyd, 2004).

Sequencing and timing of muscle contractions also influence the type and quality of movement. Some movements require sudden bursts of speed, such as swinging a bat or throwing a ball. Other motions, such as kneading bread, should be performed more slowly. Certain movements require precise control, as in writing, while other movements only need gross coordination, such as walking. The speed and precision of a muscle contraction is dependent on many variables. Variations can occur in the speed of a muscle contraction, the frequency of contractions, and the strength of the contraction. Often, one of these variables is gained at the loss of another. For example, the faster a group of muscle fibers shorten, the less force they can exert (Alexander, 1992).

The speed of muscle contractions can be affected by the diameter of the axon, the thickness of the myelin sheath, or the properties of the muscle fibers themselves. In general, as the speed of a muscle contraction increases, the potential for fatigue also increases. Conversely, muscles that are slower to contract are better suited for activities that require endurance. To help combat fatigue, different motor units are activated in sequence, rather than all units being activated at the same time. In this manner, a certain number of motor units are relaxing at all times. Some muscle fibers have a longer refractory period than others, meaning that more time passes before they can be activated and are able to produce tension again.

The strength of a muscle contraction is dependent on the number of muscle fibers recruited, the size of the muscle fibers, and the size of the axon. The larger each of these is, the stronger the contraction will be (Gench et al., 1999). Amazingly, the CNS automatically matches the speed and strength of muscle contractions to the requirements of each and every individual movement to produce efficient, smoothly executed motions. The CNS can spontaneously increase or decrease the number of motor units activated, select between types of motor units, or make numerous other adjustments. These adjustments allow us to perform the activities of our choosing without the need for any conscious input on our part.

Skeletal Functions

The skeletal system provides the framework for the body. It also gives support and protection to other systems of the body. The bones of the thorax, or trunk, protect vital organs, such as the heart and lungs, while the skull protects the brain. The skeleton consists of a series of bones connected to each other at joints. The joints allow movement to occur. In addition, the skeleton provides attachments for muscles, which enable movement at the joints. The bones of the skeleton also perform other important functions, such as blood cell formation in the bone marrow and storage of certain minerals (Thompson & Floyd, 2004).

Articulations of bones, more commonly known as joints, are of immense functional importance. All skeletal movement in the body occurs at joints. When there is disease or injury at a joint, movement will be negatively impacted. Several factors influence the amount of stability provided, or movement allowed, at each joint. Some of these factors include the type and shape of the joint, the structures surrounding the joint, and the number of degrees of freedom available at the joint.

A system of joint classification based on movement includes three types of joints, which are labeled **synarthrodial**, **amphiarthrodial**, and **diarthrodial**. Synarthrodial joints are immovable, such as the suture joints of the skull. Amphiarthrodial joints, sometimes called *cartilaginous joints*, allow for limited movement, as in the pubic symphysis. The joint classification allowing for the most movement is the diarthrodial joint, which is considered freely movable. Its movement is limited primarily by muscle, tendon, and ligaments rather than by the joint structure itself. Diarthrodial joints are enclosed within a joint capsule that secretes synovial fluid to lubricate the joint; thus, these joints are also referred to as **synovial joints**. The majority of the joints in the body are diarthrodial joints (Solomon, 2009; Thompson & Floyd, 2004).

Although diarthrodial joints allow for the most movement, there are still significant variations in movement ability from one diarthrodial joint to another. These differences are based on the number of axes a joint can rotate around and the number of planes the joint can move in. This is referred to as *degrees of freedom*. If a joint only has one axis and can move in only one plane, it is said to have one degree of freedom. An example of this would be a hinge joint, such as that found at the elbow. Similarly, if the joint has two axes and can move in two planes, it is said to have two degrees

of freedom. The metacarpophalangeal (MCP) joints in the hand represent joints with two degrees of freedom. The most freely moving joint can have a maximum of three degrees of freedom. An example of this joint type is the ball-and-socket joint of the hip. This joint can move in all three planes around three different axes. Joints with one degree of freedom provide more stability but less mobility, while joints with three degrees of freedom allow for more mobility but less stability. As noted, the trade-off for increased mobility is a loss in stability (Hall, 1999). Specific voluntary joint motions and the planes they occur in will be discussed later in this chapter.

In addition to voluntary motions, **accessory motions** increase the pain-free movement available at a given joint. Accessory movements cannot be performed voluntarily. They occur between the articular surfaces of a joint in conjunction with voluntary movement. There are three types of accessory motions, which are called *roll*, *spin*, and *glide*. Roll is sometimes referred to as *rocking*, and glide is often called *slide* or *translation*. Spin is similar to the motion of the tiny point on a toy top spinning in one location on the larger surface of the table or floor (Thompson & Floyd, 2004). Although accessory motions are available at most joints, they are readily apparent in the knee and glenohumeral (GH) joint, where one joint surface is significantly different in size than the companion joint surface. Accessory motions at these joints allow for the larger surface of one bone to remain in contact with the smaller surface of the adjoining bone, thus allowing greater range of motion (ROM). Accessory motions may also be referred to as *arthrokinematic movement*. Arthrokinematic movement related to treatment interventions is addressed in Chapter 11.

As previously noted, in order for muscles to act at joints, they must attach to the bones. These areas of attachment are generally referred to as *bony landmarks*. Interestingly, fields such as anthropology or forensic medicine use bones and bone markings to determine many things about a person, such as age, gender, race, occupation, health, or even whether or not a person had certain diseases when they died (Moore, 1985). Bony landmarks tend to be more prominent in people who performed more physical labor or were more athletic than others. Bony landmarks can be divided into two main categories: depressions (openings) and projections (bumps). In general, depressions, or openings, provide protection for softer tissue, such as nerves and blood vessels. Bony projections, bumps or extensions out from the surface, are important for two key reasons. The first reason is that they are often used as the axis for goniometric joint measurements. The second reason relates to clients who are less mobile. For these clients, certain bony landmarks need to be observed or examined periodically to inspect for decubiti. Decubiti are more commonly referred to as *bed sores*, and will often form when pressure is maintained over a bony protuberance. Certain bony landmarks, particularly those that protrude, will be discussed more in depth in subsequent chapters.

Body Structures

A brief overview of anatomical structures and their impact on movement will be presented in this section. As outlined in the OTPF-4, body structures are listed under client factors. Client factors include specific characteristics that may affect performance; however, despite their importance, these characteristics do not guarantee successful movement. Conversely, impairments in, or lack of these structures, does not necessarily indicate difficulty carrying out individual occupations of interest to the client (American Occupational Therapy Association, 2020) Body structures are just one part of the complex picture that occupational therapy practitioners must observe in order to guide the client toward increased functional performance. The World Health Organization (2001) defines body structures as the anatomical parts that support body functions. Structures include everything from microscopic cells to organs or limbs.

Nervous System

A summary of the basic functions of the nervous system was presented in the first part of this chapter. The specific structures that permit these basic functions will be further defined and illustrated in this section. There are 12 pairs of cranial nerves and 31 pairs of spinal nerves. Cranial nerves transmit information directly to or from the brain. Spinal nerves link the spinal cord with sensory receptors and with other parts of the body. The spinal nerves are all mixed nerves, transmitting sensory information to the spinal cord through afferent neurons and relaying motor information from the brain via the spinal cord to the various parts of the body using efferent neurons. Spinal nerves have two points of attachment with the spinal cord. The dorsal root contains afferent neurons or sensory fibers. The ventral root consists of motor neurons or efferent fibers (Solomon, 2009). Cranial nerves may be motor, sensory, or mixed.

Dorsal, afferent sensory receptors may be located in any organ system, including skin and muscle. Sensory receptors located in the skin are responsible for sensations such as pain, light touch, and temperature. Each dorsal nerve root receives feedback from a specific area of skin on the body. This specific area is labeled a dermatome. When injury occurs to even a single nerve root, sensation in the dermatome supplied by that nerve root will be diminished or altered (Moore, 1985). Refer to Figure 2-3 to see a representation of sensory dermatomes.

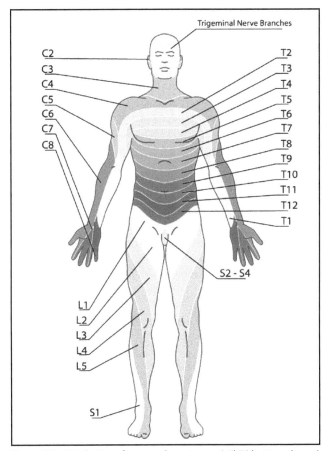

Figure 2-3. Distribution of sensory dermatomes. (stihii/shuttrstock.com)

Efferent or motor innervations can be segmental or provided by a plexus. *Segmental innervations* refer to innervations supplied directly by a single nerve root to a nearby region. In contrast, a plexus represents a network, or interconnection of nerves, that then separates into various nerves named for the region of the body they innervate. One example is the brachial plexus (Venes, 2013). Table 2-5 gives examples of nerves originating from the brachial and lumbosacral plexuses.

Most innervations of skeletal muscles in the trunk are segmental. Motor innervations to the extremities tend to be via a plexus. Plexuses are thought to provide neuromuscular protection in that if a single nerve root is damaged, muscles innervated by a plexus will continue to have some ability to function. The two plexuses this text is most interested in are the brachial plexus and the lumbosacral plexus.

The brachial plexus is composed of spinal nerve roots from the fifth cervical nerve (C5) through the first thoracic nerve (T1) and supplies the upper extremities (UEs). A representation of the brachial plexus can be seen in Figure 2-4. The lumbar plexus is formed by spinal nerve roots beginning with the first through fourth lumbar nerves (L1-L4) as shown in Figure 2-5. The sacral plexus, depicted in Figure 2-6, is made up of the fourth and fifth lumbar nerve roots (L4

TABLE 2-5

Plexuses and Nerves

PLEXUS	NERVE ROOTS	NAME OF NERVE	AREA OF BODY INNERVATED
Brachial	C5-T1	Ulnar	Medial forearm, fourth and fifth digits
		Radial	Dorsal aspect of arm, forearm, and hand
Lumbosacral	L1-L4	Femoral	Anterior thigh
	L5-S3	Sciatic	Posterior leg

Adapted from Kiernan, J. A. (2009). *Barr's the human nervous system: An anatomical viewpoint* (9th ed.). Lippincott Williams & Wilkins and Solomon, E. P. (2009). *Introduction to human anatomy and physiology*. Saunders-Elsevier.

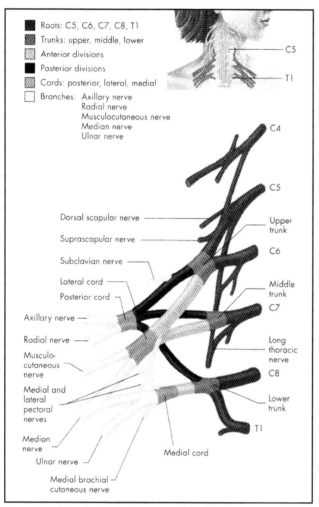

Figure 2-4. The brachial plexus, anterior view, nerve roots C5-T1. (Reproduced with permission from Seely, R. R., Stephens, T. D., & Tate, P. [2003]. *Anatomy and physiology* [6th ed.]. McGraw-Hill.)

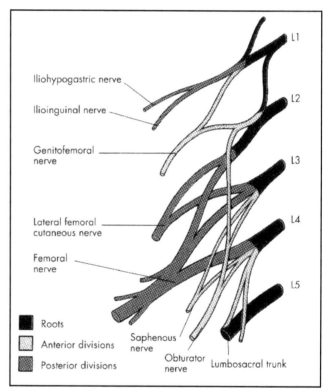

Figure 2-5. The lumbar plexus, anterior view, nerve roots L1-L5. (Reproduced with permission from Thompson, C., & Floyd, R. T. [2004]. *Manual of structural kinesiology* [15th ed.]. McGraw-Hill.)

Muscular System

According to Thompson and Floyd (2004), there are more than 600 muscles in the body, including 215 pairs of skeletal muscles. Other sources indicate a lesser number of muscles. What is important to note is that there are a lot of muscles in the body that influence multiple types of movement. Muscles can be described in many ways, such as by shape, location, fiber orientation, size, origin, insertion, or function. Regardless of how skeletal muscles are described, they all react in a similar way.

and L5) in addition to the first, second, and third sacral nerve roots (S1-S3). The lumbar and sacral plexuses are often considered together as the lumbosacral plexus. The combined lumbosacral plexus, consisting of nerve roots L1-S3, innervates the lower extremities (LEs; Moore, 1985; Venes, 2013).

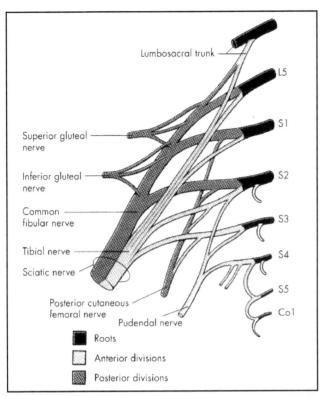

Figure 2-6. The sacral plexus, anterior view, nerve roots L5-S3. (Reproduced with permission from Thompson, C., & Floyd, R. T. [2004]. *Manual of structural kinesiology* [15th ed.]. McGraw-Hill.)

A brief review of muscle is presented here. A muscle is composed of several motor units. A motor unit is defined as one motor neuron and all the muscle fibers it innervates (Thompson & Floyd, 2004). Motor units are the building blocks of muscle tone and allow us to perform graded muscular contractions (Hall, 1999). Although the response of a motor unit is all or none, the strength of the response of the entire muscle is determined by the number of motor units activated. A motor unit is made up of fasciculi that are organized into functional groups of varying sizes. A fasciculus is several muscle fibers bundled together.

Each fasciculus, or motor unit, is made up of the same type of muscle fibers, although the entire muscle itself is usually made up of a combination of fiber types. Most muscle fibers are of the twitch type, meaning they produce tension in response to a single stimulus. Twitch-type fibers are further divided into fast twitch (also referred to as *type II*) and slow twitch (also referred to as *type I*). Fast twitch fibers are those that reach maximum tension very quickly; however, they are also prone to fatigue quickly. Fast twitch fibers allow us to complete activities that require large bursts of force, such as jumping or throwing. Conversely, slow twitch fibers take up to seven times longer to reach their peak tension. Although slower to respond to stimulation, these fibers are resistant to fatigue. Due to these factors, slow twitch fibers, such as those found in postural muscles, are well suited for sustained

activity. A single motor unit may contain anywhere from 100 to 2000 muscle fibers. Fine motor and precise movement are coordinated by motor units containing relatively few muscle fibers. On the other hand, movements requiring gross motor skills and increased force utilize motor units containing a maximum number of muscle fibers (Hall, 1999; McMillan, 2012; Oatis, 2010).

A muscle fiber is the muscle cell. *Fiber* is the name given to a muscle cell because of its narrow, elongated shape. The sarcomere is the contractile unit in the muscle cell. This is where the actin and myosin are located. Neither actin nor myosin can change in length. Rather, the length of the muscle shortens as the overlapping of the actin and myosin fibers becomes greater (Solomon, 2009).

The structural arrangement of fibers within muscle helps to determine the muscle's function. Shorter fibers, such as those in a pennate arrangement, are specialized to produce more force. Longer fibers, such as those in a parallel arrangement, seem to favor larger excursion or movement and less force (Lieber & Bodine-Fowler, 1993). The two major types of skeletal fiber arrangement are pennate and parallel. The term *pennate* is derived from the Latin word for feather. The muscle fibers in a pennate arrangement are oblique or at an angle to the tendon, similar to a feather. Examples of pennate muscles include the peroneus (fibularis) longus and peroneus (fibularis) brevis, as well as the deltoid. On the other hand, fibers in a parallel arrangement run the length of the muscle. The sartorius and biceps brachii muscles are examples of muscles with a parallel fiber arrangement. These two structural arrangements of muscle are further subdivided according primarily to the shape of the muscle. Pennate fibers can be classified as unipennate, bipennate, or multipennate depending on the number of branches. Figure 2-7 depicts the rectus femoris, a muscle with bipennate fibers, which is a subclassification of the pennate arrangement. Parallel fibers may be categorized as flat, fusiform, strap, radiate, or sphincter. Figures 2-8 through 2-10 are all examples of the parallel fiber arrangement; however, each one is slightly different, relating to the categorization of the muscle. Flat muscles are usually thin and broad. Fusiform muscles are spindle shaped with a wider belly in the middle and thin ends. An example of this is in Figure 2-8, which depicts the biceps brachii muscle, a muscle with parallel fiber arrangement, which is further categorized as fusiform. Strap muscles are usually uniform in diameter and longer than other muscles. The sartorius muscle is an example of a strap muscle and is depicted in Figure 2-9. Radiate muscles are sometimes described as fan shaped or triangular. Two examples of radiate muscles are the deltoid muscle (Figure 2-10) and gluteus maximus muscle. Sphincter muscles are circular and are basically never-ending strap muscles that surround openings. Their function is to close an opening when they contract, as in the mouth (Thompson & Floyd, 2004).

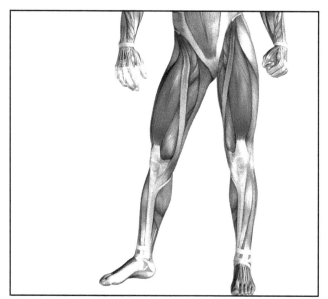

Figure 2-7. Bipennate muscle fibers can be seen in this picture of the rectus femoris muscle. The bipennate classification is a subclassification of the pennate arrangement. (design36/shutterstock.com)

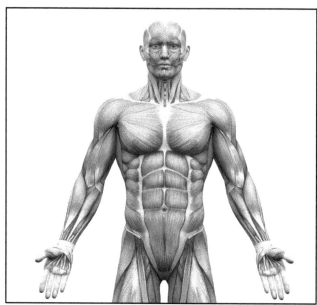

Figure 2-8. Muscle fibers in a parallel arrangement, further classified as the fusiform shape, are seen here in the biceps brachii muscle. (decade3d - anatomy online/shutterstock.com)

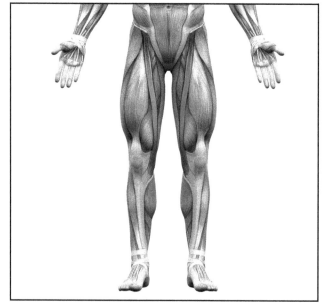

Figure 2-9. The sartorius muscle is an example of a strap-shaped muscle of the parallel fiber arrangement. (decade3d - anatomy online/shutterstock.com)

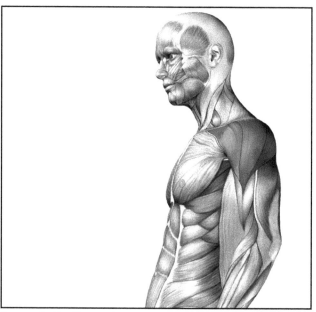

Figure 2-10. The radiate arrangement of muscle fibers, a subcategorization of the parallel fiber arrangement, is depicted here in the deltoid. (design36/shutterstock.com)

Many other terms are also used to describe muscles. Fortunately, most of these are used in the muscle's name and will give clues as to the function, location, size, or other characteristics of the muscle. When identifying a muscle, think about each component of its name. The name itself may indicate the location, action, or other characteristics of the muscle. One such example is the extensor carpi radialis longus. One action of this muscle described in its name is extension. It further designates the location, the wrist (carpi), on the radial side (radialis). Finally, it indicates that more than one muscle exists for this purpose. Because this muscle is the longus, it must have a shorter counterpart, the brevis. If there was not a shorter counterpart, longus would not be part of its name. Nomenclature used to characterize muscle includes descriptions of size, shape, location, action, direction of fibers, number of divisions, points of attachment, or a combination of these. Examples of nomenclature for certain muscles can be found in Table 2-6. Word origins for certain muscle names are listed in Box 2-4.

TABLE 2-6
Muscle Categorizations

NOMENCLATURE	EXAMPLES
Shape	Rhomboid, trapezius
Size	Teres major, teres minor
Location	Tibialis anterior, latissimus dorsi
Action	Extensor digitorum, supinator
Direction of fibers	Internal oblique, transverse abdominis
Number of divisions	Biceps brachii
Points of attachment	Sternocleidomastoid, coracobrachialis
Action and shape	Pronator quadratus
Action and size	Adductor magnus, extensor carpi radialis longus
Size and location	Vastus lateralis
Shape and location	Serratus anterior, tibialis posterior
Location and attachment	Brachioradialis
Location and number of divisions	Triceps brachii, biceps femoris

Adapted from Thompson, C. W., & Floyd, R. T. (2004). *Manual of structural kinesiology* (15th ed.). McGraw-Hill.

BOX 2-4

WORD ORIGINS FROM LATIN

Carpus: Or carpi; wrist or pertaining to the wrist.
Magnus: Large, great, denoting a structure of large size.
Pollicis: Thumb or first digit of hand.
Quadratus: Square, having four equal sides, denoting the number four.
Rectus: Straight; as in rectus femoris or rectus abdominis.
Sartor: A tailor; as used in the sartorius muscle, which allows us to sit crossing our legs, in the tailor position.
Serratus: A saw; notched, toothed.
Teres: Round, smooth, cordlike; as in teres major or pronator teres.

(Steadman, 1982)

hand, and extrinsic muscles as those that originate outside of the body part on which they cause action (Thompson & Floyd, 2004). Intrinsic muscles allow for dexterity, fine movements, and coordination, whereas extrinsic muscles provide for more gross motor skills and strength.

Skeletal System

The skeleton is divided into two parts: the axial skeleton and the appendicular skeleton. The skull and trunk comprise the axial skeleton. The trunk consists of the vertebral column, ribs, and sternum. The appendicular skeleton is composed of the shoulder and pelvic girdles, the UEs, and the LEs. Most of the long bones of the body are in the appendicular skeleton. Long bones allow for greater ROM for movement. The surface of bones is not smooth; rather, bones have bumps, depressions, and holes. As discussed earlier, there are two major categories of bony landmarks, projections and depressions or openings. Bony markings that are projections appear wherever tendons, ligaments, and fascia are attached (Moore, 1985). The long bones of the body have many such markings, as several muscles attach to long bones. Table 2-7 identifies a partial listing of bony projections, examples, and their relevance to movement or the formation of decubiti. Depressions or openings in bone, such as the obturator foramen, transverse foramen of the cervical vertebrae, or the greater sciatic notch, provide protection to vital structures.

In order to locate a muscle and know its action, one must know the origin and insertion. In general, the origin describes where a muscle begins, or originates. This point is usually proximal, or closer to the trunk or midline of the body, and is often considered to be more stable. The end point for the muscle is termed the *insertion*. The insertion is usually distal, or farther away from the trunk and midline of the body, and is considered the most movable part. Usually, during muscle activation, the insertion moves toward the origin; however, at times, the origin can move toward the insertion. This is called *reversal of muscle function*. Reversal of muscle function is when the insertion remains fixed or stable and the origin moves toward the insertion (Thompson & Floyd, 2004). Examples include stabilizing the hands during a push-up or elevating and propelling the trunk forward during crutch walking. Specific origins and insertions are not listed in this text as they can be readily found via internet search, if needed.

Still other terminology describes the general location and function of certain muscle groups. Both the LEs and UEs have intrinsic and extrinsic muscles. These terms are relative to the ankle or wrist joints. Intrinsic muscles originate distal to the joint while extrinsic muscles originate proximal to the joint. Some sources define intrinsic muscles as muscles within or acting solely on a specific body part, such as in the

Most voluntary movement occurs in the joints of the appendicular skeleton. Joints allow for different amounts of movement depending on the shape of the joint and the number of axes it rotates around. Joint axes and motions are determined by the planes in which the joint can move. The body is divided into three imaginary planes: the frontal, sagittal, and transverse. Each plane has an axis that corresponds

TABLE 2-7

Examples of Bony Projections

PROCESS	MARKING	DESCRIPTION	EXAMPLE	CONSIDERATION
Attachments for tendon, ligament, or fascia; axis for movement or risk for decubiti	Crest	Linear elevation, ridge, narrow	Iliac crest, crest of tibia	Decubitus
	Epicondyle	Rounded projection proximal to condyle	Lateral epicondyle of humerus	Axis for elbow flexion and extension, decubitus
	Process	Any notable projection	Olecranon process	Decubitus
	Spine	Sharp elevation or projection, slender	Anterior superior iliac spine	Axis for hip abduction and adduction, decubitus
	Trochanter	Very large projection, rounded or blunt	Greater trochanter of femur, malleolus	Axis for hip flexion and extension, axis for ankle plantarflexion and dorsiflexion, both—decubitus

Data source: Moore, K. L. (1985). *Clinically oriented anatomy* (2nd ed.). Williams & Wilkins and Thompson, C. W., & Floyd, R. T. (2004). *Manual of structural kinesiology* (15th ed.). McGraw-Hill.

BOX 2-5

ALTERNATE NAMES FOR PLANES AND AXES

Frontal can be referred to as coronal.
Sagittal can be referred to as anteroposterior.
Transverse can be referred to as horizontal.
Vertical can be referred to as longitudinal.

(Solomon, 2009; Thompson & Floyd, 2004)

to it. The axis is always perpendicular, or at a right angle, to the plane it is associated with. Movement occurs around the axis and is parallel to the plane. Box 2-5 identifies each plane with its alternate name.

The three planes of the body are depicted in Figures 2-11 and 2-12. Figure 2-11 is an anterior view of the body, while Figure 2-12 is a lateral view. The frontal plane (yellow) divides the body into anterior and posterior, or front and back sections. The sagittal plane (gray) divides the body into left and right sides. The horizontal plane (blue) divides the body into upper and lower portions. Movements available in each plane will now be described.

The frontal plane divides the body into anterior and posterior sections. The axis for movement in the frontal plane is called the *sagittal axis*. Rotation around the sagittal axis and parallel to the frontal plane allows for the movements of abduction, adduction, radial deviation, ulnar deviation, and lateral bending. The position of the LEs in abduction and the UEs in adduction during the beginning stance of a golf swing can be seen in Figure 2-13. The sagittal plane divides the body into left and right sides. The axis for the sagittal plane is termed the *frontal axis*. Rotation around the frontal axis, and parallel to the sagittal plane, consists of flexion and extension. Some sources identify hyperextension in addition to extension, which would also occur in the sagittal plane. Box 2-6 discusses hyperextension. A functional example of flexion, a child exiting a toy car, can be seen in Figure 2-14, whereas extension is seen in Figure 2-15. Extension is observed in the neck, trunk, hips, knees, and elbows of the girl in Figure 2-15.

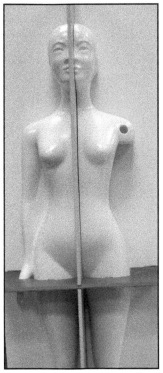

Figure 2-11. Anterior view of the planes of the body: frontal (yellow), sagittal (gray), and horizontal (blue). In this view, the frontal plane appears as the background. (© 2003 Jennifer Bridges, PhD. All Rights Reserved. Denoyer.com)

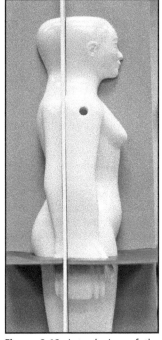

Figure 2-12. Lateral view of the planes of the body: frontal (yellow), sagittal (gray), and horizontal (blue). In this view, the sagittal plane appears as the background. (© 2003 Jennifer Bridges, PhD. All Rights Reserved. Denoyer.com).

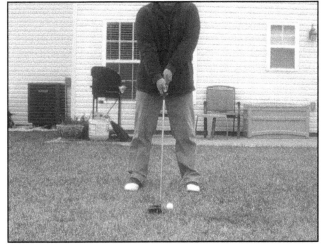

Figure 2-13. Abduction observed in the LEs; adduction demonstrated in UEs during golf stance. (Reproduced with permission from Jeremy L. Keough, MSOT, OTR/L, FAOTA.)

BOX 2-6

EXTENSION OR HYPEREXTENSION?

Roughly half of the available sources use the term *hyperextension* to describe a posterior movement from the anatomical position. The other half of the available sources use the term *hyperextension* to denote movement in the direction of extension that is beyond normal limits. While a joint may normally be able to move through its available ROM past the starting position in extension, such as the shoulder joint, this movement may be abnormal for other joints. MCP hyperextension may be an example when the MCP joint is hyperextended past the starting position due to a stretch of the involved body structures.

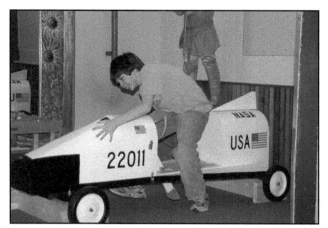

Figure 2-14. Flexion observed in the trunk, hips, knees, ankles, and left elbow of this boy. (Reproduced with permission from Angela Grussing.)

The horizontal plane divides the body into upper and lower portions. The axis for movement in the horizontal plane is the *vertical axis*. The movements about this axis are termed *internal* or *medial rotation*, *external* or *lateral rotation*, *rotation to the right* or *left*, *horizontal abduction* and *adduction*, *supination*, and *pronation*. Internal rotation and external rotation are depicted in the hand signals used by the cyclist in Figures 2-16 through 2-18. The traditional signal for a right-hand turn, in Figure 2-16, incorporates external rotation. This signal originated for vehicle drivers who could not reach across the car to point out of the passenger window toward the right. The cyclist felt it important for the reader to know that simply pointing to the right with the right hand, as seen in Figure 2-17, is the signal more commonly used by cyclists today. The signal to slow down or stop uses internal rotation as in Figure 2-18. Figure 2-19 portrays the motion of horizontal abduction with the right arm as the arm pulls the arrow back on a bow. The left arm remains in a neutral position between horizontal abduction and horizontal adduction. Supination is observed in the left hand in Figure 2-20, while pronation is observed in the right hand during the functional activity of removing cookies from a pan. Although most movements are identified as occurring in one plane, people often move in a combination of patterns and across planes. One such movement at the shoulder is referred to as *scaption*. Scaption denotes a forward movement at the GH joint that occurs approximately midway between flexion (sagittal plane) and abduction (frontal plane). Descriptions and examples of movement can be found in Table 2-8.

In addition to the degrees of freedom, the shape or type of the joint also helps to determine the movements available. Joint types include ball and socket, hinge, saddle, pivot, gliding, and condyloid. These are descriptive terms for synovial joints. Table 2-9 gives examples of each joint type in addition to the degrees of freedom available, planes, axes, and typical movements.

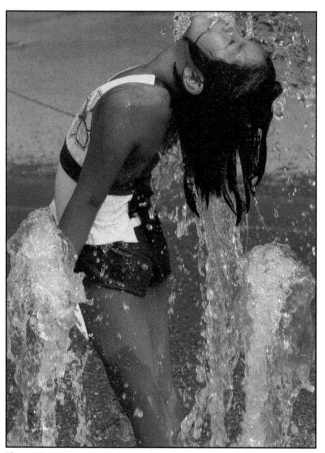

Figure 2-15. Extension observed in the neck, trunk, hips, knees, and elbows of this girl. (Reproduced with permission from Angela Grussing.)

When describing movement, it is important to be able to give an accurate description of what actions are observed. Reference positions and anatomical directional terms are used in order to do this effectively and in a manner that others will understand. Two reference positions that may be used to describe movement and illustrate planes are the **anatomical position** and **fundamental position**. The anatomical position is the reference position most widely used and is also the reference position for the definitions used in this text. For both reference positions, the subject is standing in an upright posture, eyes looking forward, feet parallel with toes pointed forward, and the arms slightly abducted at the side of the body. In the anatomical position, the palms are facing forward. If the palms face the side of the body, the person is in the fundamental position (Solomon, 2009). Commonly used anatomical directional terminology can be found in Table 2-10.

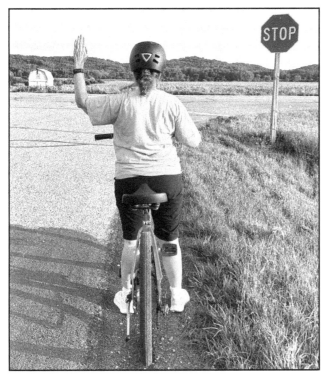

Figure 2-16. External rotation observed in the left arm, which is demonstrating the traditional hand signal for right turn. (Reproduced with permission from Carolyn L. Roller, OTR/L.)

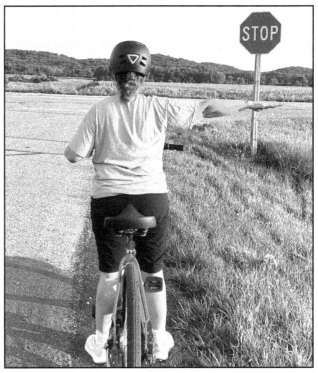

Figure 2-17. Abduction of right arm, as seen in the more commonly used right hand turn signal. (Reproduced with permission from Carolyn L. Roller, OTR/L.)

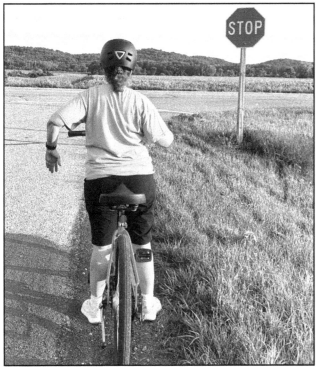

Figure 2-18. Internal rotation observed in the left arm, which is demonstrating the hand signal for stop or slow down. (Reproduced with permission from Carolyn L. Roller, OTR/L.)

Summary

It should now be evident that functional movement requires complex interactions of multiple body systems, including the nervous, skeletal, and muscular systems, as well as major organ systems. Every component or system has an effect on the other and contributes to the overall function, or lack thereof, of the body (Lieber & Bodine-Fowler, 1993). Only through the synchronization of the body's anatomical systems and structures can we use functional movement patterns in our daily lives (Whiting & Rugg, 2006).

Figure 2-19. Horizontal abduction of the right arm is demonstrated in the picture. As the girl pulls the arrow backward, her arm moves in the direction of horizontal abduction. The legs are in abduction. (Reproduced with permission from Riley Sain.)

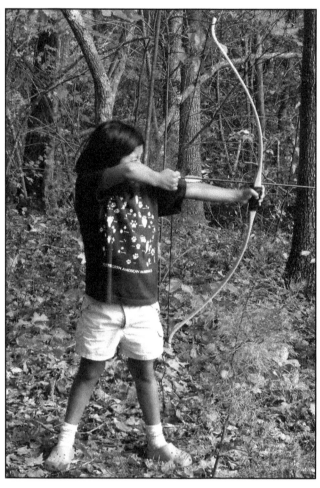

Figure 2-20. The left hand is held in supination as it stabilizes the cookie tray while the right hand is postured in pronation as it holds the spatula to remove the cookies.

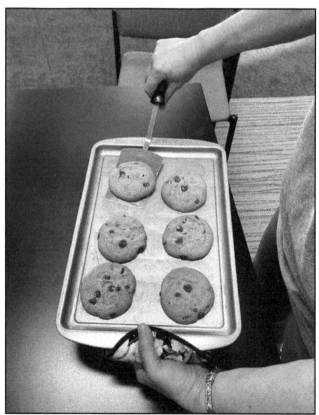

TABLE 2-8

Terms Describing General Movement

MOVEMENT	DESCRIPTION	EXAMPLE
Abduction	Lateral movement away from midline or center of body	Arm and leg position in upward stroke of jumping jack exercise
Adduction	Medial movement toward midline or center of body; opposite of abduction	Normal resting position while seated or standing with arms at side of body
Flexion	Bending of joint, usually reduces joint angle, two bones moving closer together	Occurs at elbow when bringing fork to mouth
Extension	Joint angle increases, straightening; opposite of flexion	Knee position in standing
Circumduction	Combination of flexion, extension, abduction, and adduction leading to circular motion	Stirring or churning a large vat of apple butter or molasses
Lateral (external) rotation	Rotary movement around vertical axis of bone away from midline of body	Combing back of head, fastening necklace behind neck
Medial (internal) rotation	Rotary movement around vertical axis of bone toward midline of body; opposite of lateral rotation	Reaching into pants pocket
Pronation	Position of forearm when palm is facing down	Position of hands on computer keyboard when typing
Supination	Position of forearm when palm is facing up; opposite of pronation	Position of hand when holding a handful of small candies and fingers are open, not fisted
Horizontal abduction	Humerus positioned in horizontal plane, arm raised to 90 degrees, with movement away from midline and toward back of body; opposite of horizontal adduction	Movement of arm while pulling the string back on a bow to shoot an arrow
Horizontal adduction	Humerus positioned in horizontal plane, arm raised to 90 degrees, with movement toward midline and front of body; opposite of horizontal abduction	When in driver's seat, reaching across chest with right arm to reach shoulder belt
Lateral flexion (side bending)	Movement of head, neck, or trunk laterally away from midline or center of body; abduction of the spine	Leaning over sideways while seated to pick something up off the floor
Scaption	Short for scapular plane elevation, term first made public in 1991 by Dr. Marilyn Pink; elevation of the GH joint in the plane of the scapula, in about 30 degrees of horizontal adduction from the frontal plane	Reaching upward to remove an item from a cabinet that is not directly in front of you; reaching upward to scratch your head

Adapted from Solomon, E. P. (2009). *Introduction to human anatomy and physiology.* Mosby-Elsevier; Thompson, C. W., & Floyd, R. T. (2004). *Manual of structural kinesiology* (15th ed.). McGraw-Hill; and The Free Medical Dictionary. (n.d.). http://medical-dictionary.thefreedictionary.com/scaption

TABLE 2-9

Characteristics of Synovial Joint Types

TYPE OF JOINT	JOINT EXAMPLE	DEGREES OF FREEDOM	PLANES	AXES	MOVEMENT EXAMPLES
Ball and socket	Shoulders and hips	3 (Triaxial)	Frontal	Sagittal	Hip abduction, adduction
			Sagittal	Frontal	Hip flexion, extension
			Horizontal	Vertical	Hip internal and external rotation
Hinge	Elbows and knees	1 (Uniaxial)	Sagittal	Frontal	Elbow flexion, extension
Saddle	Thumb carpometacarpals	2+ (Bi- or multiaxial)	Sagittal	Frontal	Flexion, extension
			Frontal	Sagittal	Abduction, adduction
			Multi	Multi	Opposition
Pivot	Radioulnar, atlantoaxial	1 (Uniaxial)	Horizontal	Vertical	Supination, pronation, neck rotation
Gliding	Carpal bones	Variable	Variable	Variable	Accessory motions
Condyloid	MCP joints 2 through 5	2 (Biaxial)	Frontal	Sagittal	Abduction, adduction
			Sagittal	Frontal	Flexion, extension of the lesser digits

Adapted from Gench, B. E., Hionson, M. M., & Harvey, P. T. (1999). *Anatomical kinesiology*. Eddie Bowers Publishing, Inc. and Thompson, C. W., & Floyd, R. T. (2004). *Manual of structural kinesiology* (15th ed.). McGraw-Hill.

TABLE 2-10

Anatomical Directional Terminology

TERM (Alternate name in parentheses)	ORIENTATION OR DESCRIPTION
Anterior (ventral)	Toward the front of the body, toward the belly
Posterior (dorsal)	Toward the back of the body or buttocks, relating to the back
Superior (cephalic)	Toward the head, upward, higher than another structure
Inferior (caudal)	Toward the feet, downward from another body part, below in relationship to another structure
Medial (internal)	Toward the middle of the body or midline
Lateral (external)	Toward the sides of the body, away from the midline, on or to the side
Proximal	Toward or closer to the attachment to the trunk or origin, nearer to the center of the body
Distal	Away from or farther from the midline of the body or attachment to the trunk, farther from the point of reference or origin
Superficial	Toward the surface of the body, used to describe relative depth of muscles or other tissue
Deep	Toward the inside of or within the body, below the surface
Contralateral	Opposite sides of body, right vs. left

(continued)

TABLE 2-10 (CONTINUED)
Anatomical Directional Terminology

TERM *(Alternate name in parentheses)*	ORIENTATION OR DESCRIPTION
Ipsilateral	On the same side of the body; right arm and right leg are ipsilateral to each other
Prone	Lying on stomach in a face-down position
Supine	Lying on back in a face-up position

Adapted from Solomon, E. P. (2009). *Introduction to human anatomy and physiology.* Saunders-Elsevier and Thompson, C. W., & Floyd, R. T. (2004). *Manual of structural kinesiology* (15th ed.). McGraw-Hill.

References

Alexander, R. M. (1992). *Exploring biomechanics in animals.* Scientific American Library.

American Occupational Therapy Association. (2020). Occupational therapy practice framework: Domain and process (4th ed.). *American Journal of Occupational Therapy, 74*(Suppl. 2), Article 7412410010. https://doi.org/10.5014/ajot.2020.74S2001

Angevine, J. B., & Cotman, C. W. (1981). *Principles of neuroanatomy.* Oxford University Press.

Bertoti, D. B. (2004). *Functional rehabilitation through the life span.* F. A. Davis Company.

Cronin, A., & Mandich, M. (2005). *Human development and performance throughout the lifespan.* Thomson Delmar Learning.

Dvorak, L., & Mansfield, P. J. (2013). *Essentials of neuroanatomy for rehabilitation.* Pearson Education, Inc.

Farber, S. D. (1982). *Neurorehabilitation: A multisensory approach.* W. B. Saunders Company.

Fisher, B., & Yakura, J. (1993). Movement analysis: A different perspective. *Orthopaedic Physical Therapy Clinics of North America,* 1-14.

Gench, B. E., Hionson, M. M., & Harvey, P. T. (1999). *Anatomical kinesiology.* Eddie Bowers Publishing, Inc.

Hall, S. (1999). *Basic biomechanics* (3rd ed.). WCB/McGraw-Hill.

Houglum, P. A., & Bertoti, D. B. (2012). *Brunnstrom's clinical kinesiology* (6th ed.). F. A. Davis Company.

Kiernan, J. A. (2009). *Barr's the human nervous system: An anatomical viewpoint* (9th ed.). Lippincott Williams & Wilkins.

Lieber, R. L., & Bodine-Fowler, S. C. (1993). Skeletal muscle mechanics: Implications for rehabilitation. *Physical Therapy, 73*(12), 844-856. https://doi.org/10.1093/ptj/73.12.844

McMillan, I. R. & Carin-Levy, G. (2012). *Tyldesley & Grieve's muscles, nerves and movement in human occupation* (4th ed.). Wiley-Blackwell.

Moore, K. L. (1985). *Clinically oriented anatomy* (2nd ed.). Lippincott Williams and Wilkins.

Oatis, C. (2010). *Kinesiology: The mechanics and pathomechanics of human movement* (2nd ed.). Lippincott Williams & Wilkins.

Purves, D., Augustine G. J., Fitzpatrick D., Katz, L. C., LaMantina, A.-S., McNamara, J. O., & Williams, S. M. (Eds.), (2001). *Neuroscience* (2nd ed.). Sinauer Associates.

Solomon, E. P. (2009). *Introduction to human anatomy and physiology.* Saunders-Elsevier.

Steadman, T. (1982). *Steadman's medical dictionary* (24th ed.). Williams and Wilkins.

Thompson, C. W., & Floyd, R. T. (2004). *Manual of structural kinesiology* (15th ed.). McGraw-Hill.

Venes, D. (2013). *Taber's cyclopedic medical dictionary* (22nd ed.). F. A. Davis Company.

Whiting, W. C., & Rugg, S. (2006). *Dynatomy: Dynamic human anatomy.* Human Kinetics.

World Health Organization. (2001). *International classification of functioning, disability and health.* Author.

Applications

The following activities will help you apply knowledge of the functions and structures of body systems to real-life situations. Activities can be completed individually or in a small group to enhance learning.

1. **Muscle Contractions**: The purpose of this task is to help you better understand the need for both types of contractions, concentric and eccentric, and how they work together. The area of the body where the muscles contract is listed for you. The contraction for each muscle group might be a different type. First, determine the type of contractions used while performing the activity listed. Next, hypothesize what would happen if the muscle was not contracting in the manner identified. Complete the grid in Table 2-11. In all of the examples using eccentric contractions, what is the one common force or resistance acting on the muscle?

TABLE 2-11

Muscle Contractions: Concentric or Eccentric?

MOVEMENT	MUSCLE GROUP USED	TYPE OF CONTRACTION	WHY IS THIS CONTRACTION NEEDED?
Putting book on table	Elbow flexors	Eccentric	Book would smash through table.
	Finger flexors	Concentric	You would lose grasp and drop the book.
Lowering buttocks to sit on chair	Quadriceps		
Raising hand in class	Shoulder flexors		
Stepping down to the next stair with right leg	Left quadriceps		
While seated, raising leg to tie shoe	Quadriceps		
Your example here			

2. **Determining Joint Types**: The purpose of this application is to help the reader identify types of joints in common objects to better understand how similar joints in the body function. The type of joint will determine, to some extent, the amount and type of movement allowed. Recall that the types of joints include ball and socket, hinge, saddle, pivot, gliding, and condyloid. Not all types are easily found in the environment. Complete Table 2-12.

TABLE 2-12

Types of Joints in Common Objects

OBJECT	JOINT TYPE	MOVEMENTS ALLOWED	DEGREES OF FREEDOM
Door	Hinge	Open and close or back and forth	One
Computer mouse (type with ball in base)			
Sliding side door on van			
Standard stick shift on car			
Your example here			

3. **Planes and Axes**: The purpose of this application is to enable the reader to better understand the planes of motion and the axes associated with them. Fill in the grid in Table 2-13 according to the example given.

TABLE 2-13

Planes and Axes Application

FUNCTIONAL ACTIVITY	JOINT MOVEMENTS	PLANE OF MOTION	AXES OF MOTION
Walking up stairs	Hip flexion	Sagittal	Frontal
	Knee flexion	Sagittal	Frontal
Performing jumping jacks	Shoulder _____	_____	_____
	Hip _____	_____	_____
While driving, turning head to look over shoulder before merging	Neck _____	_____	_____
	Trunk _____	_____	_____
Washing hair	Shoulder _____	_____	_____
	_____	Frontal	_____
	_____	Horizontal	_____
	Wrist _____	_____	_____
	Wrist ulnar and radial deviation	_____	Sagittal
Sitting cross-legged on the floor	Hip _____, _____, _____	_____	_____
Your example here			

4. **Bony Landmarks**: Certain bony landmarks are identified in therapy for measuring ROM. Other bony landmarks are areas of concern because decubiti can form over them. For these reasons, it is important for the practitioner to be able to find these landmarks. Use an anatomy book for reference, if needed. Working with a partner, find the following bony landmarks by palpating gently:
   a. Lateral malleolus
   b. Head of the fibula
   c. Lateral epicondyle of humerus
   d. Greater trochanter
   e. Anterior superior iliac spine
   f. Styloid process of ulna

5. **Other Body Systems**: The purpose of the following activities is to allow for a greater understanding of how other body systems affect movement. Although a person may not know what it is like to have a certain disease or disability unless they truly have it, a better understanding can be developed through simulation. The following activities will try to simulate movement as experienced with a decrease in various body systems. Follow the steps listed next:

a. Select an activity of your choice, such as walking, brushing hair, or eating a snack.

b. Select one of the body system simulations listed in the following section.

c. Equip yourself with the decreased function listed.

d. Perform your selected activity.

e. For each activity/simulation, answer the questions listed at the end.

Potential simulations for body system dysfunction include the following:

- Occlude vision using a blindfold.
- Inhibit proprioceptive and tactile feedback by wearing gloves and donning boots that are several sizes too big. Stuff the boots with newspaper or extra layers of socks.
- Spin in a circle several times to alter your vestibular system.
- Wear earmuffs or sound-eliminating headphones to occlude hearing.

Questions:

a. Could you perform the task? Could you complete your entire day with this "disability"? What overall effect would this have on your day?

b. Was the activity harder to perform? If so, how?

c. Did it take longer to perform? Why?

d. Were you less accurate in your movements? Describe how. Why do you think this happened?

e. Did you move in a different manner than usual? Why? Did you make any accommodations to your usual way of doing this? If so, what were they?

CHAPTER 3

Factors Influencing Movement

Susan J. Sain, MS, OTR/L, FAOTA

Key Terms

accessibility
active insufficiency
axis
buoyancy
center of gravity
closed kinematic chain
close-pack position
compression
contact force
contexts
decubiti
distraction
drag
force

force couple
friction
inertia
kinematic chain
lever
lift
negotiability
open kinematic chain
open-pack position
passive insufficiency
resistance
shear force
tenodesis
universal design

Chapter Outline

Introduction
Contexts
  Environmental Factors
  Personal Factors
  Forces in Nature
Related Factors
  Simple Machines
  Active and Passive Insufficiency
  Kinematic Chains
  Open- and Close-Pack Joint Positions
Summary
References
Applications

Sain, S. J., & Roller, C. L. *Kinesiology for the Occupational Therapy Assistant: Essential Components of Function and Movement, Third Edition* (pp. 51-74).

Introduction

This chapter investigates various factors that impact movement. Many of these factors are external to body functions and body structures, yet they dictate characteristics of movement. The *Occupational Therapy Practice Framework: Domain and Process, Fourth Edition* (OTPF-4) discusses **contexts** and their impact on movement. Contexts encompasses both environmental and personal factors. Subcategories of environmental factors are the natural environment and human-made changes to the environment, products and technology, support and relationships, attitudes, and services, systems, and policies. Personal factors addressed under context in the OTPF-4 incorporate things like age, education, profession, lifestyle, social background, race and ethnicity, gender identity, and cultural identification, to name a few. Concepts of **accessibility**, **negotiability**, and **universal design** are explained as they relate to movement. Forces of nature, such as gravity and Newton's laws of motion will be considered. Another factor impacting movement is **force**. Three primary external forces, fluid force, **contact force**, and gravity, are discussed. Secondary forces emerge from these primary forces and impact the body. The secondary forces addressed are joint **compression**, joint contraction, and pressure. The impact of simple machines on movement is presented. Still other factors that impact movement are internal and are related to certain aspects of joints and muscles. These factors include muscular insufficiency, **kinematic chains**, and **open-** or **close-pack joint positions**. All of these factors have the ability to enable or hinder movement and many of them can be manipulated in therapy to achieve maximal results.

People live and exist in relation to their environment and within the context of their lives. Thus, it stands to reason that contexts and environments can have a significant impact on function and functional movement. Modifying or changing the context or environment may enhance a client's ability to participate in occupations of their choice. Both the World Health Organization's (WHO) *International Classification of Functioning, Disability and Health* (ICF) and the American Occupational Therapy Association's (AOTA) OTPF-4 discuss the impact of contextual and environmental factors on function and disability. WHO (2001) essentially states that a client's disability resides within the society, and not within the individual. A client with a disabling condition or diagnosis is hindered by societal norms, expectations, environmental accessibility, and other factors. In other words, a client with a diagnosis is not disabled by the actual medical condition. In this sense, if stereotypes and stigmas did not exist and universal design was widely accepted, then the independence and functioning of a person with a disability would be no different from that of any other person.

The ICF lists two groups of contextual factors: personal and environmental. Within the ICF, personal factors are considered intrinsic, or internal to the person, while environmental factors are considered extrinsic, or external to the individual. The key is how these factors impact the person's ability to function by either facilitating or hindering performance. The OTPF-4 category of contexts encompasses environmental and personal factors. As in the ICF, *environment* refers to external situations; however, environment also includes social and attitudinal surroundings. Box 3-1 defines context and environment as presented in the OTPF-4. This chapter will follow the definitions of the OTPF-4 as they relate to the domain of contexts.

Contexts

As stated previously, the domain of contexts in the OTPF-4 is divided into two areas: environmental factors and personal factors. Environmental factors include "natural environment and human-made changes to the environment, products and technology, support and relationships, attitudes, and services, systems and policies" (AOTA, 2020, p. 10). Personal factors encompass "chronological age, sexual orientation, gender identity, race and ethnicity, cultural

BOX 3-1

Context: "Construct that constitutes the complete makeup of a person's life as well as the common and divergent factors that characterize groups and populations. Context includes environmental factors and personal factors."

Environmental factors: "Aspects of the physical, social, and attitudinal surroundings in which people live and conduct their lives."

Personal factors: "Unique features of the person reflecting the particular background of their life and living that are not part of a health condition or health state. Personal factors are generally considered to be enduring, stable attributes of the person, although some personal factors may change over time."

(AOTA, 2020, pp. 76, 81)

identification and attitudes, social background, life experiences, habits and behavioral patterns, individual psychological assets, education, profession, lifestyle, and other health conditions including fitness" (AOTA, 2020, pp. 10-11). All of these areas impact engagement and participation in occupations.

Environmental Factors

The first division of contexts is environmental factors. According to the OTPF-4, environmental factors influence functioning and disability and can have either a positive or negative impact. Negative impacts are considered barriers to occupation or something that hinders or makes engagement more difficult. Positive impacts would help to enable participation in an occupation or activity. The ICF definition of environment includes the physical, social, and attitudinal surroundings in which people carry out their lives. Items or categories included in the classification of environmental factors within the ICF are products, technology, natural and human-made features of the environment, attitudes of people, services, systems, and policies (WHO, 2001). As you can see, the environmental factors subdivisions presented in the OTPF-4 closely adhere to the framework and philosophy of the WHO. WHO states that health, function, and participation are based on external factors and are not solely based on factors within the individual. While studying these environmental variables, keep in mind that many of them can be modified by the occupational therapy practitioner to enhance functional movement. Additionally, a client's needs and movement demands will change depending on the environment and the context in which the client is performing the task. In other words, one functional movement pattern or option is not sufficient; clients will need a range of movement options to meet the ever-changing conditions encountered daily.

The environmental factor of natural and human-made changes to the environment incorporates geography, population, flora, fauna, climate, natural events, human-caused events, light, and time-related changes. Humans can impact the environment in many ways. One of these is the built or

human-made physical environment, which includes buildings, roads, bridges, communication towers, flood walls, and numerous other structures. In addition, human impact can cause widespread changes in the environment that affect our daily lives. Some examples include pollution, environmental disasters, and war. The natural physical environment includes things such as terrain; bodies of water; sensory aspects, including climate, scents, plants, and animals; and forces, such as gravity and **friction**. Some of these forces and their relationship to motion have been described by Sir Isaac Newton. Newton's three laws of motion will be described later in this chapter as they impact functional movement, including how these concepts can be applied to occupational therapy. Other factors related to gravity, the **center of gravity** (COG) in the body or in an object, and stability against competing forces will also be discussed in this chapter. Other natural phenomena can also alter the environment, often in negative ways, causing significant and lasting change that affects human performance and engagement in occupation. Some examples include hurricanes, earthquakes, mudslides, and excessive or insufficient rainfall. The impacts of these natural occurrences are beyond the scope of this text.

The built or human-made environment can have a significant impact on an individual's ability to engage in independent occupation. Structures, including buildings and roads, that are properly designed and adhere to the laws related to accessibility can enable engagement in occupation and increase functional mobility. On the other hand, structures that are not adequately constructed can have a detrimental impact on function. Accessibility is regarded as a beginning point when considering impact on function. A building or bathroom can be accessible, but not functional. Consider the bathroom that is large enough for a wheelchair, has grab bars for transfers, and has a door that is easy to maneuver. What could hinder independent functioning? Perhaps the toilet paper dispenser is out of reach once the person has transferred to the commode. This is a common occurrence impairing an individual's use of the bathroom.

The ability of the person to interact with the environment and independently use common features, such as a toilet paper dispenser, is part of a more comprehensive approach called *negotiability*. Negotiability implies that the

---

BOX 3-2

Accessibility: "Removing barriers that prevent people with activity limitations from the use of services, products, and information."
Negotiability: "The ability to access a feature of the environment and use it for its intended purpose in a manner acceptable to the person."
(Cronin & Mandich, 2005, p. 351)

Universal design: "The design of products and environments to be usable by all people, to the greatest extent possible, without the need for adaptation or specialized design."
(The Center for Universal Design, 1997, para. 7)

---

built environment is also designed so that features such as doors, soap and towel dispensers, household appliances, light switches, and sinks are usable by everyone. Negotiability is related to the concept of universal design. The intent of universal design is to simplify life for all people, regardless of age or ability, by making all environments (built, social, print, and virtual) usable by as many people as possible (The Center for Universal Design, 1997). Universal design is more valuable and cost effective if items are initially designed and constructed in a way that is usable for the most people without later having to make adaptations. The concept of universal design has been applied to many areas in addition to the construction of buildings. One such example is a professor providing handouts electronically. In this way, a student with visual deficits can independently and privately enlarge the print for enhanced personal use. Computerized lecture handouts could also benefit the student who has problems with handwriting, spelling, or grammar. If keyboarding is more efficient for this student, notes can be taken electronically with the automatic spell and grammar check activated, or the student could use voice recognition software to transcribe notes. Computerized/digital handouts may also benefit the student who has no particular deficits but would prefer to access notes from a home computer late at night. When working with clients who have movement impairments or who are not engaging in their occupations of choice, the occupational therapy practitioner needs to assess the human-made environmental features to determine what, if anything, is impeding function. Often, modifying the built physical environment will increase engagement and enhance functional movement. Accessibility, negotiability, and universal design are defined in Box 3-2, and examples of each related to specific conditions are given in Table 3-1.

The natural physical environment can also affect function in many ways. Geographic terrain can impair or enhance movement. It is easier to walk, ride a bike, propel a wheelchair, or rollerblade on a hard, smooth, flat, even surface than on uneven, rough, steep terrain strewn with rocks. Climate, especially heat and humidity levels, can decrease function in people of all abilities. For a person with cardiovascular and respiratory problems, increases in temperature and humidity can constitute a significant health risk. For the generally healthy individual, these same excesses can decrease endurance and enjoyment of an activity. Sensory aspects including aromas, plants, and animals, may pose a problem for people with allergies or asthma, while for other individuals these sensory qualities may enhance the experience.

The second environmental factor listed in the OTPF-4, products and technology, has components including food and other products for personal consumption, technology for personal use in daily living, mobility products, processes or products for communication, education, employment, sporting and recreational activities, and virtual environments. There are a wide variety of products that can be adapted to enable participation in multiple occupations. Each would need to be assessed individually with the client, the chosen occupation, and the context in which the occupation takes place. A complete discussion of products is beyond the realm of this text. The virtual environment can be described as one that occurs in the absence of physical contact. In most situations, the *virtual environment* refers to some type of communication or interaction between two or more individuals; however, the interaction could also be solely between an individual and an electronic system. There are many forms of virtual environment, which include, but are not limited to, computers; airway transmissions for handheld electronic devices; television, radio, and satellite transmissions; home environmental control systems; and video courses or conferencing. The use of the virtual context is almost limitless and can be incorporated in many areas of occupation, such as play, work, leisure, education, and health care (Cronin & Mandich, 2005). Telemedicine, or the more recent development of telehealth, represents one way that health care is becoming more virtual. Telemedicine focuses more on treatment, whereas telehealth focuses on prevention as well. These systems can monitor the status of the client in their own home. So, whether our clients are interested in the virtual world or not, it is encroaching on their lives! The virtual context requires different skills and knowledge than the real-world environment, and this must be taken into

TABLE 3-1

Definitions and Examples of Accessibility, Negotiability, and Universal Design

EXAMPLE	ACCESSIBILITY	NEGOTIABILITY	UNIVERSAL DESIGN
Wheelchair use in home	Ramps, elevators, grab bars	Automatic doors, lower light switches	Original construction with 17″ high toilet (customary is 14″ to 15″), curbless showers, stepless entrances, flexibility, ease of use
Severe visual impairments in academics	Braille, white cane, guide dog	No clutter in hallways, sound notification crosswalks	Varied and flexible means of attending, teaching, engaging students, testing
Weak grasp at mealtime	Adapted utensils, containers opened by others, pre-cut food	Lightweight utensils with easy-grip handles, lightweight glasses or use of straw to drink	In this situation, universal design principles are similar to examples in negotiability.

consideration in therapy. For some individuals, the virtual environment has greatly expanded the ability to interact with others in society.

The next two aspects of environmental factors, support and relationships and attitudes will be discussed jointly. Support and relationships includes "people or animals that provide practical physical or emotional support...in the home, workplace, or school" (AOTA 2020, p. 10). Attitudes include values and beliefs held by someone other than the client. The expectations of other people with whom the client interacts need to be considered as these greatly influence an individuals' choice of, and participation in, any given occupation. As indicated in the ICF, attitude as an environmental factor incorporates consequences of social interactions that affect the person individually and on the societal level (WHO, 2001). Societal level consequences may include limiting factors, such as stereotypes, or supportive factors, such as legislation mandating that people with differing abilities are treated equally. Real or perceived expectations of other people greatly impact a person's choice of, and engagement in, an occupation. This is often seen in parents' desires regarding their children's employment or educational occupations. For example, children may be expected to work in the family business, regardless of what the child wants. Some occupations are chosen because they encourage interaction with the social environment, such as being in a choir. Other occupations are chosen because they limit the social interactions required (e.g., reading). As with the other aspects of contexts, supports, relationships, and attitudes may enhance or impede engagement in occupation. When considering involvement in occupation, these factors must be taken into account.

The final aspect of environmental factors, services, systems and policies, often develops out of societal attitudes. Included here are economic services, health services, and legislation, such as the Americans with Disabilities Act (ADA). These are created to meet the needs of individuals, groups, and populations. For example, the ADA requires accessibility standards be met, thus enabling persons of all abilities the use of a facility.

Personal Factors

The second division of contexts is personal factors. As stated previously, personal factors include age, sexual orientation, gender identity, race and ethnicity, cultural identification and attitudes, social background, life experiences, habits and behavioral patterns, individual psychological assets, education, profession, lifestyle, and other health conditions, including fitness. Although all personal factors, or the particular background and unique features of the person, impact engagement and participation in occupations, the personal factors of race and ethnicity and cultural identification and cultural attitudes will be discussed in detail here. Culture incorporates values, ideas, behaviors, language, traditions, daily practices, expectations, and attitudes adhered to by a certain group of people, race, or ethnicity. Cultural traditions tend to be passed down from one generation to the next. Culture defines what is acceptable to a certain society. Culture shapes how many things are done. It must be noted that not all members of a certain culture will adhere to the expectations of their culture in the same manner. A person must refrain from stereotyping people based on cultural norms; however, knowledge of generalizations regarding certain cultural norms may help practitioners to provide care that is more meaningful to the client. To stereotype is to "repeat without variation" (Merriam-Webster, n.d.). As such, a stereotype is limiting, often derogatory, and usually ends any type of meaningful communication. On the other hand, a generalization serves as a place to begin discussion with a client. A generalization may include common assumptions related to a particular culture, but the person holding the assumption does not force this trait or attribute on all people within that cultural group.

For example, your client is an older Hispanic woman receiving inpatient occupational therapy. A generalization about Latin American families is that the extended family, including elders, is very important. Knowing this generalization about family values can guide discussion related to discharge planning for your older adult client. If, on the other hand, based on the generalization, you automatically assume the client will return home and be cared for by family members, that is a stereotype. The generalization leads to discussions that are sensitive to perceived cultural standards while the stereotype assumes that all people of a given culture will act the same way all the time. The practitioner should not simply assume that they know the cultural norms for a certain group of people, nor should they assume that these norms have value for a particular client. Behaving in this way would be stereotyping. Additionally, cultural norms may differ from one socioeconomic group to another, even within the same cultural group. Knowledge of cultural norms can lead to dialogue and greater understanding of the individual and how the person internalizes that cultural norm. This information can then be used to aid communication, select therapeutic activities, and tailor an intervention program best suited for the particular client. In this way, incorporating the cultural context makes the intervention more meaningful to the client.

One example of a functional activity affected by cultural standards is mealtime. Many countries in Europe and North, Central, and South America use silverware to eat. Many Asian countries, however, use chopsticks. In Morocco and India, the first three fingers on the right hand are often used for eating. All of these forms of eating require different use of the fingers and associated joints and muscles. The time of the meal also varies greatly. In Spain and several Latin American countries, the main meal is eaten at about 2 p.m. In many of these countries, businesses and schools close for 2 to 4 hours during the middle of the day to allow time to eat a large meal and rest afterwards. The evening meal is often eaten at about 10 or 11 p.m., much later than bedtime for most children from the United States! In Japan, it is customary to sit on cushions on the floor while eating at a low table. Imagine how differently this custom may impact the older adult population with limited mobility or a person in a wheelchair as compared to another custom. For these populations, the standard in the United States of sitting on a chair at a higher table might prove easier. This one activity of daily living, eating, and the skills and movements necessary to accomplish this task vary greatly from one cultural group to another.

Cultural standards can also impact child development. For example, in Guatemala, it is not uncommon for women who sell at market to carry infants and young children in a sling near their body or contain them in a box that they cannot climb out of while the women work. These practices keep the child safe and from wandering away. These children may exhibit delays in walking and crawling, primarily due to lack of experience. When given the opportunity, they usually master these gross motor skills quickly. In this situation, it is both the culture and the environment that are influencing movement. Many developmental markers that are used in the United States are not commonly used elsewhere. Examples include the pediatrician encouraging a child to play pat-a-cake or asking an older child to draw a house. For infants not from the United Sates, it is often their first exposure to the game of pat-a-cake; therefore, the game is not repeated or imitated. This should not be recorded as a lack of knowledge, or ability on the child's part. Rather, it may simply be a lack of experience or exposure. Similarly, during the draw-a-house activity, children who have been living in refugee camps may draw a tent, not a house. These children may have never lived in a house before coming to this country. Depending on the assessment instrument used, a tent drawing might not be scored as passing or age appropriate. These examples of cultural norms indicate how culture may influence behavior, affect movement, guide communication, and have an impact on what is acceptable to an individual. Occupational therapy goals and intervention must reflect the cultural context of the client in order to provide benefit and interest to the client.

Another category of personal factors, habits and behavioral patterns, was addressed under the domain of performance patterns in Chapter 1. Still other personal factors include primarily internal factors, such as age, sexual orientation, gender, behavioral patterns, and psychological assets (e.g., temperament, coping styles). Most of the internal personal factors cannot be modified or easily changed. Personal factors that are less intrinsic to the individual may include, but are not limited to, socioeconomic status and educational level. These factors may be modified during one's lifetime. Personal factors can affect a person's motivation to move or determine the selection of movement activities. Activity patterns may change over the lifespan, with younger people tending to choose activities that require more energy expenditure, such as soccer. An older individual may select a less aggressive sport, perhaps golf; however, golf is a relatively expensive sport, so a person in a lower socioeconomic group may not be able to participate, even if interested. Thus, one can see that all personal factors do indeed impact a person's ability and opportunity to function.

As you can see, contexts are interrelated. Accordingly, each area impacts the others. For example, within the virtual environment of text messaging, attitudes may change from those associated with other forms of communication. People tend to reply immediately to a text message whereas they may return a phone call, email, or letter hours, or even days, later. Considering personal factors, younger people tend to text more than those in retirement years. Additionally, cultural standards are different in the virtual realm. Behavior standards related to what is acceptable are often altered. Different behaviors are considered appropriate or acceptable in the virtual context, such as texting using abbreviations and acronyms, whereas these would not be acceptable in a real-world environment such as an English composition class. Environmental factors also impact engagement and behaviors. One acts differently in a football stadium vs. a church service. A person's engagement in any occupation is affected by all of the contexts described previously. Each factor has the potential to aid or hinder the desire to move, thus impacting involvement in occupation. Therefore, modifying or changing one factor may enhance or interfere with occupational performance overall.

Forces in Nature

Also of importance to the study of kinesiology and movement is an examination of the various forces in the natural environment that impact movement. Forces in nature can produce, stop, or modify motion. Additionally, once something is in motion, force can increase or decrease the speed of the motion or change the direction of the motion (Luttgens & Hamilton, 1997). A force can either produce a push or a pull. When referring to the body, push is also termed *compression* or *approximation*, and pull may be referred to as *tension* or **distraction**. When both force types are balanced, the object is said to be *in equilibrium*. Movement occurs when the forces are not balanced or are not in equilibrium (Smith et al., 1996). Newton developed his laws of motion while studying various natural forces.

In order to fully appreciate Newton's laws of motion, it is helpful to first have a basic understanding of some of the forces at work in nature that affect one's ability to move. Force can be generated from internal or external sources. The most common internal force is the force produced by muscles. Muscular force is discussed in other chapters of this text. There are a multitude of external forces. This chapter will only consider three primary external forces: fluid force, contact force, and gravity. These forces are considered primary because they occur first and they can lead to other effects on the body, which are referred to here as *secondary forces*. This text will discuss three secondary forces. Discussion of secondary forces will begin with joint compression, followed by joint distraction, and end with pressure on body surfaces (Luttgens & Hamilton, 1997; Smith et al., 1996). Primary forces will be presented first.

The primary external force to be discussed first is fluid force, which includes air and liquids, such as water. Water and air are both subject to the same laws and principles. Important concepts to understand include **buoyancy**, **drag**, and **lift**. Buoyancy is commonly considered a phenomenon of water as we are more aware of the effects of buoyancy in water. One definition of buoyancy is an upward force equal to the weight of the displaced liquid. Although in principle this also applies to air, the buoyancy of air has a much smaller impact on human movement. Due to the increased buoyancy

in water relative to air, water can support a body more easily than air. For example, a client whose muscles are not strong enough to overcome the effects of gravity in order to stand independently may be able to do so while in waist- or chest-deep water. Occupational therapy practitioners may also use the medium of water to unload weight from painful joints, such as occurs with arthritis, in order to allow the client to experience pain-reduced or pain-free movement. However, due to the increased drag, or **resistance** to forward motion, of water over air, water can also be used to increase resistance and, therefore, be used for strengthening purposes. Increasing the speed of a movement in water increases drag and will make the movement more difficult to complete; it will also require more energy expenditure. Another way to increase drag is to increase the surface area of an object. The final principle, lift, refers to a change in fluid pressure as a result of differences in air or liquid flow velocities around an object. Lift is produced when flow over one side of the object is faster than the flow over the opposite side of the same object. Lift acts perpendicular to the direction of fluid flow and is best exemplified in the ability of heavy planes to remain in the air, as described in the Bernoulli principle (Luttgens & Hamilton, 1997). Drag and lift can only occur if there is velocity occurring either in the object or in the fluid. The greater the velocity, the greater the effects of drag and lift.

Drag and lift can be felt if you place your hand out of a car window while the car is in motion. If your elbow is flexed to 90 degrees and your hand is perpendicular to the ground, you experience drag; pressure is felt on the surface of the hand facing the front of the car, and turbulence is felt on the opposite side. Streamlining reduces drag, allowing for easier and faster movement through the fluid. If you gradually lower your hand toward a position parallel to the ground, the drag decreases as the contact surface area lessens, and less pressure is felt on the hand. When the hand is parallel to the ground, you experience much less drag or resistance because the surface area of your fingertips is much less than that of the palm of your hand. However, before your hand reaches the parallel-to-the-ground position and is tilted with the fingers slightly upward, you will feel lift—the air flow is faster under your fingers and, thus, tends to push them upward, the effect of lift. Because fluid forces have a greater impact on movement as velocity increases, they present less of an impact on daily occupations than do the other forms of force discussed here. Contact forces, such as normal reaction and friction, have a greater impact on functional movement and are easier to manipulate in daily life activities.

Contact force occurs when one object comes in contact with another, creating force between the objects. There are many categories of contact force including normal reaction and friction. In normal reaction, each object must contact the other with the same magnitude or amount of force. Normal reaction is related to the idea that forces must be paired and opposite to each other. The two opposing forces are sometimes called *interaction pairs* or *action-reaction forces*. A child hanging from a jungle gym pulls down on the

BOX 3-3

Examples of ways to *increase* friction to enable client participation and independence include using gloves for wheelchair propulsion, placing gripper pads under throw rugs, using Dycem or gripper pads under dishes while eating or cooking, and using sticky or tacky finger cream to count or separate money or turn pages in a book.

Examples of ways to *decrease* friction to enable client participation and independence include placing a plastic bag in the seat of a chair to help the client slide forward or pivot in the chair; placing tennis balls over the feet of a walker or on chair legs to make them easier to slide across the floor; and placing heavier items (e.g., a pan of water) on a smooth cloth or pillowcase before sliding them over the counter, floor, or other surface.

BOX 3-4

"A pressure [injury] is localized injury to the skin and/or underlying tissue, usually over a bony prominence, as a result of pressure, or pressure in combination with shear. A number of contributing and confounding factors are also associated with pressure [injury]; the significance of these factors has yet to be elucidated."

(European Pressure Ulcer Advisory Panel, 2009; National Pressure Injury Advisory Panel, 2009)

equipment at the same time and with the same force (action) as the equipment pushes back up on the child (reaction). This concept is represented in Newton's third law of motion: for every action, there is an equal and opposite reaction. This law and its applications to functional movement will be discussed later in the chapter.

Another type of contact force, friction, is described as force acting in the opposite direction to the desired movement and occurring at the area of contact between the two surfaces. Friction can also be described as a force that opposes the efforts of one object to slide or roll over another object. Considering movement or resistance in opposite directions, friction can either enable the activity or make it more difficult to complete depending on the desired outcome. Friction is preferred during the push-off phase of walking so the foot does not slip across the floor, causing a fall. Friction in this case can be increased by wearing rubber-soled shoes. On the other hand, too much friction is undesirable for the dancer trying to glide across the floor. In this example, friction is decreased by the smooth leather sole of the ballet shoe moving against the polished surface of the hardwood dance floor. Yet another example is observed when using the hands to grasp an object. Friction is desired on a tennis racquet so that the racquet does not fly out of the hand. A gymnast decreases friction with the use of chalk so both hands will rotate easily around the uneven bars. The amount of friction is often manipulated in therapy to enable functional movement. As friction has an impact on every motion, the applications in therapy are endless. Refer to Box 3-3 for examples of how to modify friction to enable participation. Friction and pressure can lead to **shear force** or shearing force. Pressure acts at a right angle, or perpendicular, to the skin's surface. Shear force is a frictional force acting parallel to the skin's surface

that may cause the body to slide against the resistance of the skin and the surface it is resting on. This in turn may lead to the skin remaining stationary (due to friction between the skin and the supporting surface) but deeper fascia moving with the skeleton. This movement creates distortion, or shearing (Venes, 2013). Shear forces are important to consider in therapy as they can cause **decubiti**, also referred to as *pressure injuries* or, more commonly, *bed sores*. Pressure injuries are defined in Box 3-4. One cause of shearing is if a client is not properly positioned in a wheelchair and the buttocks are sliding forward toward the front of the chair. Friction and pressure due to body weight will keep the skin from moving forward in the seat. However, the underlying tissues and bones will tend to slide forward, causing distress between the skin and deeper tissues. This damages small blood vessels, eventually leading to skin and tissue breakdown. Refer to Box 3-5 for further discussion of shear force.

The final external force mentioned is a force that affects absolutely every movement and occupation in which we engage. It is known as gravity. The direction of the force of gravity is always toward the center of the earth. The COG of an object is the point around which the body's mass is evenly distributed. Mass and weight are not the same thing. Mass is defined as the quantity of matter contained in an object, whereas weight is the amount of gravitational force exerted on a body or object (Hall, 1999). It is true that weight is proportional to mass, or stated another way, the greater the mass, usually the greater the weight, especially on Earth. However, if a person were to travel to the moon, the body mass would remain the same while the body weight would decrease as a result of the decreased effects of gravity at that distance from the center of the earth. Even though gravity exerts a constant, unchanging force on our bodies, one can modify its effects.

BOX 3-5

Shearing occurs when underlying tissue and bone move one way and the skin moves another way. Risk of injury caused by shearing may increase when:

- The head of the bed is elevated above 30 degrees. (Note: Any angle between erect sitting and lying supine may cause shearing; however, the risk is particularly high at a 45-degree angle.)
- Patient is rolled side to side with repositioning.
- Skin is stretched or pulled.
- Massaging or rubbing red areas or areas over bony landmarks.

Risk of injury caused by shearing may be reduced by:

- Lowering the head of the bed as tolerated prior to repositioning the client.
- Flexing and elevating the knees before elevating the head of the bed while it remains elevated.
- Keeping the head of the bed raised for short periods only.
- Lifting patients when repositioning them—never drag or slide them over a surface.
- Performing more frequent but smaller shifts in position for clients who cannot tolerate major changes in position.
- Decreasing the chance of sliding in a chair with proper positioning, hip belts, elevating knees with wedges.

(Northwest Regional Spinal Cord Injury System, n.d.; Royal Children's Hospital Melbourne, 2022)

For example, an occupational therapy practitioner may have an extremely weak client begin exercises in a gravity-reduced position. If the movement is elbow flexion, gravity-reduced options may include having the client place the upper extremity (UE) on a table and positioning the arm horizontal to the floor or using a mobile arm support. Figure 3-1 shows a client working in a gravity-reduced plane. In addition, a cloth is placed under the client's arm to reduce friction, thus making the activity even easier to complete.

All of the external forces discussed, as well as the internal force provided by muscles, share some common features. Force is a **vector** quantity, which means that it has qualities of both magnitude and direction. Force is also considered to have a specific point of application or area where the force contacts the object. The **magnitude** of a force refers to its size or the amount of force exerted. The direction of a force is the path the force follows. The path of movement can be either a linear or rotary motion. **Linear motion** may be categorized either as moving along a straight line or curvilinear, moving along a curved line. **Rotary motion** occurs around an **axis**. Combinations of linear and rotary movements occur together for most functional human movements. This is called *general motion*. In many situations, the direction of movement is a downward direction following the pull of gravity. Forces other than gravity often have a different direction vector; for example, a toy car pushed across the floor would follow a perpendicular path to, or move horizontal to, the direction vector for gravity. For muscles, the direction of force is the line of pull of the muscle. The **point of application** of a force in the body is at the point of insertion of the muscle tendon. For objects, the point of application is through the COG for linear movements. If the point of application is not through the COG, a rotary movement will occur (Luttgens

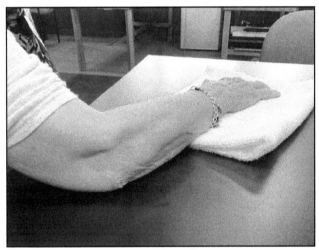

Figure 3-1. Client performing an elbow flexion exercise in a gravity-reduced plane. A cloth is placed under the client's arm to reduce the effects of friction, further grading the exercise to meet the client's weakened state.

& Hamilton, 1997). An example of both linear and rotary movement can be observed during the activity of pushing a heavy box. If the box is pushed in the middle, through its COG, it will slide across the floor in a straight line, or in a linear fashion. If the box is pushed at a point toward one of the ends and not through its COG, it will rotate. Rotary movement also occurs under the conditions of a **force couple**. A force couple is defined as two or more forces with similar magnitude but opposite or significantly different direction vectors. These forces must be applied to the same object at the same time and produce rotation. The forces act on opposite sides of the axis of the object. The axis is the center, or point, around which the object rotates. A force couple allows for greater strength in movement. A common example

BOX 3-6

Axis: A real or imaginary line point or line passing through the center of a body, about which the body may rotate.

Force couple: Two or more forces of equal magnitude, but opposite direction, applied to the same object but at different points of application, working together to cause movement; increases strength of movement, produces rotary motion.

Linear motion: Movement along a path pertaining to or representing a line that may be straight or curved; all parts of the object move in the same direction at the same speed.

Magnitude: Size, amount, and dimension; the basic unit of measurement in the United States for the magnitude of force is the pound.

Point of application: The point on the object where the force is applied; for a muscular force, this is commonly considered to be at the insertion of the muscle to the bone.

Rotary motion: Turning or movement about an axis; parts of the object further from the axis move at a greater speed than those close to the axis.

Torque: The turning or rotary effect of a force.

Vector: A physical quantity or force possessing both magnitude or size and direction; can be represented by a straight line.

(Hall,1999; Venes, 2013)

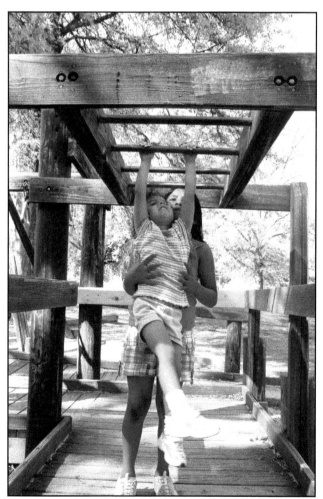

Figure 3-2. Naturally occurring joint distraction (mild separation of the bony ends of the joint) of the UEs as a child plays on the monkey bars. (Reproduced with permission from Angela Grussing.)

in daily life of a force couple is a steering wheel. While one hand pulls in a downward direction, the other hand is pulling in an upward direction. These opposite, but combined, movements cause the wheel to turn with more power than if only one hand is used. This is especially evident when the power steering mechanism is not working. In the case of the steering wheel, the axis is the steering column. The forces are provided in opposite directions on each side of the steering wheel by the UEs. The rotary force generated is called **torque** (Levangie & Norkin, 2005). Greater torque is created when turning the wheel without power steering than when the power steering is functioning. Definitions of terms in bold are located in Box 3-6.

The primary forces discussed previously include fluid force, contact force, and gravity. These forces in turn lead to secondary forces that act on the body, including joint compression, joint distraction, and pressure on body surfaces (Luttgens & Hamilton, 1997; Smith et al., 1996). Joint compression is the pushing together of both sides of the joint toward the center of the joint. Joint compression occurs naturally in the ankles, knees, and hips during walking or jumping and in the joints of the UE when doing a push-up. Joint distraction, a pulling apart of the two joint surfaces, is also sometimes referred to as *traction*. Joint distraction is often produced by external forces, such as in the use of an external fixator, to help a broken bone realign for proper healing. Joint distraction occurs naturally in the shoulder, elbow, and wrist joints, as seen in a child swinging across the monkey bars (Figure 3-2). Lower extremity (LE) knee and hip joint distraction can be observed in the child hanging upside down with legs wrapped around a jungle gym.

Pressures on body surfaces pose a potentially serious problem. Repeated pressure over a small surface area, such as the back of the heel for a bed-ridden client, can easily lead to decubiti. In the fabrication of splints, the therapist needs to be exceedingly careful to avoid areas of pressure as this can also cause pain, discomfort, and skin breakdown. In general, if the pressure can be distributed over a larger point of application (surface area), the likelihood of skin breakdown, tissue death, or bruising is lessened. The concept of diffusing pressure over a larger surface area is evident when comparing high-heeled shoes that have a very small heel size to tennis shoes. If someone steps on your toe with a spiked heel, it will hurt much more than if that same person steps on your toe while wearing tennis shoes. This is because the pressure exerted by the weight of the person wearing tennis shoes is distributed through the much larger surface area of the entire bottom of the shoe. Refer back to the discussion on shear force for other causes of decubiti.

When considering a client's functional movement, the practitioner must always consider the forces at work that impact movement. Just as primary forces can be manipulated during occupational therapy treatment, secondary forces are also important to consider. Two examples of manipulation of primary forces discussed include increasing or decreasing friction and reducing the effects of gravity to aid movement. Secondary forces such as joint manipulation, including compression or traction, may also be used or modified by the practitioner to enhance range of motion (ROM). Additionally, the effects of pressure need to be continually monitored to avoid skin breakdown and tissue damage.

Newton's laws of motion stem from his observations of the forces at work in nature. His laws describe the forces that produce, modify, and stop motion. Newton published his findings in 1687 in a book called *Philosophiae Naturalis Principia Mathematica (Mathematical Principles of Natural Philosophy)* commonly known as the *Principia*. Newton's laws, as he originally penned them, are printed here (Ravilious, 2010).

- Newton's law of inertia: Every object persists in its state of rest or uniform motion in a straight line unless it is compelled to change that state by forces impressed upon it.
- Newton's law of acceleration: Force is equal to the change in momentum (mV) per change in time. For a constant mass, force equals mass times acceleration (expressed in the famous equation F = ma).
- Newton's law of action and reaction: For every action, there is an equal and opposite reaction.

To better understand *Newton's first law of motion*, the concept of **inertia** needs to be addressed. Inertia is defined as "the tendency of a body to remain in its state (at rest or in motion) until acted upon by an outside force" (Venes, 2013, p. 1232). If an object is at rest, a force must act on the object to initiate movement. If, however, an object is already in motion, it will remain in motion, moving at the same speed and progressing in the same direction unless a force modifies or stops its motion. A skateboarder demonstrates the impact of this law as it acts on the skateboard as well as on the skateboarder. The skateboard will stop abruptly when it hits the curb (outside force); however, the skateboarder will not stop because their body did not have a force act on it. The skateboarder will continue moving forward, through the air, at the same speed and in the same direction until the force of gravity pulls the direction of their movement downward and, ultimately, contact with the ground stops their motion. The use of seat belts in cars, lap belts on wheelchairs, and straps in baby strollers help provide the force needed to stop the body's forward motion when the moving object the body is riding in stops abruptly.

The law of acceleration, commonly referred to as *Newton's second law*, describes why an object with less mass will move faster than an object with greater mass, given the same push or force. Inversely, this law states that a greater force or push is required to move (or stop) an object of larger mass than what is required to move (or stop) an object of smaller mass. You may have experienced this while driving if you have ever towed a heavy trailer, camper, or boat. It will take longer to stop your vehicle as compared to when you are not towing anything. It will also take longer to accelerate to the speed limit when towing the item. Acceleration may be defined as "the rate in change of velocity with respect to time" (Merriam-Webster, n.d.). This law can be observed easily in the health care setting. One example is that it takes less force or, simply stated, is easier, to propel a small, lightweight person (less mass) in a wheelchair than it does to propel a heavier person (more mass). The practitioner needs to keep this law in mind when working with clients who have general weakness. If a greater force is required to move something that has more mass, or is heavier, the practitioner needs to exhibit caution when using assistive devices, adaptive equipment, or splints. These devices increase the weight of the extremity being moved, thus requiring more force to produce and maintain movement for a functional activity. For example, if a client uses a splint to improve grasp and also needs a built-up handled utensil, self-feeding will require greater force or effort from the client, which may not be desirable. If, however, for safety reasons, a client propelling their own wheelchair or walker needs to decrease their speed, adding weight would help.

Newton's third law, the law of action and reaction, implies that there must be two forces present. Each force acts on the other, with the direction of the forces being opposite and the magnitude of the forces being equal. This concept is observed when a person leans against a wall. The wall supports the person by "pushing" back with equal force to the weight and pressure of the person pushing against the wall. Otherwise, the wall would cave in. In relation to functional movement, this concept can enable or hinder client independence. For example, it is much harder for a person to walk on a sandy beach, in which some sand is displaced prior to the equal and opposite reaction taking effect, than when the person walks on a paved sidewalk. Similarly, it is more difficult for a weak client to stand from a soft chair or sofa than it is to rise from a hard-surfaced chair.

BOX 3-7

Inclined plane: Used for elevating objects; a flat surface or plane that is at an angle to the horizontal surface it is placed upon.

Lever: A rigid bar that rotates about an axis or fulcrum; downward motion at one end causes upward motion at the opposite end.

Pulley: Used to change the direction of force or the point of application of force; consists of a rope around a small wheel that has a grooved rim to keep the rope in place.

Screw: Technically, a type of inclined plane, converts rotary motion into linear motion, either forward or backward.

Wedge: Converts downward force into perpendicular force, separating or splitting the object; a tool that is wide at one end and narrow at the other.

Wheel and axle: Used to move things over a greater distance; a circular object that rotates around a shaft.

(Free Dictionary Online, 2022; Merriam-Webster, n.d.)

When considering functional movement, it is essential for the occupational therapy practitioner to consider Newton's laws of motion in relation to client performance. Understanding these laws allows the practitioner to assess movement and make adjustments to the environment, objects in the environment, or the activity itself in order to increase independence or to create the right challenge for the client. Additionally, recognizing the ever-present consequences of these laws will enhance safety awareness and compliance.

Related Factors

Further factors that can influence functional movement and the practice of occupational therapy are included here. Simple machines, created to lessen the amount of effort required to perform a task or movement, will be discussed. Aspects of joint and muscle properties not discussed elsewhere in the text will also be addressed. These include active and **passive insufficiency**, kinematic chains, and open- or close-pack joint positions.

Simple Machines

There are six types of simple machines: wheel and axle, pulley, screw, wedge, inclined plane, and **lever**. Simple machines alter the magnitude or direction (or both) of an applied force (Collins & Mandich, 2014). These machines cannot reduce the amount of work required, but they do lessen the effort needed to perform the task. Work consists of both the amount of force needed and the distance over which the force is applied. Work is defined by Merriam-Webster (n.d.) as "the transference of energy that is produced by the motion of the point of application of a force and is measured by multiplying the force and the displacement of its point of application in the line of action." There is, however, a trade-off when using simple machines. Even though the effort or force

required is lessened, the distance over which a person must apply the force is increased. Machines can also allow us to change the direction of the force applied, such as in the use of a pulley. Box 3-7 describes the six simple machines. An example of the use of an inclined plane in therapy, or for functional movement, is a wheelchair ramp. The ramp requires the walker or wheelchair to move over a greater distance but requires less effort than moving in a vertical direction, such as that of a step. Inclined planes are sometimes presented as slant boards in occupational therapy and can be used to grade activities. If a client is unable to lift an object straight up from its resting surface, the activity can be made easier by sliding the object up the slant board. The wheel and axle and the pulley may be used in therapy with exercise equipment, scooter boards, arm boards, mobile arm supports, and other devices to aid movement. The screw and wedge are tools used more often in construction-type activities to either hold things together or to separate them. The simple machine that is most significant related to the practice of occupational therapy is the lever.

A lever functions using torque or rotation. All levers consist of a rigid bar rotating about an axis. The lever has three main components. These include the axis, the point at which force or effort is applied, and the point at which resistance is encountered. Also of importance is the length of the bar, or arm, from the axis to either the force or resistance. These are labeled *force arm* and *resistance arm*. The length of these arms can be altered, which, in turn, will make a task either easier or harder to complete. In general, lengthening the force arm makes the task easier, while shortening the force arm would render the task more difficult. Similarly, shortening the resistance arm makes the task easier, whereas lengthening the resistance arm causes the task to be more difficult to complete. Refer to Box 3-8 for further description of these parts. In the body, the axis is generally considered to be the joint, the force or effort is produced by muscles, and the resistance is the weight of the limb or body in addition to any external load, such as a bag of groceries or a textbook.

Levers can serve various functions. They can overcome a large resistance with less effort, use balance, increase the speed of the motion, or increase the distance the resistance is

BOX 3-8

Axis: Also called *fulcrum* or *pivot*; the point about which the rigid bar turns.
Force: The effort or energy used to move or hold the object.
Force arm: Also called *effort arm* or *movement arm*; distance from the axis to the point of application of the force.
Resistance: Sometimes referred to as *weight* or *load*; the object one is trying to move.
Resistance arm: Distance from the axis to the point of application of the resistance or load.

(Dail et al., 2011)

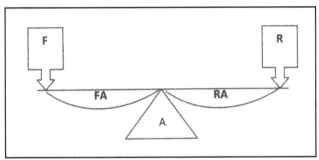

Figure 3-3. Graphic representation of first-class lever where the axis is in the middle. A represents axis, F represents force, and R represents resistance. The arrows depict the direction of the force and resistance. RA indicates the length of the resistance arm, and FA indicates the length of the force arm. First-class levers are designed for balance.

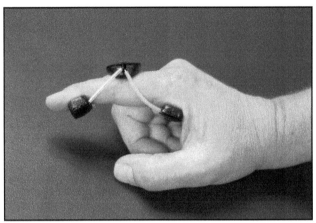

Figure 3-4. A finger splint designed using the principles of a first-class lever. The axis in this situation is the joint. Pressure (force and resistance) is balanced on both sides of the joint to encourage extension at the joint. (Reproduced with permission from Carolyn L. Roller, OTR/L.)

moved. There are three classes of levers, and each class is designed to better serve one of these functions. The difference in the classes of levers is dependent on the relationship of the three components to each other.

In a first-class lever, the axis is between the force and the resistance. A common example of this is a seesaw. The first-class lever can supply balance or change the direction of a force, such as converting a downward force into upward movement. In a seesaw, the axis is in the middle and is the point of rotation for the board resting on it. The force and resistance are the children at either end of the seesaw. In the case of the first-class lever, the direction of the force and direction of the resistance are the same, downward toward the pull of gravity. The force arm and resistance arm, however, move in opposite directions; as one goes up the other goes down. In this class of lever, the length of either the force arm or resistance arm can be changed. A crowbar is also an example of a first-class lever. In this case the crowbar converts

a downward force, say a rock, into upward movement (raising the rock to move it). Examples of first-class levers in the body are limited. Dail et al. (2011) refer to the head balancing on the vertebral column as a first-class lever. The axis is the vertebrae, the resistance is the weight of the head, pulled forward by gravity, and the force is supplied by the posterior muscles contracting to keep the head erect. First-class levers used for balance in occupational therapy can be seen with devices such as the mobile arm support balancing the forearm for functional use and in splinting a finger to decrease deformity. The axis or balance point for the splint is over the joint, while effort and resistance are applied equally on either side of the joint axis. Refer to Figures 3-3 through 3-5 for pictures of first-class levers.

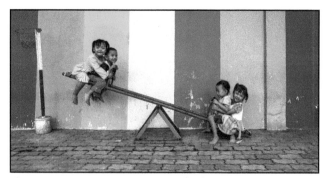

Figure 3-5. A seesaw is an example of a first-class lever. When both children are approximately the same weight, balance occurs. If the children are of different weights, the length of the force arm, the resistance arm, or both can be changed to facilitate balance. (evanttravels/shutterstock.com)

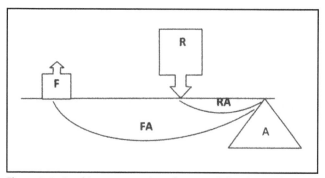

Figure 3-6. Graphic representation of a second-class lever where the resistance is in the middle. A represents axis, F represents force, and R represents resistance. The arrows depict the direction of the force and resistance. RA indicates the length of the resistance arm, and FA indicates the length of the force arm. A second-class lever is designed so that less force or strength is required to move a heavy item.

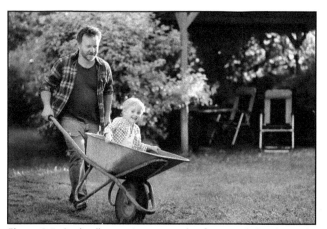

Figure 3-7. A wheelbarrow is an example of a second-class lever. The weight or resistance is between the axis and force, in this case inside the bucket. A heavy load is easier for a person to move due to the longer force arm (handles) in comparison to the short resistance arm (distance from weight in bucket to wheel axle). (Maria Sbytova/shutterstock.com)

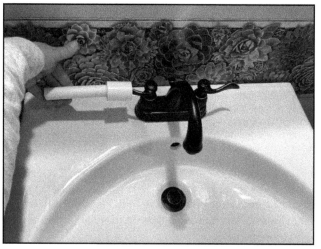

Figure 3-8. Extending the force arm on this lever-type faucet makes it easier to move the handle to turn the water on. This faucet is also a second-class lever.

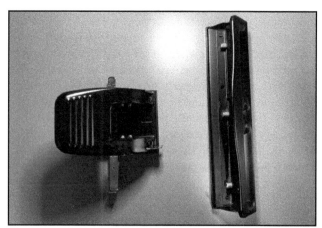

Figure 3-9. In this example of another second-class lever, a three-hole punch, the example on the left has a longer resistance arm, making it easier to punch holes in a large stack of paper.

Second-class levers give the mechanical advantage of force. With a second-class lever, a person can move a large resistance with a relatively small amount of force. In the second-class lever, the axis is at one end, the resistance is in the middle, and the force is at the end opposite the axis. In this type of lever, the force arm must always be longer than the resistance arm. As stated earlier, a longer force arm makes the task easier to perform. Unlike the first-class lever, the direction of force and the direction of resistance are opposite. Additionally, the force arm and resistance arm in the second-class lever move in the same direction. A common example of this type of lever is a wheelbarrow. The force exerted is in an upward direction moving the force arm upward while at the same time lifting the resistance or load, thus also moving the resistance arm upward. Whether or not second-class levers exist within the body is debatable. Some sources say that there is an example of this; others insist it is not so. This debate will be left to the researchers. Second-class levers are often used in therapy to make a task easier. If the occupational therapy practitioner lengthens the force arm on various devices, less energy is needed for the client to use the device. This principle can be observed in extending the handles on a nutcracker, a lever faucet, or a three-ring hole punch. Examples of second-class levers can be seen in Figures 3-6 through 3-9.

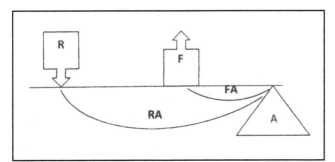

Figure 3-10. Graphic representation of a third-class lever where the force is in the middle. A represents axis, F represents force, and R represents resistance. The arrows depict the direction of the force and resistance. RA indicates the length of the resistance arm, and FA indicates the length of the force arm.

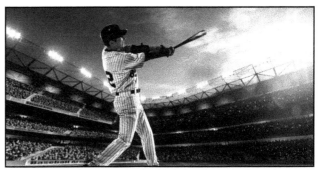

Figure 3-11. In this example of a third-class lever, the batter's torso is the axis, the point of application of force is the hands on the bat, and the force is the batter's muscle strength. The resistance is the ball. The third-class lever gives advantage to ROM and speed, as observed in the trajectory of a well-hit ball. (Eugene Onischenko/shutterstock.com)

In third-class levers, force or effort is between the axis and the resistance. As such, the resistance arm always needs to be longer than the force arm. A longer resistance arm requires more effort or force to use; however, the pay-off is increased speed and ROM. Similar to the second-class lever, the directions of the force and the resistance are opposite. Both arms move in the same direction. Unlike second-class levers, there are fewer external examples and more examples within the human body. In fact, most of the levers at work in the human body are third-class levers. External examples of third-class levers include a golf club and a baseball bat. The athlete's body is the axis, the force is applied through muscular action where the hands grasp and swing the club or bat, and the resistance is the ball. An internal example within the body occurs when a person uses the biceps brachii and other elbow flexors to overcome the resistance of a full glass of water as it is lifted to the mouth. In this case, the elbow is the axis, the point of insertion of the muscles is the force, and the resistance is the pull of gravity or the weight of the forearm plus the weight of the glass and water. This class of lever does require a fair amount of force or effort, but in turn it allows a person to move the distal segment of a limb across a wide ROM, to do so with speed, or both. These factors are necessary in order to carry out most functional activities. An example of a third-class lever commonly used in occupational therapy is the reacher. A reacher may be used by clients when they have decreased ROM and cannot reach items (e.g., items dropped on the floor). Basically, the reacher extends the resistance arm. This makes the item feel heavier or harder to pick up; however, the greater ROM granted does allow the client to retrieve the dropped item. A word of caution: Because extending the resistance arm makes the object seem heavier, only relatively light-weight items should be picked up with a reacher. Once again, the axis is the elbow, the force is the point of muscle insertion, and the resistance is the weight of the reacher plus the sock or other item being picked up. Examples of third-class levers can be found in Figures 3-10 through 3-12.

While working with clients, remember to use the lever class that matches the desired outcome. Keep in mind that one attribute is gained at the expense of another; for example,

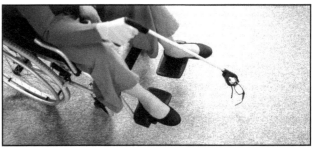

Figure 3-12. The reacher is an example of a third-class lever. In this situation, the axis is the elbow joint, the force is composed of the action of the elbow flexor muscles, and the resistance is the glasses, the weight of the limb, and the weight of the reacher combined. In this case, the resistance arm is lengthened by the distance from the hand to the end of the reacher. The advantage gained is ROM; the cost is increased effort or energy and strength required to pick up the glasses. (Andrey Popov/shutterstock.com)

if you increase ROM by lengthening the resistance arm, you will also increase the force needed to pick up the item. If balance and stability are desired, the first-class lever is appropriate. If the goal is to make a task easier to do, requiring less force or effort to complete the task, then the second-class lever is the better choice.

Active and Passive Insufficiency

Certain aspects of joints and muscles that affect movement will be included here. One such aspect is that of insufficiency. Many muscles in the human body cross or act at two or more joints simultaneously. These muscles can affect motion at all the joints they cross. The amount and type of motion occurring at each joint crossed is dependent on several factors, such as location of attachment or other muscles acting on the same joint. Insufficiency indicates that the muscle is not able to work to its full potential at all joints at the same time. Insufficiency is defined as "inadequacy for a specific purpose" (Venes, 2013).

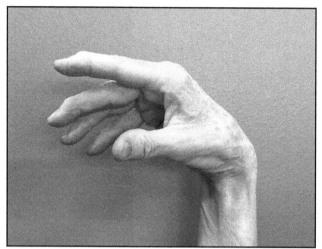

Figure 3-13. When the wrist is positioned in full flexion, passive insufficiency of the extrinsic finger extensor muscles can be observed in lack of complete finger flexion.

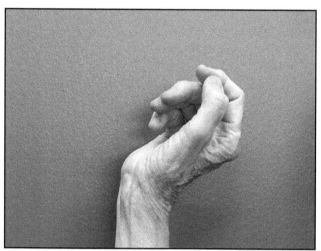

Figure 3-14. When the wrist is positioned in full extension, passive insufficiency of the extrinsic finger flexor muscles can be observed in lack of complete finger extension.

Insufficiency can occur in two different ways. **Active insufficiency** occurs when a muscle cannot shorten or contract any further and fails to shorten to the extent required for simultaneous full ROM at all joints crossed. Conversely, passive insufficiency occurs when a muscle cannot be stretched any further, yet it has not stretched the amount required for full ROM at all joints crossed at the same time. Active insufficiency occurs when the client is actively contracting a muscle to cause movement. The muscle cannot actively contract enough to cause full ROM at all joints. Often, the client feels a cramp in the muscle when nearing active insufficiency. Passive insufficiency occurs without active muscular contraction by the client in response to a stretch. The muscle cannot be stretched enough to allow full ROM at all joints crossed. In this case, the client often feels more of a burn or heat in the muscle, not a cramp. Consider the wrist and fingers as an example. If you actively and fully flex your wrist, it may be difficult to close your fingers into a tight fist. If you feel a cramping in your anterior forearm, it is due to active insufficiency of the extrinsic finger flexors, which cross several joints, including the wrist. Or the lack of full finger flexion could be due to passive insufficiency of the extrinsic finger extensors; in this case you will feel a stretch or pull across your posterior wrist and forearm. If you fully extend your wrist and relax your fingers, your fingers tend to flex on their own. This is an example of passive insufficiency of the extrinsic finger flexors. The second example, passive insufficiency of the finger flexors, can be used to the advantage of a client with a weak or insufficient grasp. This is referred to as a *tenodesis grasp*. **Tenodesis** literally means tendon binding or fixation of a tendon. Related to grasp, tenodesis is defined as "flexing of the fingers through tendon action of the extrinsic finger flexor muscles…during wrist extension. This mechanism is used for functional grip in the quadriplegic individual when paralysis is due to loss below the sixth cervical vertebra" (Venes, 2013, p. 2293). In some clients, shortening of the extrinsic finger flexors is actually encouraged to enhance the effects of passive insufficiency. Tenodesis grip strength is increased by placing the wrist in extension, causing the fingers to flex. Tenodesis splints have been designed to take greater advantage of this effect of passive insufficiency. Refer to Figures 3-13 and 3-14 to note the positioning of the fingers related to passive insufficiency of the extrinsic finger extensors and extrinsic finger flexors respectively.

Kinematic Chains

Functional movement occurs in a sequence influenced by a concept referred to as a *kinematic chain*, sometimes called a *kinetic chain*. This text will use Levangie and Norkin's (2005) terminology of a kinematic chain. The term *kinematics* is derived from the Greek word for things that move. Another term for movies, cinema, is derived from this same word. In relation to the human body, *kinematics* refers to movements of each part of the body, body movements in relation to one another, and the form or pattern of movement in relation to time. A chain is generally a linear structure composed of rigid segments interconnected with movable joints or parts. In a chain, motion in one area leads to motion in subsequent areas causing a type of ripple effect along the entire chain. A kinematic chain, therefore, depicts a combination of these two concepts. The human kinematic chain may be defined as the bones and joints moving in sequence following a specified pattern depending on whether the chain is open or closed. In an **open kinematic chain**, the distal segment is freely moving and, therefore, one joint can move without impacting movement of the other joints. Using the UE as an example, holding the hand in the air would position the distal segment, the hand, to be freely movable. In this case, the person can greet a friend by making waving motions at the wrist or fingers without having to also move the elbow or shoulder. Similarly, the person could move at the elbow, such as in chopping, and not move the wrist or shoulder joints. The idea is that one joint can move in isolation, or independently, from other joints. In contrast, in a **closed kinematic chain**, the distal segment is fixed or stabilized so movement in one joint will automatically necessitate movement at connecting joints. In standing with both feet on the floor, the LEs are in a closed kinematic chain. In this closed system, movement at one joint necessitates movement at all related joints. For example, when a person squats from a standing position, the flexion at the knee also causes hip flexion and ankle dorsiflexion. Open and closed kinematic chains in relation to human movement also describe non–weight-bearing or weight-bearing conditions. Simply stated, the open chain represents non–weight-bearing, whereas the closed chain is the weight-bearing position. In general, during most functional movement, the LE is weight bearing and in a closed-chain position, providing stability, while the UE is in an open-chain position, allowing freedom of movement of the hand to perform tasks (Hall, 1999; Levangie & Norkin, 2005).

When analyzing and prescribing activities in therapy, it is important to note the type of kinematic chain needed. If a client has reduced balance and equilibrium reactions, it would be beneficial to begin with closed-chain activities. As the client progresses, open-chain activities can be incorporated to provide mobility superimposed on stability. This is a precursor to functional movement and activity, as many life activities require dynamic motion.

Open- and Close-Pack Joint Positions

Joints can also be positioned in an open- or close-pack position. These positions refer to the stability of the joint structure. *Joint stability* is often described as the ability of the joint to resist one bone end from sliding off the other bone end, or displacing. Many factors influence joint stability, such as muscles, tendons, and the shape of the joint. In addition, the position of the joint affects its stability. Because articulating joint surfaces are not all symmetrical or of the exact same size, there is typically one position in which the joint fits together best or in which the contact between both sides of the joint is optimal. When the fit is optimal, the two sides of the joint are in the closest contact possible over the greatest surface area. This optimal fit is referred to as the close-pack position and generally is the position that offers the most stability. The open-pack position is sometimes referred to as *loose pack*. In this position, the joint is not as stable because there

is less total contact area of the joint surfaces. This position occurs any time the joint is not in the close-pack position. Some joints are shaped such that they have a greater amount of contact between articulating surfaces regardless of position and thus provide better stability overall. One such joint is the hip joint, due to the large and deep articulating surface of the acetabulum (Hall, 1999). Injury is more likely to occur in the open-pack position. Clipping, a common football injury, is caused when a player is stationary with knees bent and is hit with force on the side of the leg. In this flexed, open-pack position, the knee is twisted or dislocated relatively easily. Adding to the problem is the fact that the LE is in a closed kinematic chain in this position. As such, the foot and ankle are planted or stabilized on the ground and do not move with the impact. The next joint in the kinematic chain is the knee, which suffers the force of the impact.

When considering functional movement for clients, kinematic chains and pack positions need to be analyzed and addressed. For example, if a client is unable to fully extend the knee during a standing pivot transfer, it is important to remember the knee will be less stable than if in the extended, close-pack position. The client would need to be educated about this, and precautions might be needed to avoid twisting the knee during the transfer. If the practitioner is aware of the effects of the kinematic chain or joint position, an activity or task can be modified to either enhance stability or enable mobility depending on the need of the client. It is important to remember that all functional movement involves a combination of the positions discussed. The client must be able to fluidly move from open-pack to close-pack and vice versa, as well as change between an open and closed kinematic chain. The gait cycle offers a good example of this rapid and repeated changing of positions. Gait will be discussed further in Chapter 6.

Summary

Functional movement requires complex interactions of multiple factors in addition to the actual body components discussed in the previous chapter. Context, environment, and other related factors can enable or impede movement, as well as participation in daily activities. Often, these factors have more influence on movement than the underlying body functions; therefore, it is essential that the occupational therapy practitioner consider these various factors when working with clients. Only through the unity of all factors is participation achieved.

References

American Occupational Therapy Association. (2020). Occupational therapy practice framework: Domain and process (4th ed.). *American Journal of Occupational Therapy, 74*(Suppl. 2), 7412410010. https://doi.org/10.5014/ajot.2020.74S2001

The Center for Universal Design. (1997). Center for Universal Design. NC State. https://design.ncsu.edu/research/center-for-universal-design/

Collins English Dictionary (12th ed.). (2104). Harper Collins Publishers.

Cronin, A., & Mandich, M. (2005). *Human development and performance throughout the lifespan*. Thomson Delmar Learning.

Dail, N. W., Agnew, T. A., & Floyd, R. T. (2011). *Kinesiology for manual therapies*. McGraw-Hill.

European Pressure Ulcer Advisory Panel. (2009). Prevention and treatment of pressure ulcers: Quick reference guide. https://www.epuap.org/news/the-first-official-pressure-injury-prevention-and-treatment-quick-reference-guide-mobile-app/

Free Dictionary On-line. http://www.thefreedictionary.com

Hall, S. J. (1999). *Basic biomechanics* (3rd ed.). WCB/McGraw-Hill.

Levangie, P. K., & Norkin, C. C. (2005). *Joint structure and function: A comprehensive analysis* (4th ed.). F. A. Davis Company.

Luttgens, K. E., & Hamilton, N. (1997). *Kinesiology: Scientific basis of human motion* (9th ed.). Brown & Benchmark Publishers.

Merriam-Webster. (n.d.). *Merriam-Webster.com dictionary*. http://www.merriam-webster.com/dictionary

National Pressure Injury Advisory Panel. (2009). *Prevention and treatment of pressure ulcers: Quick reference guide*. www.npuap.org

Northwest Regional Spinal Cord Injury System. (n.d.). SCI pamphlets: Staying healthy after a spinal cord injury. University of Washington. http://sci.washington.edu/info/pamphlets/pressure_sores.asp

Ravilious, K. (2010). Isaac Newton: Who he was, why Google apples are falling. *National Geographic News*. https://www.nationalgeographic.com/culture/article/100104-isaac-newton-google-doodle-logo-apple

The Royal Children's Hospital Melbourne. (2022). Pressure injury prevention and management. https://www.rch.org.au/rchcpg/hospital_clinical_guideline_index/Pressure_Injury_Prevention_and_Management/

Smith, L. K., Weiss, E. L., & Lehmkuhl, L. D. (1996). *Brunnstrom's clinical kinesiology* (5th ed.). F. A. Davis Company.

Venes, D. (2013) *Taber's cyclopedic medical dictionary* (22nd ed.). F. A. Davis Company.

World Health Organization. (2001). *International classification of functioning, disability and health*. Author.

Applications

The following activities will help you apply knowledge of the factors influencing movement in real-life situations. Activities can be completed individually or in a small group to enhance learning.

1. **Contexts**: Contexts can greatly impact function or participation in activity. The purpose of this application is for the student to explore various ways in which selected contexts impact the individual.

   a. Select two holiday traditions in which you engage. Analyze these traditions using the four selected contexts and determine how each one impacts the tradition. Examples are provided for you. Refer to Table 3-2 to complete this application.

TABLE 3-2

Holiday Traditions

CONTEXTS	Christmas—opening presents	Thanksgiving dinner	Your example here	Your example here
PERSONAL FACTORS Habits and current behavior patterns	My family gives gifts very early on Dec. 25.	Certain family members always arrive at least 1 hour late, to everyone else's dismay.		
PERSONAL FACTORS Upbringing and life experiences	We open gifts Christmas morning as soon as the children are awake.	We have dinner late in the day so people can eat the noon-time meal at the in-laws' home.		
ENVIRONMENTAL FACTORS Products and technology	My parents always videotape the gift opening.	Phone calls, Facebook posts with pictures, and sometimes video greetings are sent to those far off who could not attend.		

b. Contexts can impair participation or enable it. This activity will help identify ways in which this can happen.

i. Select several significant events from different times in your life related to a specific activity or occupation. List these at the top of the columns in Table 3-3. For each of the selected contexts, try to list one component that interfered with this activity or occupation and one that enhanced it. A personal example is provided.

TABLE 3-3	Significant Life Events			
CONTEXTS	Adoption of child from a different country	Your example here	Your example here	Your example here
ENVIRONMENTAL FACTORS Support and relationships, attitudes	Enhance—diversity enriches all of our lives, travel to foreign country Impede—some family and community members not accepting of child of a different race			
ENVIRONMENTAL FACTOR Services, systems, and policies	Enhance—tax credit for adopting a child Impede—many rules, expenses, paperwork required for international adoption			
PERSONAL FACTORS Age	Older parent. Enhance—financially secure, more patience Impede—no cohort group, "grandparent" age			
PERSONAL FACTORS Individual psychological aspects	Enhance—openness to experience, confident, readily adaptable to various situations Impede—stress and anxiety related to additional child in family			

ii. Select a personal movement-related life event in which you were successful or pleased with the outcome. Determine the contexts that enabled this successful outcome. Next, imagine if the contexts were different, what the outcome might have been. An example is provided in Table 3-4. Complete the table with your own experiences.

TABLE 3-4
Positive and Negative Potential Effects of Contexts on Significant Movement-Related Life Events

CONTEXTS	High school volleyball		Your example here	
	Positive Attributes	*Potential Negative Attributes*	*Positive Attributes*	*Potential Negative Attributes*
ENVIRONMENTAL FACTORS Support and relationships	Peer group of athletes, family history of athleticism	Peers, family places little or no value on athleticism; time spent at home more important		
ENVIRONMENTAL FACTORS Natural environment and human-made changes	Volleyball court in yard, access to community center gymnasium	No yard, park area, or gymnasium to learn and practice in		
PERSONAL FACTORS Social background status and socioeconomic status	Middle-class family able to pay for private leagues	Low-income family unable to afford team uniforms and fees		
PERSONAL FACTORS Other health conditions and fitness	Good physical health, active lifestyle	Exercised-induced asthma		
EFFECTS ON PERFORMANCE	Increased desire to excel, to prove skill to family, self, older players	Did not try out for team, did not set goals for self, minimal identity of roles		

2. **Accessibility, Negotiability, Universal Design**: The purpose of this activity is to raise awareness of the concepts of universal design and how they benefit all people. Certain structures or places may meet ADA legal requirements for accessibility but lack negotiability for the user. For this activity, you will need to borrow a wheelchair or take a child in a stroller and visit several area attractions and public buildings (e.g., restaurants, playgrounds, museums, libraries). It is suggested to work in pairs or small groups with each pair or group assessing a different location. The information gathered can then be shared with the entire class.

   a. Determine the accessibility of the location visited. It is suggested to print and use a checklist designed for this purpose. Accessibility checklists can be found in Appendix A.

   b. Determine the negotiability of each location. Once you enter the area (accessibility), see if you can easily use it for the purposes it was created. For example, if the purpose of the location is dining, can you reach the table? Are the silverware and drinking glass easy to grasp and lift, and is the lighting ample to read the menu? If you are at an ice cream shop, can you see the tubs of ice cream in the cooler? Generate your own checklist for this or list items that you discover are not negotiable during your visit. Remember to consider things such as ease of use of handles on doors and faucets, height and location of towel and toilet paper dispensers, weight of doors, weight of eating utensils or glasses, steepness or unevenness of terrain, and so forth.

c. Summarize your findings from a and b. Make suggestions as to how the location could be made more accessible and negotiable. Discuss how designing new locations with these concepts in mind would support the concepts of universal design and access for all.

d. Consider sharing this information with the appropriate people at the location, with building associations, or with students in other programs as a community service. Perhaps some simple changes could be made that would enable more people to enjoy the location.

3. **Newton's Laws**: After this activity, you should be able to apply Newton's laws to everyday movements and motions. Review the three laws of motion. Decide which law best fits the activity or situation described. In some cases more than one law may apply. Be prepared to defend your answers. Complete Table 3-5.

TABLE 3-5
Application of Newton's Laws of Motion

ACTIVITY OR MOTION	NEWTON'S LAW	HOW DOES THIS LAW IMPACT CLIENT PERFORMANCE?
Maintaining same speed while walking to dining hall	Law of inertia	It is easier to move at same speed than to start and stop; it takes more energy to initiate movement or to stop movement.
You are jumping from a boat to a pier, the boat moves backward as you push off		
It takes more effort to continue pushing a heavier person in wheelchair down the hallway than a lighter person		
Jumping on a trampoline		
Pushing off from starting blocks for a race		
Rising from a chair		
Sitting up in bed		
Propelling wheelchair on sand (compared to concrete)		
Wheelchair coming to abrupt stop		
A fish propels its fins backward but moves forward through the water		
Your example here		
Your example here		

4. **Levers**: The goal of this exercise is to familiarize yourself with the three types of levers and their uses.
   a. Find as many examples of levers in the environment as you can. Determine the class of lever the item is. Note the type of advantage the lever gives the user. This information can be recorded in Table 3-6. An example is provided.

TABLE 3-6

Application Exercise: Levers

LEVER/ITEM	CLASS OF LEVER	ADVANTAGE OF LEVER *(Speed, ROM, less force needed, balance)*	USES FOR LEVER	LABEL OR DESCRIBE THE AXIS (A), FORCE (F), AND RESISTANCE (R)
Crowbar	First	Requires less force or effort to move object	Moves large rocks, pries things open	A—pivot point that crowbar rests on and rotates over, may be smaller rock or stump F—your strength pushing down R—rock or item being moved
Your example here				
Your example here				
Your example here				
Your example here				

   b. Practice picking things up with a long-handled reacher.
      i. Are items harder to pick up than they would be if you simply used your hand? Why or why not?
      ii. How can you make an item easier to pick up? Which arm are you changing, force or resistance?
      iii. What recommendations would you make to a client who you are suggesting should use reacher?

5. **Active and Passive Insufficiency**: The following activities will increase understanding of the concepts of active and passive insufficiency and how they affect movement. These activities can be performed individually; however, you might want a partner to observe for subtle changes in movement.
   a. **Active Insufficiency**: First, define active insufficiency in your own words; then, complete the activities that follow.
      i. Stand holding onto something for support. Bend your knee and raise that same leg as far as you can toward your chest. Notice how much hip flexion you have. Keeping your leg elevated, straighten your knee. Consider what happens.
         • Does the amount of hip flexion you have change? How? Why do you think this occurs?
         • Do you feel something in your anterior thigh? Describe the feeling.
         • You are experiencing active insufficiency of what muscle group?
      ii. Stand holding onto something for support. Keeping your leg straight, extend it as far backward as possible. Notice how much hip extension you have. Flex your knee as far as possible. Consider what happens.
         • Does the amount of hip flexion you have change? How? Why do you think this occurs?
         • Do you feel something in your posterior thigh? Describe the feeling.
         • You are experiencing active insufficiency of what muscle group?

iii. Is active insufficiency dependent on the muscle group used?

iv. For those of you who experienced a stretch or passive insufficiency, which muscle group did this occur in for i and ii?

b. **Passive Insufficiency**: First, define passive insufficiency in your own words. Then, complete the activities that follow.

i. Squat and touch your toes. Notice how much hip and knee flexion you have. While keeping your hands on your toes, extend or straighten your knees as much as possible. Consider what happens.

- Does the amount of hip flexion you have change? How? Why do you think this occurs?
- Do you feel something in your posterior thigh? Describe the feeling.
- You are experiencing passive insufficiency of what muscle group?

ii. Stand holding onto something for support. Flex your hip and knee on the same side. Hold your foot against your buttocks with your free hand. Notice how much knee flexion you have. Slowly move your hip into extension. Consider what happens.

- Can you achieve full hip extension if the knee maintains full flexion? Why or why not?
- What do you feel in your anterior thigh?
- You are experiencing passive insufficiency of what muscle group?

iii. Rest your right elbow on a table with your hand pointing toward the ceiling. Now, relax your right wrist, and allow it to drop into flexion.

- Describe the position of your fingers when they are relaxed and the wrist is in flexion.
- Using your left hand, manually extend the right wrist while keeping the right fingers relaxed.
- Describe the position of your fingers.

6. **Open and Closed Kinematic Chains**: Work with a partner or in small groups.

a. Walk slowly across the floor while your partner or group observes. Determine when each leg is in a closed kinematic chain and when it switches to an open chain. Discuss the stability and mobility of these two positions.

b. Perform this next activity while eating or drinking. Begin with eating and drinking the way you usually do. Observe the ease and fluidity of your movements. In most cases, your UEs will be in an open kinematic chain. Now, support your upper body weight on your elbows, as if you had no trunk control and needed to hold yourself up. This places the upper portion of the arm in a closed chain. Eat and drink again.

i. How did this closed-chain position at the elbow affect your ability to cut your food, feed yourself, and drink? Note all differences or changes.

ii. Referring to the differences or changes you noticed, why do you think these occurred?

iii. Discuss how eating or performing oral motor hygiene in this position might impact a client with general weakness.

7. **Open- and Close-Pack Joint Positions**: Working with a partner, place your knee and elbow joints in varying positions. In each position, gently move your partner's joint in all directions.

a. Determine which seems to be the most stable position. This is your close-pack position. Describe the close-pack position for the joint.

i. Knee

ii. Elbow

iii. Interphalangeal joints of fingers

b. Place your joint in an open-pack position. Describe how it feels when your partner tries to gently move your joint from side to side.

i. Knee

ii. Elbow

iii. Interphalangeal joints of fingers

c. Are there any similarities in between joints in the close-pack position? If so, list them.

d. Was it easier to determine these two positions in certain joints? Why do you think this is? Review the bony structures of the joint, especially the articulating surfaces, for clues.

CHAPTER 4

Introducing Body Movement

Susan J. Sain, MS, OTR/L, FAOTA

Key Terms

abnormal atypical movement

active range of motion

adaptive motor behaviors

anticipatory postural movements

body functions

body structures

end feel

hemiparesis

line of gravity

motor behaviors

motor control

motor development

motor learning

motor skills

normal atypical movement

normal typical movement

passive range of motion

performance skills

postural control

posture

praxis

stability

Chapter Outline

Introduction

Human Movement for Function

Occupational Therapy Practice Framework: Domain and Process, Fourth Edition

Motor Behavior

Movement Characteristics

Posture and Anticipatory Postural Movements

Assessment of Body Movement

Measuring Movement

Introduction to Gross Range of Motion

Introduction to Gross Manual Muscle Testing

Summary

References

Applications

Sain, S. J., & Roller, C. L. *Kinesiology for the Occupational Therapy Assistant: Essential Components of Function and Movement, Third Edition* (pp. 75-96).
© 2024 Taylor & Francis Group.

Introduction

This chapter provides an overview of human movement related to function including various approaches for assessing movement. **Motor behaviors**, **motor learning**, and **motor control** are defined with examples provided to help differentiate these concepts. Movement characteristics ranging from abnormal atypical movement patterns through the continuum to normal enhanced typical movement are described. Client behaviors depicting various movement patterns are provided. The impact **posture** and **postural control** have on movement is considered, as is the relationship between center of gravity (COG), base of support (BOS), and **stability**, which all contribute to balance. It is essential to be able to maintain balance during movement and functional activities. Considering that movement is a multi-faceted, complex activity, there are many variables that can impact its success. Therefore, a wide variety of assessment tools exist to help the practitioner determine in what areas the client needs assistance to improve movement capabilities. Two of the assessments often used in occupational therapy include measuring range of motion (ROM) and assessing muscle strength via manual muscle testing (MMT). Rationale for and how to perform these procedures are presented. Tips for increasing standardization and consistent results are also provided. Finally, contraindications to the procedures will be discussed.

Human Movement for Function

Occupational Therapy Practice Framework: Domain and Process, Fourth Edition

The *Occupational Therapy Practice Framework: Domain and Process, Fourth Edition* (OTPF-4) is a good place to start in describing the overwhelming concept of human movement. As presented earlier in Chapter 1, particular aspects of occupational therapy's domain have been identified that relate to kinesiology. The aspect of client factors that impact movement can include values, beliefs, spirituality, **body structures**, and **body functions**. Body structures responsible for movement refer to anatomical parts of the body, such as joints, bones, muscles, and structures of related body systems. Similarly, body functions are physiologic functions of the body and include neuromusculoskeletal and movement-related functions. Table 4-1 identifies some of the neuromusculoskeletal and movement-related functions listed in the OTPF-4. Occupational therapy realizes, though, that human movement is composed of much more than just minimization of movement to the smallest components of body structures and body functions. Within the OTPF-4, the domain aspect of **performance skills** provides another avenue to view human movement.

TABLE 4-1
Neuromusculoskeletal and Movement-Related Functions

FUNCTIONS OF JOINTS AND BONES	
Joint mobility	Joint ROM
Joint stability	Maintenance of structural integrity of joints throughout the body; physiological stability of joints related to structural integrity
MUSCLE FUNCTIONS	
Muscle power	Strength
Muscle tone	Degree of muscle tension (e.g., flaccidity, spasticity, fluctuating)
Muscle endurance	Sustainability of muscle contraction
MOVEMENT FUNCTIONS	
Motor reflexes	Involuntary contraction of muscles automatically induced by specific stimuli (e.g., stretch, asymmetrical tonic neck, symmetrical tonic neck)
Involuntary movement reactions	Postural reactions, body adjustment reactions, supporting reactions
Control of voluntary movements	Eye–hand and eye–foot coordination, bilateral integration, crossing of the midline, fine and gross motor control, oculomotor function (e.g., saccades, pursuits, accommodation, binocularity)
Gait patterns	Gait and mobility in relation to engagement in daily life activities (e.g., walking patterns and impairments, asymmetric gait, stiff gait)

Data source: American Occupational Therapy Association. (2020). Occupational therapy practice framework: Domain and process (4th ed.). *American Journal of Occupational Therapy, 74*(Suppl. 2), Article 7412410010. https://doi.org/10.5014/ajot.2020.74S2001

Performance skills are defined in the OTPF-4 (2020) as "observable, goal directed actions that result in a client's quality of performing desired occupations" (p. 80). Body structures and body functions impact a client's performance skills, as does context, specific occupation or activity demands, and multiple other factors. The OTPF-4 includes the category motor and process skills under performance skills. Table 4-2 provides examples of **motor skills** from the OTPF-4. This category helps to describe motor and muscular movements. **Praxis** is the ability to plan and perform purposeful movement. Movement varies as it can include all of these actions or only some of these actions.

Body functions and performance skills have been introduced as one approach to describing movement. An example is presented in Figure 4-1, which displays David playing a piano. Neuromusculoskeletal and movement-related body functions used by David to play the piano include ROM to reach the playing keys, strength to lift up and maintain his arm against gravity, muscle endurance to play a whole song, and his involuntary movement reactions sitting or standing during engagement in this activity. Motor and performance skills used by David to play the piano include paces of movements for tempo of the appropriate keys, coordinates fingers, and positions body to reach the keys, endures needed standing or sitting balance, and manipulates the key cover board. As can be seen, multiple aspects can affect human movement in engagement in a functional activity.

Quite often, within the medical model, occupational therapy practitioners address those specific aspects that enable or hinder movement for a client to maximize health and participation in life. While at times these aspects are more readily observable, a skilled practitioner trained on how the body moves is necessary to provide the appropriate approaches and treatments needed to achieve the optimal outcome. This vagueness is unavoidable without further clarification of the margins of human movement that this text is able to cover. In particular, this text emphasizes a kinematic view of human movement with emphasis on functional movement important to occupational therapy practitioners. A review of human motor behavior is essential.

TABLE 4-2
Performance Skills: Motor Skills

EXAMPLES OF MOTOR SKILLS

Aligns posture and body position: In response to environmental circumstances to complete a task.

Bends: As in reaching for a toy or tool in a storage bin.

Coordinates: Body movements to complete a job or task, such as putting a pillowcase on a pillow.

Manipulates: Keys or a lock to open a door.

Paces: Tempo of movements needed to vacuum a room or fold clothes.

Walks and stabilizes: Balance while walking on an uneven surface or standing while showering.

Figure 4-1. David playing a piano. (Pixel-Shot/shutterstock.com)

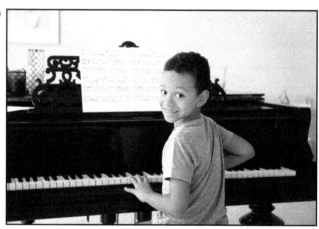

BOX 4-1

MOTOR BEHAVIOR AREAS

Motor control: Events that occur over short time intervals.
Motor development: Events that occur covering months, years, or decades.
Motor learning: Events that occur over hours, days, and weeks.

(Pendleton & Schultz-Krohn, 2006; Whiting & Rugg, 2006)

Motor Behavior

Spaulding (2005) identifies motor behavior as observable and measurable movement. More specifically, Whiting and Rugg (2006) define *motor behavior* as a term that describes how the similar concepts of **motor development**, motor learning, and motor control combine to typify muscular control and movement. Motor development identifies the changes in movement behavior that occur as the client progresses through the lifespan from infancy until death (Whiting & Rugg, 2006). Motor learning is defined as the acquisition or modification of learned movement patterns over time (Pendleton & Schultz-Krohn, 2006). Lastly, motor control is defined as the outcome of motor learning involving the

ability to produce purposeful movements of the extremities and postural adjustments in response to activity and environment demands (Pendleton & Schultz-Krohn, 2006). Box 4-1 represents how each concept relates over the lifespan. Each concept, while different, is important to understand in order to develop an understanding of human movement.

Whyte and Morrissey (1990) identify motor development as "a process of continuous modification caused by neurologic growth and maturation, residual effects of previous experiences, and effects of new motor experiences" (p. 45). Motor development, then, continuously occurs from birth until death. Motor development is often associated with motor milestones of the developmental sequence. The development sequence is beneficial for viewing the sequential

TABLE 4-3
General Motor Stages of the Developmental Sequence

1. Prone	9. Stands with support	17. Stands on one foot
2. Reaches for objects	10. Pulls sit-to-stand	18. Rides tricycle
3. Sits with support	11. Walks with support	19. Skips on one foot
4. Rolls prone to supine	12. Stands alone	20. Hops on one foot
5. Crawls	13. Climbs stairs holding railings	21. Climbs stairs with one foot per step
6. Palmar grasp	14. Climbs stairs alone	22. Skips on both feet
7. Rolls supine to prone	15. Jumps on both feet	23. Runs on toes
8. Sits unsupported	16. Walks on tips of toes	24. Walks heel-to-toe
		25. Kicks, throws, climbs

Adapted from Lippert, L. S. (2017). *Clinical kinesiology for physical therapy assistants* (6th ed.). F. A. Davis Company; Simon, C. J., & Daub, M. M. (1993). Human development across the life span. In H. Hopkins & H. Smith (Eds.), *Willard and Spackman's occupational therapy* (8th ed., pp. 95-130). J.B. Lippincott Co; and Whyte, J., & Morrissey, J. (1990). Motor learning and relearning. In M. B. Glenn & J. Whyte (Eds.), *The practical management of spasticity in children and adults* (pp. 44-69). Lea & Febiger.

attainment of motor milestones; however, it does not explain motor development that follows through adulthood and later life. Table 4-3 identifies general motor stages of the developmental sequence. These stages help us to see the sequential nature of the developmental sequence.

The developmental sequence is hierarchical, where one motor milestone builds on the development of the previous motor milestones. While they are sequential, there is no specific time frame for acquisition of skills, and, at best, a range of typical motor behavior norms for milestone acquisition may be provided. The developmental sequence provides an explanation for how the human body develops motorically and provides information on the building blocks of skilled movement. Initially, responses of infants are reflexive and involuntary but later lead to voluntary controlled movement. Whyte and Morrissey (1990) suggest that movement initially sequences from mobility to stability and then to controlled mobility to distal skilled movement with proximal stabilization. Other types of developmental sequences for motor development have been suggested. They include proximal to distal development, cephalocaudal direction, and reflex-dominated activity to reflex-inhibited activity. The developmental sequence, while beneficial, may not be the only method for explaining how the human body organizes motor movements throughout the lifespan.

Motor learning is defined as the acquisition and modification of learned movement patterns over time (Pendleton & Schultz-Krohn, 2006). Motor learning takes into consideration the client, task, and environment. Motor learning has provided valuable information on the development of treatment approaches, such as the task-oriented approach and constraint-induced movement therapy (Pendleton & Schultz-Krohn, 2006). Further description of motor learning is outside the focus of this text; however, it is an important concept to help understand human movement behavior.

Motor learning explains how people move and develop motor skills over time with practice and experience. Motor skills are defined as voluntary movements used to complete a desired task or achieve a specific goal (Whiting & Rugg, 2006). Motor skills are goal directed and observable as a client interacts with the environment and task. Examples may include writing your name, drinking from a cup, or turning a key. Motor skills may be synonymous with motor control; however, there are subtle differences in their definitions.

Motor control is the outcome of motor learning involving the ability to produce purposeful movements of the extremities and postural adjustments in response to activity and environment demands (Pendleton & Schultz-Krohn, 2006). The definition of motor skills includes voluntary movements, which may exclude the use of reflexes and automatic reactions as motor skills. Not only does motor control include purposeful movements, but it also recognizes postural adjustments. In occupational therapy, reflexive and automatic reactions may be used to enable function or achieve a desired goal.

Steve, in Figure 4-2, illustrates another example of how the different concepts of motor behavior can influence movement. In Figure 4-2, Steve, who is recovering from a motor vehicle accident, is playing with an electronic game console as a therapeutic activity. This is the first time Steve has played with this particular console, so he is using his motor control to provide the proper outcome while manipulating the game controllers. As Steve continuously uses the game over days and weeks, motor learning is occurring, which allows him to achieve improved outcomes for the desired movements required. Steve must have integrated early reflexive patterns and progressed along the developmental sequence to sit upright or stand when needed to participate in the game. The developmental sequence would have started years earlier at birth. All three concepts of motor behavior collaborate to allow purposeful, goal-directed motor behavior to occur.

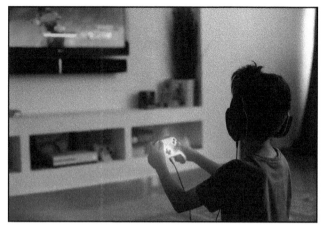

Figure 4-2. Steve is playing with an electronic game console as a therapeutic activity during therapy. (Evgeniy pavlovski/shutterstock.com)

Shumway-Cook and Woollacott (2001) identify key aspects of skilled movement to include the ability to adapt and move efficiently and consistently in a variety of environments. Motor control and motor skills are aspects that are important for the production of skilled movements. Both motor skills and motor control consider the person, activity, and context. Motor learning and motor development, while important, include topics outside the scope of this text and will be covered more in other courses. Developing an understanding of normal movement is essential to apply the concepts of motor behavior in the OTPF-4 in occupational therapy.

Movement Characteristics

Martin (1977) describes human movement as a change in position and object that passes through a series of positions. Movement for the sake of movement is not functional and is not reflective of what consists of normal or typical motor behavior. Movement is inexplicably linked to function. Merriam-Webster (n.d.) describes function as "any of a group of related actions contributing to a larger action; especially: the normal and specific contribution of a bodily part to the economy of a living organism." As such, functional movement correlates well with the definitions already provided of motor control and motor skills. Functional movement, however, may not be synonymous with normal movement.

Normal movement may be a misnomer in that there may be a wide variation of movements that could be considered normal as cited in Latash and Anson (1996, p. 3). Varying movements may be identified as "normal," "normality," and "normal movement patterns." Spaulding (2005) supports this by stating that there are many different functional abilities in the well population as well as in those with disabilities. People can often function at high levels without ever meeting optimum levels of ability, depending on the strategy

used (Fisher & Yakura, 1993). The Functional Movement Continuum, as described in Table 4-4, was created to help characterize the variety of functional movement available.

The Functional Movement Continuum is based on Latash and Anson's (1996) presentation of "normal movement patterns to span a broad range of patterns from clumsy and impaired movements to uniquely specific movements" (p. 2). This continuum has been expanded upon to reflect function and those characteristics important in occupational therapy. The Functional Movement Continuum describes **adaptive motor behaviors** that occur over the four common categories in the continuum.

Adaptive motor behaviors are defined as follows:
- Certain ways the body acts in a situation (Horak, 1987).
- Appropriate and efficient movement strategies used by the body (Horak, 1987).
- The body's ability to apply normal movement strategies to achieve functional goals (Landel & Fisher, 1993).

Adaptive motor behaviors reflect the body's ability to select and choose from a variety of movement options. These movement options may roughly be categorized into four groups:
1. Abnormal atypical movement
2. Normal atypical movement
3. Normal typical movement
4. Normal enhanced typical movement

Functional movement characteristics are provided for each category to reflect the functional capabilities and quality of movement that can be found in each section (Horak, 1987).

At one end of the continuum is **abnormal atypical movement**. This category is characterized by the inability to produce the desired movement strategy necessary to complete an activity within generally accepted parameters. Impairments that may prevent or limit movement strategies may include increased or decreased spasticity, pathological movement synergies, decreased interjoint coordination, incorrect timing of motor sequence, or muscle weakness (Roby-Brami et al., 2003). Abnormal postural adjustments, muscle weakness, and a lack of mobility may also limit movement strategies (Cirsea & Levin, 2000). Functional examples might include a person with severe rheumatoid arthritis who is no longer able to sit-to-stand from a commode or is no longer able to grasp due to severe ulnar deviation of the wrist. Another example might include a client with a high complete cervical injury who is no longer able to complete a functional task independently with adaptations. Individual impairments may affect movement patterns over time and lead to nonfunctional maladaptive movement behaviors.

The abnormal atypical movement category reflects a lack of movement options and significantly impaired motor movements that prevent the participation and completion of functional tasks even with adaptive approaches. Accepted parameters for performance may be individual or environmental, depending on the task and context of movement application. An example might include a client who is able to

TABLE 4-4
Functional Movement Continuum

ADAPTIVE MOTOR BEHAVIORS	MOTOR BEHAVIOR CHARACTERISTIC
Abnormal atypical movement	• Inability to produce the desired movement strategies and characteristics necessary to complete an activity/occupation in generally accepted parameters
Normal atypical movement	• Awkward • Uncoordinated • Inefficient • Conscious thought • Limited movement options • Low complexity • Increased time • Low joint angle • One joint motion • Low velocity • Low acceleration
Normal typical movement	• Smooth • Coordinated • Efficient • Automatic • Variety of movement options • High complexity • Decreased time • High joint angle • Multiple joint motions • High velocity • High acceleration
Normal enhanced typical movement	• Highly trained motor skills or motor control that allow for high efficiency, adaptability, and consistency in a variety of environments

self-dress completely, but the task takes more than 2 hours to complete. Ultimately, there is a lack of movement strategies for the task and environment, which may lead to permanent disability if the activity cannot be completed adequately (Shumway-Cook & Woollacott, 2001).

Perhaps the majority of human motor behaviors can be characterized as either **normal typical movement** or **normal atypical movement**. Normal atypical movement reflects the motor behavior response of an individual when typical movement strategies are temporarily or permanently no longer feasible. Additionally, a new task may require novel or previously inexperienced motor behaviors, which may be characterized within this category. As motor development and motor learning occur, movement for the new task may adapt to be more reflective of normal typical movement. Movement characteristics, as presented in Table 4-4, change from the description of normal typical motor behavior possibly due to a lack of or loss in the repertoire of movement options available. McPherson et al. (1991) support this when

they identified that individuals with cerebral palsy displayed a need for greater ROM components in reaching as compared to individuals without cerebral palsy. There continues to be movement options available to complete a task but the number of movement options may be reduced.

An example of normal atypical movement may include a client with flaccid **hemiparesis** in the dominant upper extremity (UE) following a stroke. The individual may be able to use their nondominant arm to enable self-feeding or use the flaccid dominant UE as a secondary assist to complete a functional task. Figure 4-3 shows Aisha, who had a peripheral nerve injury in her right dominant arm, writing with her left nondominant UE. Figure 4-4 illustrates Mary, who was diagnosed with a cerebrovascular accident engaging in functional mobility with a wheelchair. In each case, the client is unable to complete the purposeful activity of writing or ambulation as she would have prior to onset of the injuries. With adaptive motor behaviors, however, these clients are still able to complete writing and functional mobility.

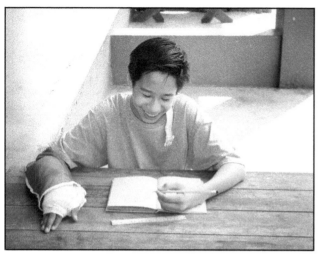

Figure 4-3. Client using normal atypical movement to write using nondominant UE. (Thongchai S/shutterstock.com)

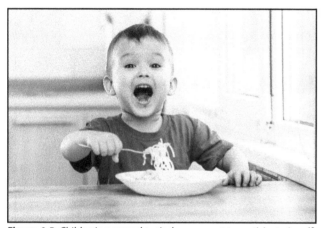

Figure 4-5. Child using normal typical movement to participate in self-feeding. (komokvm/shutterstock.com)

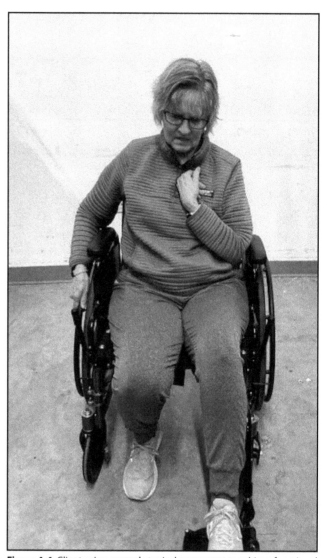

Figure 4-4. Client using normal atypical movement to achieve functional mobility.

In the well population, an example of normal atypical movement may include learning to play video games on a different game console. Prior experience from playing video games on a Playstation (Sony Computer Entertainment America) game console is helpful with adapting motor behaviors; however, motor behavior with a different game console may be characterized as normal but atypical until mastered.

Fisher (1987) reported that normal typical movement may be reported by a person as being easier and feeling like the limb is lighter. Normal typical movement may be able to access and select from numerous movement possibilities to produce multi-planar, complex combinations of movement (Greene & Wolf, 1989). Movement may occur efficiently and effectively with no undue stress or injury production (Fisher & Yakura, 1993). Table 4-4 identified movement characteristics that might be found in normal typical movement. Examples of normal typical movement may include writing with your dominant hand, smiling at a joke, or bringing a utensil to your mouth during eating. Figure 4-5 demonstrates a child participating in self-feeding. He is initiating normal typical movement required in that context to eat.

Normal typical movement is different for each person. As each person's motor behavior has the capacity to adapt, normal typical movement is always changing. As a child loses their front baby teeth or has a loose tooth, the child adapts motor behavior for chewing. Another example of adaptation may include the multiple ways to wave hello. All may be correct depending on the person, task, and environment (or context). A focus on function and the task must be maintained due to the infinite number of movement combinations that may be considered normal and typical.

Lastly, normal enhanced typical movement is reflective of highly trained motor skills and motor control. This motor behavior allows for high efficiency, adaptability, and consistency in performance of a task in a variety of environments. Quite often, normal enhanced typical movement does not occur naturally. It is also very specific to the individual, task,

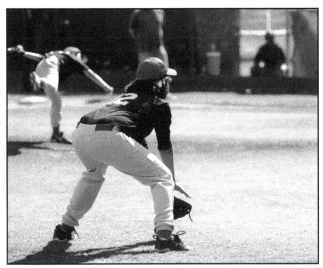

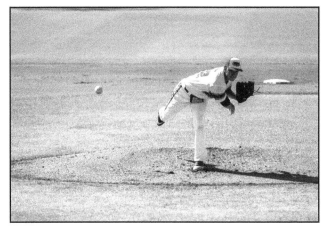

Figure 4-7. Baseball player pitching a baseball, demonstrating normal enhanced typical movement. (YES Market Media/shutterstock.com)

Figure 4-6. Baseball player in the ready position at third base demonstrating normal enhanced typical movement. (Brent Reeves/shutterstock.com)

and context and can be found in many different situations. One example might include a baseball player playing the position of pitcher or third base in the infield. While any person might be able to play these positions, by the end of the baseball season, a player may develop high efficiency and consistency with movements required above what may be accepted of any person. Figure 4-6 illustrates a baseball player in the ready position at third base in the infield. Figure 4-7 illustrates a baseball player pitching the ball.

Posture and Anticipatory Postural Movements

Functional movement occurs simultaneously with posture and **anticipatory postural movements**. Box 4-2 presents definitions of posture, postural control, and anticipatory postural movements. Posture is a separate aspect of movement that can be typified by particular positions, such as static standing, squatting, static sitting, and lying. Posture has to change when the body moves in transitions (e.g., when moving from static sitting to dynamic sitting or static standing to dynamic standing). Postural control and anticipatory postural movements are descriptions of posture that more specifically relate to changes in position relative to the person, task, and environment or context.

Postural movements and changes are important because they do the following:

- Contribute to the development of motor ability (Kanbur et al., 2005).
- Precede limb movement for increased function (Horak, 1987; Tyldesley & Grieve, 2002).
- Maintain stability, COG, and BOS.
- Prepare the body for movement (Martin, 1977).

Anticipatory postural movements occur automatically and precede voluntary limb movement (Horak, 1987). Postural adjustments may occur in sequence and may be difficult to identify through observation, possibly due to their subtleness (Horak, 1987). Martin (1977) identifies that this difficulty may be attributed to the inability to identify when automatic behavior ends and becomes volitional movement. Additionally, while postural adjustments may be similar for a particular movement, changes in the environment or context may require further adaptation for functional movement. An example may include standing on a sandy beach. Differing postural adjustments may be needed if you are standing in the surf as the sand washes away from around your feet. Another example occurs when a client sits on the edge of a mat or sits all the way back on a mat. Sitting on the edge of a mat requires much more trunk control and postural adjustments vs. sitting comfortably back on a mat, which is less challenging. Certainly, the inability to appropriately sequence, initiate, or adequately produce desired anticipatory postural movements can affect UE movement and engagement in functional tasks.

Maintaining stability, BOS, and COG are key aspects of posture. *Stability* refers to the ability to maintain the body in equilibrium. Stability is essential to movement to prevent falls and enable distal mobility of the extremities to occur. Tyldesley and Grieve (2002) identify that a stable equilibrium is created when the **line of gravity** (LOG) lies within the BOS. COG refers to the balance point of an object where all sides are equal (Lippert, 2006). COG can include the body as a whole or individual parts of the body. Due to the differences in weight, height, and body distribution among clients, the COG is always moving and may not be the same among clients. LOG is the vertical line from the COG to the earth, and BOS is contained within the area of the body parts in contact with the ground (Lippert, 2006).

Box 4-3 identifies six principles that demonstrate the relationship between balance, stability, and motion (Lippert, 2006). First, lowering the COG will result in increased stability. A person who is sitting is more stable than a person

---

BOX 4-2

Anticipatory postural movements: "Reflect movements of the trunk or posture in response to changes in task or environmental demands."

Postural control: "The regulation of the body's position in space for the dual purpose of stability and orientation."
(Shumway-Cook & Woollacott, 2001)

Posture: "State of the body in relationship to gravity, the ground and to its body parts or extremities."
(Martin, 1977)

BOX 4-3

PRINCIPLES OF STABILITY

1. Lowering the COG will increase stability.
2. COG and LOG must remain in the BOS for stability.
3. Increasing the mass will increase the stability.
4. Increasing the BOS will increase the stability.
5. Increasing friction between the object and surface will increase stability.
6. Focusing on a spot will increase stability.

(Lippert, 2006)

---

who is standing. Additionally, lying down has a lower COG and even more stability. The second principle states that the COG and LOG must reside in the BOS for stability. This can be seen when leaning forward in sitting or standing. At some point, you will have to stop leaning forward or increase the BOS or risk falling and experiencing a loss of stability as the LOG moves outside the BOS. As a client engages in dynamic sitting balance activities and reaching, they may be at increased risk that the LOG will fall outside of the BOS.

Assessment of Body Movement

Measuring Movement

The occupational therapy assistant is quite often expected to identify functional movement during therapeutic intervention and grade therapeutic activities and exercises to maximize the benefit for the client. Examples include training a client to use a reacher or shoehorn, increasing or decreasing resistance to an arm bike, or altering the reaching distance to an object. The occupational therapist may establish a movement goal through the occupational therapy evaluation and treatment planning process. Occupational therapy assistants can assist through documenting their observations of the client's performance as well as administering standardized

evaluations for which they have displayed service competency. The occupational therapy assistant then can assist in the assessment of movement from the occupational therapy evaluation throughout treatment with the collaboration of the occupational therapist. As movement in function is difficult to describe simply, one approach alone may not adequately identify how the human body moves.

Lieber and Bodine-Fowler (1993) recommended that each component of the system should be identified to evaluate the complex phenomenon of movement. Gentile identified three levels of goal-directed functional behaviors that can be evaluated, as described in Shumway-Cook and Woollacott (2001). They include action, movement, and neuromotor process. *Action* refers to the area of occupation that is being performed by the client. Ultimately, can the client complete an activity of daily living task of interest to them? Remember, functional movement includes the interaction of the individual, activity, and environment or context.

The second level of analysis, *movement*, refers to the movement strategies used to complete a functional task. This may include transitional movements, such as sitting to standing or supine to sitting, bed mobility, and reaching to complete a task. This level of analysis fits well with aspects found in the performance, motor, and praxis skills of the OTPF-4 (see Table 4-2). The Motor Activity Log (MAL) is a good example of an assessment that identifies movement that fits in this category. The MAL is a structured interview used

---

BOX 4-4

ASSESSMENT TOOLS FOR THE IDENTIFICATION OF MOVEMENT

- Bennett Hand Tool Dexterity test (H-TDT)
- Berg Balance scale
- Box and Block test
- Bruininks-Oseretsky Test of Motor Proficiency (2nd ed.; BOT-2)
- Children's Handwriting Evaluation scale (CHES)
- Crawford Small Parts Dexterity test (CSPDT)
- Erhardt Developmental Prehension Assessment (EDPA)
- Functional Dexterity test
- Fine Motor Task Assessment
- Fugl-Meyer Assessment

- Grooved Pegboard test
- Jebsen-Taylor Hand Function test
- Lincoln-Oseretsky Motor Development scale
- MMT
- Minnesota Rate of Manipulation test
- MAL
- Nine-Hole Peg test
- Purdue Pegboard
- ROM testing

(Crepeau et al., 2009)

---

to assess a client's perception of movement strategies chosen to complete a task. Taub and colleagues (1993) created the MAL to assess movement changes following constraint-induced movement therapy. The MAL identifies the client's perceived amount of movement and quality of movement during a functional task. Amount of movement is identified by the percentage of motion created from no movement to 100% of available movement. Quality of movement is identified through a sequential scale from poor to fair to normal quality of movement.

The *neuromotor process* is the last category for analysis. Shumway-Cook and Woollacott (2001) identify that this process includes sensation, perception, strength, and motor coordination. Body functions, such as neuromusculoskeletal and movement-related functions (see Table 4-1), provide more examples of components that can be analyzed by this process. Overall, many assessment tools may be needed to provide specific information on functional movement. Some assessment tools that provide information on body functions and performance skills relative to movement are identified in Box 4-4. ROM and MMT are two common assessment tools used by occupational therapy practitioners and will be covered in greater detail throughout this text.

Introduction to Gross Range of Motion

ROM and MMT are two of the most common assessments used by occupational therapy practitioners in the physical disability setting. During the occupational therapy evaluation, ROM and MMT help to identify problems with movement, assist in developing treatment goals, and aid in the overall analysis of occupational performance. During the intervention process, ROM and MMT aid in intervention planning, treatment implementation, and treatment review necessary to modify the treatment plan as needed. ROM and

MMT are also useful in identifying progress and achievement of occupational therapy goals and in providing a measurement for functional outcomes.

ROM is defined as the arc of motion through which a joint moves. Articles on ROM techniques and recommendations can be traced back to the first issues of the *American Journal of Occupational Therapy* in 1947 and 1948 (Hurt, 1947a, 1947b, 1948).

ROM is used by occupational therapy practitioners to:
- Determine available mobility.
- Identify client strengths and impairments.
- Establish a baseline.
- Document improvements in mobility.
- Aid in selecting effectiveness of interventions.

Active range of motion (AROM) and **passive range of motion** (PROM) are different types of measurements used by occupational therapy practitioners. AROM describes the joint movements as the client alone moves a joint through the available ROM. At times, **active assist range of motion** (AAROM) is used by the clinician. AAROM identifies that the therapist manually assisted the client to move the joint; however, the client also activated some joint motion. PROM, on the other hand, refers to joint movement created by the occupational therapy assistant moving the extremity. With PROM, the client does not activate muscles and does not participate in joint motion. Sabari et al. (1998) identified that AROM measurements may be more reliable than PROM measurements due to the variability in force that can be applied by the examiner. This also means that PROM may be slightly more difficult to measure due to variations of force that can be applied at the end range of movement. **End feel** describes how the joint movement feels at the end of ROM. End feel may influence the amount of force a clinician uses to identify available ROM. Table 4-5 describes the different types of end feel that may be experienced.

TABLE 4-5

Types of Joint End Feel

End feel: The feel experienced by a clinician at the end ROM for a joint.	
TYPES OF END FEEL	**EXAMPLES**
Abnormal: The feel experienced when the typical quality of feel is different.	Spasticity, muscle guarding, or springy sensation
Firm: The feel experienced when a normal joint or ligament is stretched.	Wrist flexion or extension
Hard: The feel experienced when two bones block motion.	Elbow extension
Soft: The feel experienced when two muscle groups are compressed.	Knee and elbow flexion

Adapted from Thomas, C. L. (Ed.). (1993). *Taber's cyclopedic medical dictionary* (17th ed.). F. A. Davis Company.

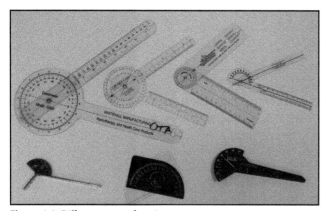

Figure 4-8. Different types of goniometers.

Gajdosik and Bohannon (1987) stressed that identification of movement through visual observation is unreliable when precision and accuracy is needed. As such, assessing AROM and PROM in the clinic is most often achieved with the use of a goniometer. A goniometer is a tool used to measure joint movements and angles. A goniometer has a stable or stationary arm on one side that usually includes numbers around a circle on the central part of the arm. Like a protractor, the circular numbers represent degrees of angular measurement. The other arm of the goniometer is called the *moving* or *movement arm*. The moving arm rotates around the stationary arm of the goniometer at a central point called the *fulcrum*. As can be seen in Figure 4-8, many types of goniometers exist to increase the accuracy and ease of measuring different joints of the body.

The goniometer measures joint angle changes in one plane. Wrist flexion is an example of a movement that occurs in one plane. A goniometer, however, does not measure joint movement in multiple planes. Wrist flexion and ulnar deviation, for example, could not be measured together or similarly, as these movements occur in different planes. A different joint axis would be needed due to the different planes. A joint axis is defined as the fixed center point that the joint moves around. Usually, landmarks at the joint are used to align the fulcrum

of the goniometer to the joint axis point to provide an accurate joint ROM measurement. Exceptions may occur when the landmark cannot be identified.

ROM is usually recorded using the neutral zero method (Rondinelli et al., 2008). The starting point for joint measurement is the neutral position, or 0 degrees, ending at the degree of available ROM. An example of the neutral zero measurement for the elbow joint might be 0 to 165 degrees. In this example, the client can move the elbow joint from full extension all the way to 165 degrees of elbow flexion. If the client is not able to reach the starting position, the measurement may be recorded differently. For example, a measurement of 20 to 165 degrees identifies that the elbow joint cannot reach the neutral position or starting point of zero. This can also be recorded as –20 degrees of elbow extension, meaning a loss of 20 degrees of ROM. *Extension lag*, or –, refers to the incomplete extension ability to return to the starting position (Rondinelli et al., 2008). Additionally, some settings may also use + to reflect a joint's ability to move into hyperextension. Often, the documentation will be determined by the setting, third-party requirements, and the experience of the therapists. ROM for each joint of the body can be found in Appendix B.

In assessing ROM, clinicians often first assess gross ROM. If a client appears to display atypical movement, the clinician may then assess formal AROM. PROM may be performed if impairments are noted with AROM. Collaborating with the occupational therapist may provide further insight into the causes of ROM impairments and their overall impact on occupational performance.

When assessing AROM, the clinician positions the client in the most supportive position to conduct ROM testing. Other joints may be stabilized while the joint being measured is isolated and moved to the neutral position for the start of goniometric testing. The fulcrum of the goniometer is placed over the landmark representing the axis of the joint being measured. The stationary arm is usually positioned proximal to the joint being measured and parallel to or along the plane being measured. The moving arm is usually placed distal to the joint being measured and, again, parallel to or

TABLE 4-6
Measures to Increase Standardization for Range of Motion

- When possible, have the same clinician perform repeated ROM measurements or at least ensure the client performs procedures in the same manner (some measurements can be done in different ways).
- Have the client in the same position (e.g., seated, prone, supine) when performing the assessment.
- Use the same type and size of goniometer as prior measurements.
- Practice using a goniometer to establish service competency with goniometer placement.
- Control contextual considerations to limit impact on ROM measurements (i.e., the temperature of the room, effects of gravity).
- Use the most appropriate goniometer for the size and shape of the joint being measured. Select the client position that will not limit joint ROM.
- Document any factors that may have influenced ROM measurements (i.e., pain, edema).
- When possible, assess AROM first to identify need for PROM or isolated ROM measurements.
- Observe and measure the unaffected extremity first to provide insight into the typical movement capability of the other extremity.

along the plane being measured. Landmarks of the body will also be used for alignment of the goniometer arms. While maintaining the fulcrum of the goniometer over the joint axis, the moving arm follows the motion of the joint, and the stationary arm stays aligned proximal to the joint where no movement occurs. The client only moves the joint through the available ROM.

If impairments are noted with AROM, PROM may be required. In PROM, the clinician again positions the client in such a manner as to support and facilitate PROM testing. The fulcrum of the goniometer is placed over the landmark representing the axis of the joint being measured. The stable arm is usually positioned proximal to the joint being measured and parallel to or along the plane being measured. In positioning the stable arm, the clinician can provide stabilization proximal to the joint to eliminate compensatory movement and multiple joint motions. The moving arm is usually placed distal to the joint being measured and, again, parallel to or along the plane being measured. While positioning the moving arm of the goniometer, the clinician should be able to grasp just distal to the joint being measured to provide the force needed for joint movement. With PROM, the clinician provides the force needed for joint motion instead of the client.

While repeated measurements from the same therapist are most reliable, measurements from different therapists can also be reliable if standardized procedures are followed (Rothstein et al., 1983). Table 4-6 provides measures to increase standardization for ROM by occupational therapy practitioners. Gajdosik and Bohannon (1987) also identified that one ROM measurement is just as effective as finding the average of repeated measurements. One last consideration is

that some clients may have contraindications or precautions with ROM. Possible contraindications and precautions for ROM and MMT are identified in Table 4-7. The UE chapters in this text will allow for practice of ROM applications found in occupational therapy.

Introduction to Gross Manual Muscle Testing

Quite often, MMT accompanies ROM testing within the clinical setting. While ROM tests for available joint range, MMT assesses the accompanying muscles' abilities to generate force. MMT is defined as a manual technique used to identify the relative strength of specific muscles (Thomas, 1993). Isolated MMT attempts to identify strength of individual muscles while gross MMT is used to assess the strength of muscle groups required to create a joint motion. This text focuses on allowing students to develop service competency with ROM and gross MMT. It is important to recognize, though, that particular occupational therapy settings may require the occupational therapy assistant to develop service competency with isolated MMT. In many settings, gross MMT techniques provide an adequate testing procedure to meet client needs. MMT is the most common method of testing muscle strength in the clinic (Bohannon, 2005; Dvir, 1997; Knepler & Bohannon, 1998).

The purpose of MMT is to:
- Determine strength and identify impairments.
- Establish a baseline.
- Document improvements in strength.
- Aid in selecting effective interventions.

TABLE 4-7

Range of Motion and Manual Muscle Testing Contraindications and Precautions

CONTRAINDICATIONS AND PRECAUTIONS	EXAMPLES
Inflammation	Significantly swollen hand or UE
Pain	Pain with joint movement, to touch, or resistance
Recent surgery	Surgery for shunt placement or to treat a fracture
Myositis ossificans	Bony growth at the joint or bone affecting muscles
Bone cancer	Compromised bone function and structure
Osteoporosis	Compromised bone function and structure
Dementia	Inability to follow commands due to agitation/cognitive impairments
Chronic obstructive pulmonary disease	Shortness of breath, inability to move extremity adequately
Cardiovascular conditions	Recent heart surgery, cardiac precautions
Multiple sclerosis	Increased fatigue unwarranted
Arthritis	Compromised joint function and structure

Adapted from Latella, D., & Meriano, C. (2003). *Occupational therapy manual for evaluation of range of motion and muscle strength.* Delmar Cengage Learning and Pendleton, H. M., & Schultz-Krohn, W. (2006). *Pedretti's occupational therapy: Practice skills for physical dysfunction* (6th ed.). Mosby-Elsevier.

As different testers may apply varying levels of resistance, MMT, like ROM testing, is most effective when the same therapy practitioner completes repeated tests. Resistance is only provided when assessing isometric grades of 3+ through 5. Resistance is a concentric force provided by the therapy practitioner in the direction opposite to the contracting muscle or muscles. It is also very important that each therapy practitioner apply their **maximal** resistance each time an isometric test is given, regardless of the client's strength, age, gender, etc. If maximal resistance is not applied, how can the practitioner accurately assess the amount of resistance used and use the exact same amount of resistance the next time the test is performed? In effect, not using maximal resistance renders the test inaccurate. Maximal resistance is defined as the maximum amount of force the therapy practitioner can exert using only their arm. Other factors that can affect MMT include gender, strength of the tester, service competency level, and spasticity or fluctuating tone. Like ROM, MMT should be performed with precautions and contraindication in mind. Table 4-7 identifies ROM and MMT contraindications and precautions.

MMT is graded on a scale from 0 to 5 where 0 is equivalent to no muscular contraction or movement and 5 is equivalent to normal MMT strength.

Table 4-8 displays the MMT scale, and it is important for each student to memorize. Of significance, isometric MMT grading techniques are used if the client demonstrates a minimal MMT strength grade of 3 or higher. Dvir (1997) identified that no more than 35% of maximal strength is required to support the arm in an antigravity position. Also, MMT grading techniques are conducted in the gravity-eliminated position if the client demonstrates an MMT strength grade of 2 or less. The gravity may be eliminated by positioning the joint perpendicular to the pull of gravity. Shoulder flexion in a gravity-eliminated position can be achieved in side-lying, and shoulder abduction gravity can be eliminated when supine on a mat.

The steps of MMT include positioning the client and extremity to be tested, stabilizing the joint, palpating appropriate joint muscle groups, observing muscle contractions, resisting muscles, and grading strength (Killingsworth & Pedretti, 2006). If gravity-eliminated MMT is indicated, the clinician will follow the same steps; however, resistance is not applied and the client will be positioned differently (i.e., the gravity-eliminated position). The occupational therapy assistant practitioner will follow these steps for gross MMT:

1. **Positioning the client and extremity**: First, the occupational therapy assistant will position the client in the optimum position to perform MMT. Quite often, the client will be positioned in a wheelchair. MMT can be performed if the client is supine in bed or lying on a mat; however, the effects of gravity may be different from that experienced in a sitting position. Quite often, it is useful to observe how the client moves. This may help to identify intact body structures and body functions and possible impairments. The occupational therapy assistant may also refer to the occupational therapy evaluation for a baseline status or rely upon prior occupational therapy treatment and observations.

TABLE 4-8

Isometric Manual Muscle Testing Grades

	NUMERICAL GRADE	ALTERNATIVE GRADING SCALE	DESCRIPTION OF MOVEMENT *(The client…)*
Isometric grading	5	Normal (N)	Maintains the testing position against gravity and maximal resistance.
	4	Good (G)	Maintains the testing position against gravity and moderate resistance.
	4-	Good- (G-)	Maintains the testing position against gravity and less than moderate resistance.
	3+	Fair+ (F+)	Maintains the testing position against gravity and minimal resistance.
Screening test	3	Fair (F)	Moves the joint through full available ROM against gravity or maintains the testing position.
	3-	Fair- (F-)	Moves the joint through greater than half but less than full available ROM against gravity.
	2+	Poor+ (P+)	Moves the joint through less than half of the available ROM against gravity.
Gravity eliminated	2	Poor (P)	Moves the joint through full ROM with gravity eliminated.
	2-	Poor- (P-)	Moves the joint through greater than half but less than full available ROM with gravity eliminated.
	1+	Trace+ (T+)	Moves the joint through less than half of the available ROM with gravity.
	1	Trace (T)	Demonstrates no joint movement, but there is a slight observable or palpable muscle contraction.
	0	Zero (0)	Demonstrates no joint movement and no palpable or observable muscle contraction.

Adapted from Latella, D., & Meriano, C. (2003). *Occupational therapy manual for evaluation of range of motion and muscle strength.* Delmar Cengage Learning and Pendleton, H. M., & Schultz-Krohn, W. (2006). *Pedretti's occupational therapy: Practice skills for physical dysfunction* (6th ed.). Mosby-Elsevier.

At this point, the occupational therapy assistant is able to identify if the client needs isometric testing or gravity-eliminated testing. In isometric testing, the joint is typically positioned at about half the available ROM, which allows the muscle to ideally be positioned to maximize the force production for the muscle contraction. Muscles have lower force generation capability when there is a small joint angle as well as when the joint angle is closer to the available end range of movement.

2. **Stabilizing the joint**: The clinician needs to stabilize the joint being measured. The occupational therapy assistant will place one hand, called the *stabilizing hand*, just proximal to the joint being measured to stabilize the joint. Positioning the client may also provide methods to stabilize other parts of the body and avoid compensatory movements, or compensation. *Compensation* is defined as the use of other muscles by the client to achieve joint movement. While stabilizing the joint, the occupational therapy assistant can often palpate the muscles responsible for the joint movement.

3. **Palpating appropriate joint muscle groups**: Many muscles may be able to be palpated due to their location close to the surface of the body. Muscle characteristics that may be observed include the size of the muscle contraction, muscle striations or directional pull of the muscles, response upon muscle activation, and response once resistance is applied. The skilled practitioner will feel for when the contraction begins and ends. Is there a smooth build-up in force or is the contraction an all or nothing response? What is the effect of hypotonicity, or decreased tone, if present? Additionally, in the case of increased tone, can the practitioner identify when the voluntary contraction ends and when the involuntary movements begin? Hypotonicity and hypertonicity may provide inaccurate results for MMT. Care must also be provided to ensure that the muscle contraction is not impeded by palpation.

BOX 4-5

By assessing MMT of the uninvolved intact extremity, the clinician will be able to gain information of typical normal movement that may be characteristic of the involved impaired extremity.

Occupational therapy practitioners are often required to place their hands on clients in assessment and preparatory methods to facilitate a client's engagement in occupations. In addition to MMT, examples include hand-over-hand assistance with activity of daily living tasks to help a client experience the movement required for dressing, and AAROM or PROM assessment before or after occupational therapy services to identify any changes. Important considerations during muscle palpation include:

a. Take your time.

b. Visualize the muscle and muscle contraction.

c. Be aware of the typical muscle fiber positioning.

d. Soft touch may be better than heavy pressure that blunts the sensation.

e. Use the pads of the fingertips for smaller muscles and whole hand for larger muscles.

f. Anticipate that your touch may produce a response on the body or muscle.

g. Muscle origin and insertion will help you identify the direction of the muscle fibers.

h. If the muscle is contracting, keep your hand still over the muscle.

i. If the muscle is stationary, you can move your fingers over the muscle.

j. Muscle tendons will usually have a different feel compared to the muscle.

4. **Observing muscle contractions**: Observing muscle contractions may also provide evidence of muscle activation and joint movement. Quite often, observation of muscle contractions occurs simultaneously with palpation of the muscles, causing joint movement. Observing muscle movement occurs when the occupational therapy assistant first meets the client and observes functional movement. The first observations provide clues on movement and what adaptations to the approach need to be incorporated to standardize MMT. Observation of muscles during testing may also provide evidence of muscle contraction when palpation is not possible. Box 4-5 provides a good suggestion to increase service competency with application of MMT.

5. **Resisting muscles**: Resistance is only applied for isometric MMT (muscle grade of 3+ or higher). The occupational therapy assistant has already positioned the client, positioned the extremity, and stabilized the joint by placing a stabilizing hand just proximal to the joint. The

occupational therapy assistant is also observing and palpating available muscle contractions. The occupational therapy assistant then places their other hand just distal to the joint being tested halfway to the next distal joint in the extremity. This is the location for placement of resistance and provides a standard location for repeated tests. The palmar surface of the hand provides a uniform application of force for the application of resistance. Use of fingertips for force application should be avoided due to discomfort to the client from poking the muscle and possible inconsistent application of force, not to mention poor ergonomics for the practitioner.

The occupational therapy assistant asks the client to maintain their arm in the position of roughly half available ROM as force is applied to the arm to cause joint movement. Force is briefly applied for just enough time to assess resistance to the force produced by the therapist. The therapist builds up the application of force as the client provides resistance, and in such a manner as to not surprise the client. It is important to remember precautions to MMT with force application. For example, arthritic joints and weak bones may not have the structure necessary to resist typical applications of force. Refer back to Table 4-7 for examples of precautions and contraindications of MMT.

6. **Grading strength**: The occupational therapy assistant will use the isometric MMT grades presented in Table 4-8 to assess muscle strength. Quite often, the occupational therapy assistant will first identify whether the client has a MMT strength grade of 3, or fair (F). The client will demonstrate this grade if the joint moves through the full available ROM against gravity or is able to maintain the testing position.

If the client demonstrates MMT strength of at least 3, the occupational therapy assistant will then perform the isometric grading test procedures. Resistance is applied for all muscle grades above 3. The amount of resistance determines the MMT strength grade.

If the client demonstrates a MMT strength of less than 3, then the occupational therapy assistant will perform the gravity-eliminated grading test procedures. The MMT grade is determined by the amount of joint movement in the gravity-eliminated position. If joint movement is not possible in the gravity-eliminated position, then the MMT grade is determined by the presence or absence of a muscle contraction.

TABLE 4-9
Measures to Increase Standardization for Manual Muscle Testing

- When possible, have the same clinician perform repeated MMT measurements or at least ensure the client performs procedures in the same manner (some measurements can be done in different ways).
- Have the client in the same position (e.g., seated, prone, supine) when performing the assessment.
- Practice applying MMT to develop service competency.
- Control contextual considerations to limit impact on MMT (i.e., the temperature of the room, effects of gravity, temperature of mat or occupational therapy assistant's hands).
- Document any factors that may have influenced MMT measurements (i.e., pain, dementia, edema, age, gender, weakness, command following).
- Observe and measure the unaffected extremity first to provide insight into the typical movement capability of the other extremity.
- Gain information prior to the MMT through reviewing medical records, observing the client move and perform a functional task, and assessing the intact bilateral extremities first.
- Minimize variations to MMT and identify when variations exceed standardization to the point that accurate MMT may not be possible.

One of the focuses of this text is to aid the development of service competency for both ROM and MMT. Table 4-9 provides suggestions to increase service competency for MMT. (Table 4-6 lists suggestions for improving service competency in ROM measurement.) In order to develop service competency, it is also important to memorize the isometric MMT grading scale to easily and appropriately apply muscle strength grades. This textbook only provides one norm for ROM and one scale for MMT; however, numerous scales exist. The occupational therapy clinic protocols, service provider, and third-party payer requirements may determine which ROM norms and MMT scale will be used.

Summary

As discussed previously, motor control builds on motor learning and motor behaviors, allowing an individual to perform purposeful movements voluntarily. These movement patterns fall into a continuum of function, ranging from least functioning to optimal functioning. In general, most of the time, we perform in the typical movement range; however when impacted by disease or disability, we may need to employ abnormal atypical or normal atypical movement patterns. More often than not, in therapy, we work with individuals who perform in the atypical movement categories. Maintaining one's balance and postural control are also essential for functional, voluntary movement to occur. This chapter discussed six principles we can use with clients that enhance the interplay between balance, stability, and motion.

Therapy practitioners often need to quantify movement and strength. ROM and MMT can be reliable and effective methods of assessing movement and strength in the clinic, especially when the occupational therapy assistant displays service competency. ROM and MMT assess very specific aspects of movement. The body functions of joint motion and strength are particularly needed for movement, and have, historically, been widely assessed within the medical model. Yet, these body functions do not shed light on the numerous other body functions affecting movement. Minimum needed ROM angles and MMT strength required to adequately be within functional limits or within normal limits are purposefully not stressed in this text as so many other variables impact function. The redundancy of human movement and infinite ability to compensate or substitute motions can lead to infinite possibilities for acceptable functional movement to complete a task.

92   *Chapter 4*

References

American Occupational Therapy Association. (2020). Occupational therapy practice framework: Domain and process (4th ed.). *American Journal of Occupational Therapy, 74*(Suppl. 2), Article 7412410010. https://doi.org/10.5014/ajot.2020.74S2001

Bohannon, R. W. (2005). Manual muscle testing: Does it meet the standards of an adequate screening test? *Clinical Rehabilitation, 19*, 662-667.

Cirsea, M. C., & Levin, M. F. (2000). Compensatory strategies for reaching in stroke. *Brain, 123*, 940-953.

Crepeau, E. B., Cohn, E. S., & Boyt-Schell, B. A. (2009). *Willard and Spackman's occupational therapy* (11th ed.). Lippincott Williams & Wilkins.

Dvir, Z. (1997). Grade 4 in manual muscle testing: The problem with submaximal strength assessment. *Clinical Rehabilitation, 11*, 36-41.

Fisher, B. (1987). Effect of trunk control and alignment on limb function. *Journal of Head Trauma Rehabilitation, 2*(2), 72-79.

Fisher, B., & Yakura, J. (1993). Movement analysis: A different perspective. *Orthopaedic Clinics of North America, March*, 1-14.

Gajdosik, L., & Bohannon, R. W. (1987). Clinical measurement of range of motion: Summary of goniometry emphasizing reliability and validity. *Physical Therapy, 67*(12), 1867-1872.

Greene, B. L., & Wolf, S. L. (1989). Upper extremity joint movement: Comparison of two measurement devices. *Archives of Physical Medicine & Rehabilitation, 70*, 288-290.

Horak, R. (1987). Clinical management of postural control in adults. *Physical Therapy, 67*(12), 1881-1885.

Hurt, S. P. (1947a). Joint measurement. *American Journal of Occupational Therapy, 1*(4), 209-214.

Hurt, S. P. (1947b). Joint measurement: Part II. *American Journal of Occupational Therapy, 1*(5), 281-285.

Hurt, S. P. (1948). Joint measurement: Part III. *American Journal of Occupational Therapy, 2*(1), 13-15.

Kanbur, N. Ö., Düzgün, I., Derman, O., & Baltaci, G. (2005). Do sexual maturation stages affect flexibility in adolescent boys aged 14 years? *Journal of Sports Medicine and Physical Fitness, 45*(1), 53-57.

Killingsworth, A. P., & Pedretti, L. W. (2006). Evaluation of muscle strength. In H. Pendleton & W. Schultz-Krohn (Eds.), *Pedretti's occupational therapy: Practice skills for physical dysfunction* (pp. 469-512). Mosby-Elsevier.

Knepler, C., & Bohannon, R. W. (1998). Subjectivity of forces associated with manual muscle testing grades of 3+, 4-, and 4. *Perceptual and Motor Skills, 87*, 1123-1128.

Landel, R., & Fisher, B. (1993). Musculoskeletal considerations in the neurologically impaired patient. *Orthopaedic Physical Therapy Clinics of North America, 2*(1), 15-24.

Latash, M. L., & Anson, J. G. (1996). What are "normal movements" in atypical populations? *Behavioral and Brain Sciences, 19*(1), 55-106. https://doi.org/10.1017/S0140525X00041467

Lieber, R. L., & Bodine-Fowler, S. C. (1993). Skeletal muscle mechanics: Implications for rehabilitation. *Physical Therapy, 73*(12), 844-856.

Lippert, L. S. (2006). *Clinical kinesiology and anatomy* (4th ed.). F. A. Davis Company.

Martin, J. P. (1977). A short essay on posture and movement. *Journal of Neurology Neurosurgery and Psychiatry, 40*, 25-29.

McPherson, J. J., Schild, R., Spaulding, S. J., Barsamian, P., Transon, C., & White, S. (1991). Analysis of upper extremity movement in four sitting positions: A comparison of persons with and without cerebral palsy. *American Journal of Occupational Therapy, 42*(2), 123-129.

Merriam-Webster. (n.d.). *Merriam-Webster.com dictionary*. http://www.merriam-webster.com/dictionary

Pendleton, H. M., & Schultz-Krohn, W. (2006). *Pedretti's occupational therapy: Practice skills for physical dysfunction* (6th ed.). Mosby-Elsevier.

Roby-Brami, A., Feydy, A., Combeaud, M., Biryokova, E. V., Bussel, B., & Levin, M. F. (2003). Motor compensation and recovery for reaching in stroke patients. *Acta Neurologica Scandinavica, 107*, 369-381.

Rondinelli, R. D., Genoverse, E., Katz, R. T., Mayer, T. G., Mueller, K., & Ranavaya, M. (2008). *Guides to the evaluation of permanent impairment* (6th ed.). American Medical Association.

Rothstein, J. M., Miller, P. J., & Roettger, R. F. (1983). Goniometric reliability in a clinical setting. *Physical Therapy, 63*(10), 1611-1615.

Sabari, J. S., Maltzev, I., Lubarsky, D., Liszkay, E., & Hanel, P. (1998). Goniometric assessment of shoulder range of motion: Comparison of testing in supine and sitting positions. *Archives of Physical Medicine & Rehabilitation, 79*, 647-651.

Shumway-Cook, A., & Woollacott, M. H. (2001). *Motor control: Theory and practical applications* (2nd ed.). Lippincott Williams & Wilkins.

Spaulding, S. J. (2005). *Meaningful motion: Biomechanics for occupational therapists*. Elsevier-Churchill Livingstone.

Taub, E., Miller, N. E., Novak, T. A., Cook III, E. W., Fleming, W. C., Nepomuceno, C. S., & Crago, J. E. (1993). Technique to improve chronic motor deficit after stroke. *Archives of Medicine & Rehabilitation, 74*, 347-354

Thomas, C. L. (Ed.). (1993). *Taber's cyclopedic medical dictionary* (17th ed.). F. A. Davis Company.

Tyldesley, B., & Grieve, J. (2002). *Muscles, nerves and movement in human occupation* (3rd ed.). Blackwell Publishing Company.

Whiting, W. C., & Rugg, S. (2006). *Dynatomy: Dynamic human anatomy*. Human Kinetics.

Whyte, J., & Morrissey, J. (1990). Motor learning and relearning. In M. B. Glenn & J. Whyte (Eds.), *The practical management of spasticity in children and adults* (pp. 44-69). Lea & Febiger.

Applications

The following activities will help you apply knowledge of movement in real-life applications. Activities can be completed individually or in a small group to enhance learning.

1. **OTPF-4: Body Functions—Neuromusculoskeletal and Movement-Related Functions**: Many body functions affect movement. The purpose of Application #1 is to help the reader become more familiar with body functions identified in the OTPF-4 and how they impact function and movement. The body functions identified in the OTPF-4 and particularly involved in movement (i.e., neuromusculoskeletal and movement-related functions) are listed next. For Application #1, identify two activities and explain how each body function impacts the ability to participate in that functional activity.

BODY FUNCTIONS	ACTIVITY EXAMPLE	ACTIVITY #1	ACTIVITY #2
	Getting dressed		
Joint mobility: ROM	To doff and don clothes		
Joint stability	For pain-free smooth ROM		
Muscle power: Strength	For picking up clothes and body parts		
Muscle tone	To activate UE reaching movements		
Muscle endurance	To complete dressing in timely manner		
Involuntary movement reaction	Righting reactions, protective reactions		
Gait patterns	Needed to get clothes to wear		

   a. Why do you think that ROM and MMT have historically been assessed more regularly in the clinic than the other body functions identified in the OTPF-4?
   b. Are all body functions identified as important in each activity? Why or why not?
   c. Are all the body functions identified incorporated in the activities listed previously? Minus a body function, can the activity still be performed?

2. **OTPF-4: Performance Skills—Motor Skills**: Many performance skills in the OTPF-4 can also affect movement. The purpose of Application #2 is to help the reader become more familiar with some of the performance skills identified in the OTPF-4, particularly motor skills, and how they impact function and movement. The examples of the performance skills—motor skills identified in the OTPF-4 are listed in the following section. For Application #2, use the same two activities from the previous application, and explain how each performance skill impacts the ability to participate in that functional activity.

MOTOR SKILLS	ACTIVITY EXAMPLE	ACTIVITY #1	ACTIVITY #2
	Getting dressed		
Bends	For socks and shoes, pick up items		
Paces	Timely sequence of arm in dressing		
Coordinates	UE, holding sleeve while putting other arm in sleeve		
Aligns	Balance on foot to put other leg in pants		
Stabilizes	Changing body posture when needed, like when standing on pants when pulling pants up		
Manipulates	To fasten pants or belt buckle		
Gait patterns	Needed to get clothes to wear		

a. When reflecting on performance skills, do you think that multiple body functions can influence how a performance skill is related to movement?

b. Are body functions more important than performance skills in enabling movement for the activities you have chosen? Explain your decision.

c. Are all of the performance skills identified incorporated in the activities listed previously?

d. Minus a performance skill, can the same activity be performed?

3. **Functional Movement Continuum**: Most functional movement can be described as normal atypical movement or normal typical movement. This application is designed to help accentuate both aspects of adaptive motor behaviors. At some point in your life, you have probably performed one of the tasks that follow. For this application, refer back to that experience, and select one of the activities to answer the following questions.

- Dribble a basketball with your dominant arm.
- Throw a ball with your dominant arm.
- Brush your teeth, brush your hair, or apply make-up with your dominant arm.
- Write a sentence with your dominant arm.
- Dribble a basketball with your nondominant arm.
- Throw a ball with your nondominant arm.
- Brush your teeth, brush your hair, or apply make-up with your nondominant arm.
- Write a sentence with your nondominant arm.

Select one of the previous activities. For this activity, circle the descriptors in the following table that best characterize the movement produced.

NORMAL ATYPICAL MOVEMENT	NORMAL TYPICAL MOVEMENT
Awkward	Smooth
Uncoordinated	Coordinated
Inefficient	Efficient
Conscious thought	Automatic
Limited movement options	Multiple movement options
Low complexity	High complexity
Increased time	Decreased time
Low joint angle	High joint angle
One joint motion	Multiple joint motions
Low velocity	High velocity
Low acceleration	High acceleration

a. If the activity selected was with the dominant arm, are more characteristics circled under the Normal Typical Movement column?

b. Likewise, if the activity was performed with the nondominant arm, are more characteristics circled under the Normal Atypical Movement column? If not, why do you think this occurred?

4. **Motor Behavior**: The human body continuously learns and adapts movement to the activity being performed. First, identify an activity. Next, identify the best descriptor of motor behavior (motor learning, motor control, or motor development) for each activity/task. Try to give an example of each motor behavior.

ACTIVITY	MOST APPLICABLE MOTOR BEHAVIOR
1.	
2.	
3.	
4.	
5	
6.	

5. **Range of Motion**: The purpose of this application is to gain experience using a goniometer to measure an angle. Choose an object in the room to find an example of an angle that you can measure. If you are not able to identify an object in the room, intersecting two lines on paper will create an angle that you can measure with a goniometer. An example might include a hardcover book standing on its end. Align the goniometer arms along the top edge of the front and back cover of the book. The fulcrum of the goniometer may not be directly over the spine of the book but that is okay. Appropriately aligning the goniometer arms will center the fulcrum of the goniometer in the proper position that is parallel to the apex of the angle produced by the open book. For your example, identify the following:

   a. What are you trying to measure?

   b. What is the apex of the angle?

   c. Are the goniometer arms aligned?

   d. What is the joint angle measurement?

6. **MMT Grade Scale**: Match the MMT grade to its description of movement.

MMT GRADES	DESCRIPTION OF MMT GRADE MOVEMENT
5	Maintains testing position against gravity and minimal resistance
4	Moves the joint through full ROM with gravity eliminated
4-	Moves joint through less than half of available ROM and no gravity
3+	Moves joint through less than half of available ROM and gravity
3	No joint movement and no palpable muscle contraction
3-	Maintains testing position against gravity and maximal resistance
2+	Moves joint through full available ROM against gravity
2	No joint movement but slight observable muscle contraction
2-	Maintains testing position against gravity and moderate resistance
1+	Moves joint through more than half ROM but less than full ROM in gravity
1	Moves joint through more than half ROM but less than full ROM, no gravity
0	Maintains test position against gravity and less than moderate resistance

   a. Which MMT grades are included in isometric grading?

   b. Which MMT grades are included in gravity-eliminated testing?

   c. Which MMT grades are not included in either isometric grading or gravity-eliminated testing?

7. **Palpating Muscles**: Using anatomical pictures of muscles, muscle models, and other materials, attempt to see how many different muscles you can palpate on the UE, individually or in groups. Identify the muscle, location, and joint motion it produces.

CHAPTER 5

Function and Movement of the Trunk and Neck

Maribeth P. Vowell, PT, MPH, EdD and Susan J. Sain, MS, OTR/L, FAOTA

Key Terms

anterior pelvic tilt

atlas

axis

backward pelvic rotation

base of support

center of gravity

cervical retraction

dynamic balance

forward pelvic rotation

intervertebral disk

kyphosis

lateral pelvic tilt

lordosis

muscle imbalance

neutral pelvic tilt

nonstructural scoliosis

pelvic obliquity

posterior pelvic tilt

scoliosis

static balance

structural scoliosis

syndesmosis

Valsalva maneuver

vertebral column

Chapter Outline

Introduction

Occupational Profile

Body Functions of the Trunk and Neck

   Motions of the Trunk and Neck

   Motions of the Pelvic Girdle

   Observation of Posture of the Trunk and Pelvic Girdle

   Observation of Balance and Postural Control

   Common Problems Associated With the Spine and Pelvis

Body Structures of the Trunk and Neck

   Body Structures of the Spine and Rib Cage

   Body Structures of the Pelvic Girdle

   Ligaments

   Muscles of the Trunk and Neck

Summary

References

Applications

Sain, S. J., & Roller, C. L. *Kinesiology for the Occupational Therapy Assistant: Essential Components of Function and Movement, Third Edition* (pp. 97-121).
© 2024 Taylor & Francis Group.

Introduction

The focus of this chapter is on motions of the neck and trunk and the underlying anatomy that allows for these motions. Joint motions, spinal curves, and movement characteristics are identified. Their relationship to posture, movement, and function is presented. The **vertebral column** and its attachment to the pelvis provide the basis for trunk movement and support all other movement. Pelvic positioning is key to positioning of the spine. Pelvic positioning and normal curvature of the spine are introduced early in the chapter as functional movement depends on these. How these parameters impact balance and postural control is also addressed. Subsequently, abnormal curvature of the spine and its impacts are described. Body structures, including the various types of vertebrae, ligaments, and muscles, are presented. Unique characteristics of vertebrae at each spinal level (cervical, thoracic, lumbar, sacral, coccygeal) are pointed out. Roles of the ligaments are defined. Muscles are divided into categories related to the body region they act upon—pelvis, trunk, neck. Muscles of the neck and trunk are paired; if they contract bilaterally they will cause different movements than if they contract unilaterally. Descriptions of these motions are included. Throughout this chapter references will be made to the client in the occupational profile and his functional problems, goals, and treatment.

Occupational Profile

The following occupational profile is provided to demonstrate how posture, positioning, and stability are all related to occupational performance. Terrence, the client in the following occupational profile, will be referred to in this chapter in order to apply the kinesiological and anatomical principles involved with posture and trunk movements. The following data were gathered during the occupational therapy evaluation.

Subjective: Terrence states that he has difficulty raising his arms overhead while sitting in his wheelchair. Additionally, the occupational therapist identifies that Terrence has difficulty with swallowing and seems short of breath. Terrence has used a manual wheelchair since his admission to an assisted-living facility 6 years ago. He reports a decrease in his ability to perform any overhead activity (recently increased trouble combing his hair and retrieving items above him in the refrigerator). As of late, Terrence has been experiencing increased fatigue and difficulty swallowing, especially when drinking from a cup or glass.

Terrence is able to propel his lightweight manual wheelchair to the dining area approximately 50 feet from his apartment. He confirms, however, that this has been more difficult than usual as he feels tired by the time he gets to the dining area. He has not been able to finish his meal without needing frequent rest breaks. Terrence also reports difficulty raising his glass and tilting his head back to finish his beverages. Due to fatigue, Terrence has to return to his room after meals rather than staying in the lobby to read the newspaper with his friends.

Terrence moved to the assisted-living apartment 6 years ago from his downtown apartment after his retirement from the university where he taught economics for nearly 25 years. He was diagnosed with secondary progressive multiple sclerosis 14 years ago. Terrence enjoys reading, playing chess, listening to music, playing the piano, and engaging in social groups at the university and the assisted-living center. He uses a rolling walker in his apartment, but states that he becomes very tired after walking to the bathroom from his living room. He spends much of his day napping to recuperate from the activities that he has completed. He expresses fear of falling, especially in the bathroom, and as a result he has learned to limit his fluid intake to avoid unnecessary trips to the bathroom. He is 5'9" and weighs 190 pounds.

Objective: Terrence has no complaint of pain at rest but does state that his endurance is more limited than it was 3 months ago. He was recently evaluated for a power wheelchair for mobility and positioning. The areas addressed during the wheelchair assessment included the following:

- Skin integrity
- Trunk mobility
- Presence of orthopedic abnormalities and whether each is flexible or fixed
- Presence of abnormal tone
- Adequate joint range of motion (ROM) for the seated posture
- Adequate ROM, endurance, and strength for the mode of propulsion or drive control
- Balance and the presence of asymmetries and orthopedic deformities (Davis, 2007)

An improper wheelchair may create limitations in mobility, health issues, and/or decreased participation in activities of daily living (Bolin et al., 2000; Brubaker, 1986; Guerraz et al., 2003; Herman & Lange, 1999).

The evaluation highlighted the following.

Functional skills: Terrence experiences fatigue and shortness of breath when he ambulates more than 10 feet using the rolling walker. He uses a manual wheelchair for distances greater than 10 feet, but fatigues when propelling the wheelchair to the dining room and other areas within the assisted-living facility. Terrence is independent and uses modifications with his activities of daily living. He utilizes a grab bar, tub bench, and handheld shower for bathing. Terrence requires moderate assistance for instrumental activities of daily living, such as shopping and meal preparation, and eats two of his three meals in the dining room at the assisted-living facility. He is able to complete simple meal prep for breakfast but requires assistance for shopping, as he is unable to propel his manual wheelchair to the local grocery store two blocks away. He is independent with a modified stand pivot transfer using his rolling walker, but complains of anxiety when performing transfers due to a fear of falling. It is for this reason he schedules his day to limit the number of times he gets into and out of his manual wheelchair. Additionally, he limits the number of times per day that he uses the restroom and the number of days per week that he takes a shower due to a fear of falling. He has recently developed a urinary tract infection and is taking antibiotic medication.

Range of motion: Active range of motion of the extremities is grossly within normal limits with the following exceptions:

- Glenohumeral (GH) joint flexion:
  Right: 0 to 75 degrees   Left: 0 to 70 degrees
- GH joint abduction:
  Right: 0 to 60 degrees   Left: 0 to 65 degrees
- GH joint external rotation:
  Right: 0 to 25 degrees   Left: 0 to 45 degrees

- GH joint internal rotation:
  Right: 0 to 35 degrees   Left: 0 to 40 degrees
- Hip flexion:
  Right: 15 to 80 degrees   Left: 15 to 80 degrees
- Knee flexion:
  Right: 0 to 120 degrees   Left: 0 to 115 degrees

Strength: Strength is 4/5 (Good) with the following exceptions:

- GH joint flexion:
  Right: 3/5   Left: 3/5
- GH joint abduction:
  Right: 3+/5   Left: 3+/5
- GH joint external rotation:
  Right: 3+/5   Left: 3+/5
- GH joint internal rotation:
  Right: 3/5   Left: 3/5
- Hip extension:
  Right: 3+/5   Left: 3+/5
- Hip flexion:
  Right: 2+/5   Left: 2+/5
- Knee extension:
  Right: 3+/5   Left: 4/5

Balance: Static sitting balance is fair and dynamic sitting balance is poor. Static standing balance is fair and dynamic standing balance is poor.

Posture: The client sits with a flexible posterior pelvic tilt, slight pelvic obliquity to the right, and minimal trunk rotation on the right side. He exhibits mild increased thoracic kyphosis and mild increased cervical lordosis.

Assessment: The client is at risk for falls, pressure injury development, and impaired orthopedic limitations. A power wheelchair is recommended with the following features:

- Tilt and recline, seat elevator and elevating leg rest, and angle-adjustable foot plates
- Seat cushion with good pressure-relieving attributes
- High-contour back with headrest attached
- Pelvic positioning belt
- Joystick control—retractable swing away
- Height-adjustable desk-length arm rest

Short-Term Goals:

1. Client will demonstrate safe and independent use of power seat functions of tilt, recline, elevator, and leg elevation by 2 weeks.

2. Client will demonstrate safe and proficient use of power mobility device including on and off, steering, and navigating doorways and areas where furniture is in close proximity by 2 weeks.

3. Client will be safe and independent in sit-to-stand transfers using the seat elevator to assist by 2 weeks.

TABLE 5-1
The Planes and Axes of the Body and Their Locations

PLANE	AXIS	DESCRIPTION
Sagittal or median plane	Frontal	Divides the left and right sides of the entire body
Frontal or coronal plane	Sagittal	Divides the front and back halves of the entire body
Horizontal or transverse plane	Vertical	Divides the body at the waist (top and bottom halves of the body)

4. Client will demonstrate improved endurance with use of power mobility device by 2 weeks in order to finish eating meal in dining area without need for breaks.

5. Client will demonstrate improved sitting posture by 2 weeks in order to raise arms overhead for hair grooming.

Long-Term Goals:
1. Client will prevent the development of pressure injuries and orthopedic deformities by discharge.

2. Client will be independent in pressure relief with power wheelchair features after instruction by 4 weeks.

3. Client will be independent and safe in sit-to-stand transfers using appropriately placed grab bars in the bathroom by discharge.

4. Client will demonstrate improved respiration with appropriate use of tilt and recline position by 4 weeks in order to improve endurance for simple meal preparation.

5. Client will demonstrate improved social interactions secondary to improved endurance and improved posture by 4 weeks in order to engage in groups at the university and assisted-living center.

6. Client will demonstrate decreased risk for falling during transfers by discharge.

Body Functions of the Trunk and Neck

The neck and trunk provide essential stability for the extremities as they accomplish the needed tasks of daily living. During activities like reaching or walking, the trunk and neck muscles are quietly contracting to maintain posture. Anytime the body is upright, and especially when the limbs are active, the trunk muscles are engaged. Sometimes the word "core" is used to describe the trunk. This is an excellent analogy because it identifies the trunk as being the center of support for the limbs. *Loading* and *dynamic loading* describe the activation of trunk muscles as the limbs assume postures and movements away from the central axis of the body. As

the intensity of the load on the limbs increases, and as the limb ROM varies, muscles of the trunk intensify and volley their contractions in a coordinated and synchronous fashion. Through an amazing system of sensory receptors, trunk reflexes, and motor control mechanisms, trunk stability is maintained for an infinite combination of limb movements.

Motions of the Trunk and Neck

The vertebral column is considered functionally as a tri-axial joint, which allows for movement in the three planes (sagittal, frontal, and horizontal). As a review from Chapter 2, Table 5-1 identifies the planes and axes associated with each spinal movement. Flexion, extension, and hyperextension occur in the sagittal plane around the frontal axis. Lateral flexion occurs in the frontal plane around a sagittal axis, and rotation occurs in the horizontal plane around a vertical axis. Rotation specifically does not occur at the joint between C1 and the skull. Motions of the spine are limited by the strong supporting ligaments as well as bony approximations at the end of normal ROM. Spinal ROM may become abnormally limited when the ligaments and muscles around the spine lose their flexibility. Sedentary individuals or individuals unable to move through the normal ROM due to impairments in strength or function, such as some wheelchair users, are at increased risk for loss of normal spinal motion.

Motions of the Pelvic Girdle

Stability and function of the vertebral column are provided indirectly from the lower extremities (LEs) and pelvic girdle. The pelvic girdle unites the sacrum and the two hip bones at three different joints. The two posterior joints are the right and left sacroiliac (SI) joints and the anterior joint is the pubic symphysis. Active motions are not available at these joints and passive movements are so small that they cannot be easily or reliably measured (Arab et al., 2009; Robinson et al., 2007).

The pelvic girdle also unites with the vertebrae at the lumbosacral joint. The lumbosacral joint is the most important articulation in the pelvic girdle, as all pelvic movements

TABLE 5-2		
Movements of the Pelvic Girdle and Associated Landmarks, Planes, and Axes of Motion		
MOVEMENT	**LANDMARKS**	**PLANE/AXIS OF MOTION**
Anterior pelvic tilt	ASIS moves anterior relative to pubic symphysis and inferior relative to PSIS	Sagittal/frontal
Posterior pelvic tilt	ASIS moves posterior relative to pubic symphysis and superior relative to PSIS	Sagittal/frontal
Forward pelvic rotation	ASIS moves forward relative to contralateral side	Transverse or horizontal/vertical
Backward pelvic rotation	ASIS moves backward relative to contralateral side	Transverse or horizontal/vertical
Lateral pelvic tilt	Iliac crest moves superior or inferior compared to contralateral side	Frontal/sagittal

---

BOX 5-1

REACHING TASKS

The ability to perform reaching tasks while seated is fundamental to occupational performance, self-care, independence, and quality of life.

(Dean et al., 1999)

---

involve this joint, specifically the motions of **anterior pelvic tilt**, **posterior pelvic tilt**, **lateral pelvic tilt**, **forward pelvic rotation**, and **backward pelvic rotation**. These movements are summarized in Table 5-2, and their definitions and relationships of these movements to the rest of the trunk and to stationary posture assessment are further explained in the sections that follow. Pelvic motions always occur in coordination with movements of the trunk and LEs. Box 5-1 supports the importance of the movements of the trunk and pelvis in the performance of daily tasks.

Observation of Posture of the Trunk and Pelvic Girdle

Observation of the stationary posture of the trunk and pelvis should occur simultaneously with observation of the posture of the UEs and LEs. The goals of the postural analysis are to determine how each postural abnormality affects the other, how postural findings relate to other objective and subjective findings, and how to address the findings within the patient intervention. The postural observation can be performed in the sitting position, standing position, or both. The patient should be viewed from the anterior, posterior, and lateral views. The following sections will focus on the most important components of the postural assessment of the trunk and pelvis.

The Normal Vertebral Curves

The bony vertebrae are named by their location and are referred to as either *cervical, thoracic, lumbar, sacral,* or *coccygeal vertebrae*. The vertebral column is divided into segments associated with the names of the vertebra and is arranged to form normal anterior/posterior (concave/convex) curves. An *anterior* or *concave curve* refers to a curve that extends inward. A bowl or cup has a concave curve. A *posterior* or *convex curve* refers to a curve that extends outward in relation to the body. A ball has a convex curve. In a healthy spine, the three natural curves are flexible and occur at the cervical, thoracic, and lumbar vertebrae. The cervical curve is considered anterior (concave) when viewed laterally. The thoracic curve is associated with the rib cage, projects posteriorly (convexly), and is located in the middle section of the spine. The thoracic (convex) curve is referred to as a **kyphosis**. The lumbar curve in the lower back is concave when viewed laterally and is sometimes referred to as **lordosis**. More frequently, the term lordosis is used for an abnormally increased lumbar curvature. Kyphosis is discussed in more detail in the section Common Problems Associated

TABLE 5-3

Vertebral Segments

SEGMENT	NUMBER	SAGITTAL CURVE	FIXED OR FLEXIBLE
Cervical	7	Concave	Movable/flexible
Thoracic	12	Convex	Movable/flexible
Lumbar	5	Concave	Movable/flexible
Sacral fused with the coccyx	5 and the coccyx	Convex	Fixed

Adapted from Lippert, L. S. (2023). *Clinical kinesiology and anatomy* (7th ed.). F. A. Davis Company.

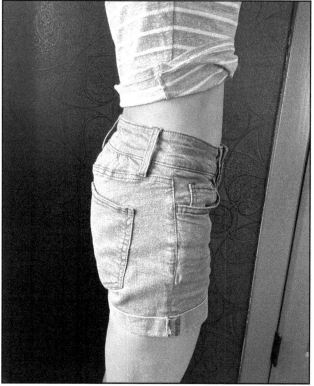

Figure 5-1. Neutral pelvic tilt. (Reproduced with permission from Carolyn L. Roller, OTR/L.)

With the Spine and Pelvis. The change from concave to convex and back again adds to the structural support, stability, and strength of the vertebral column. Other purposes of the spinal curves are to provide balance, movement, shock absorption, and an upright posture. While there is movement between each of the spinal segments or curves, the vertebral curves also move in unison with the vertebra near them. Normal curves of the spine can be compromised due to weakness, loss of flexibility, pain, loss of stability, or poor postural habits. Table 5-3 summarizes the normal curves of the vertebral segments.

The Pelvic Girdle

For the pelvis, the same terminology used to describe the pelvic girdle motions previously described are used to describe the stationary position of the pelvis during postural assessment. From the lateral view, the pelvis can be observed to be tilted anteriorly or posteriorly relative to the lumbar spine. In both the sitting and standing positions, a **neutral pelvic tilt** achieves ideal spinal alignment and decreased stress on the spinal structures. It is characterized by a pelvic position in between anterior and posterior pelvic tilt. Figure 5-1 shows a neutral pelvic tilt in the standing position. In the seated position, a neutral pelvic tilt is further characterized by equal weight distribution across the femurs and an erect spine with the lumbar spine in a normal lordosis. This natural and functional position for activity participation allows weight shifting across the stable **base of support** (BOS) offered by the ischial tuberosities (ITs) and allows the large muscle groups attached to the pelvis to move weight from behind to in front of the ITs with forward trunk movements. This allows people to reach out in front of them without falling forward. A lack of trunk stability during reaching can cause a person to fall. Additionally, during a lateral reach, a person must be able to maintain the pelvis in a stable way while shifting weight to one of the ITs, while at the same time elongating the weight-bearing side of the trunk. This lateral weight shift with trunk elongation allows people to functionally access their environment. The landmarks used for points of reference to determine the position or movement of the pelvis relative to a neutral pelvic tilt are the anterior superior iliac spines (ASIS) and posterior superior iliac spines (PSIS) of the ilium. In the standing position, the neutral pelvic tilt achieves an ideal balance of strength and flexibility between the anterior and posterior trunk musculature. Performance for nearly any upright activity, especially those that require balance, will be enhanced with the pelvis in a neutral pelvic tilt.

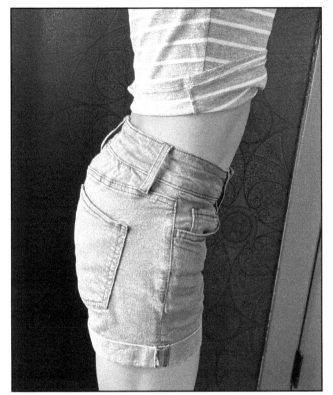

Figure 5-2. Anterior pelvic tilt. (Reproduced with permission from Carolyn L. Roller, OTR/L.)

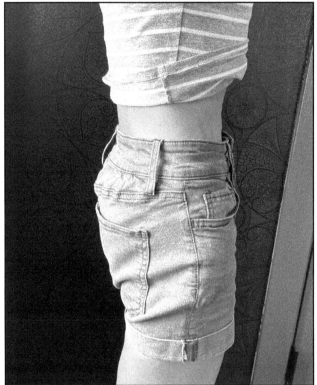

Figure 5-3. Posterior pelvic tilt. (Reproduced with permission from Carolyn L. Roller, OTR/L.)

An anterior pelvic tilt is characterized as the pelvis dipping forward, lifting the buttocks upward, and creating an increased lordosis in the lumbar spine, which is a more exacerbated curve than what is typical in normal standing or sitting. Anterior pelvic tilt is illustrated in Figure 5-2 and is characterized by the ASIS shifting inferiorly and the PSIS shifting superiorly. This posture is sometimes observed in people who are pregnant or in people who carry excessive weight in the abdomen. This weight imbalance also causes the **center of gravity** (COG) to shift forward. Another common cause of anterior pelvic tilt is a **muscle imbalance** in the abdomen, lower limbs, and pelvis; for example, a combined weakness in the abdominal muscles with tightness in the erector spinae muscle group can cause anterior tilting of the pelvis in standing.

A posterior pelvic tilt is the opposite of an anterior pelvic tilt and is characterized by the tailbone tucking beneath the body, or the PSIS shifting inferiorly and the ASIS shifting superiorly. Posterior pelvic tilt is illustrated in Figure 5-3. This posture will cause the lumbar spine to flatten and the thoracic spine to flex or increase thoracic kyphosis. Often, the increased thoracic kyphosis also results in an increase in normal cervical lordosis. When one curve changes, it impacts all of the other curvatures. These postural problems are all commonly associated with the individual confined to a seated posture, such as a wheelchair.

A lateral pelvic tilt, also referred to as **pelvic obliquity**, is characterized by one side of the iliac crest being higher than the other, as illustrated in Figure 5-4. *Pelvic obliquity* is more commonly referred to when describing a static posture and lateral tilt of the pelvis and generally refers to pelvic girdle movement in the frontal plane. Lateral pelvic tilt may be accompanied by rib cage displacement and lateral spinal flexion, and may be caused by, or can accompany, **scoliosis**, which is described in the section Common Problems Associated With the Spine and Pelvis. The pelvic motions and associated postures are summarized in Table 5-2.

Because posture and motion of the trunk are related to the kinematic chain movements of the LEs, and because movements of the pelvis are dynamic vs. fixed, changes in LE position and a variety of LE orthopedic conditions can affect the relationships and posture of the trunk and pelvis, especially when the trunk is viewed in the standing position.

Observation of Balance and Postural Control

Balance of the trunk is defined as maintenance of the body's COG over a BOS. To describe a position as being balanced, it is implied that the position offers a maximal degree of stability while using a relatively low amount of energy to maintain the position. **Static balance** can be differentiated from **dynamic balance** in that static balance is the ability to maintain a position while dynamic balance is the ability to

Figure 5-4. Pelvic obliquity. (SciePro/shutterstock.com)

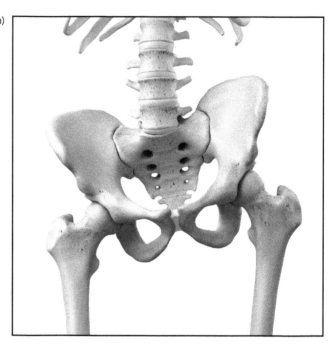

BOX 5-2

STABILITY IN SITTING VERSUS STANDING

In sitting, the COG is lower and the BOS is greater than that of standing. The increased stability of the body with proper support for the buttocks, feet, and back will increase one's ability to perform fine motor activities with the hands.

(Zacharkow, 1988)

move or function within a position. Observation of balance of the trunk, pelvic girdle, neck, and extremities can be performed in the standing or seated position. Balance involves the ability to maintain a seated or standing posture without falling (static), but it also refers to the ability to reach by extending the arm or by leaning the trunk (dynamic). In other words, a person moves their upper extremity (UE) over a BOS during functional activities that require reaching. The BOS is provided by the pelvis, thighs, and feet in sitting (Dean et al., 1999) and the feet and any ambulatory device used in standing. The ability to reach while maintaining balance is essential to independence. Individuals with movement disorders or trunk weakness have difficulty with coordinating the movements of the extremities while also maintaining balance. Poor trunk balance has also been associated with poor functional outcomes of rehabilitation efforts (Dean et al., 1999). Box 5-2 describes why a seated posture may provide a more stable position for clients to use during functional activities.

Balance, or postural control, is a complex interaction of coordinating numerous factors involving the central nervous system. Kyvelidou et al. (2009) suggest that postural control can be explained using dynamic system theory. According to dynamic system theory, the development of postural control is a product of cognitive information, as well as the synergistic organization of the neuromuscular system and morphologic, biomechanical, and environmental information. Postural control also requires the integration of several processes. Westcott and Burtner (2004) describe these processes as motor processes, sensory processes, and musculoskeletal components. The *Occupational Therapy Practice Framework: Domain and Process, Fourth Edition* (OTPF-4) refers to these processes as *performance skills* and *body functions*. Motor processes fall under the category of performance skills and include the emergence of neuromuscular response synergies to maintain the stability of the neck, trunk, and legs. Sensory processes, which are described under body functions in the OTPF-4, include the visual, vestibular, and somatosensory systems, as well as the central sensory strategies of limb orientation. Musculoskeletal components, also within the domain of body functions, consist of things such as soft tissue, muscle strength, and ROM. Additionally, sensory processes incorporate proprioception, which was first described in 1906 by Sherrington as sensations arising from deep areas of the body that contribute to conscious sensations, postural equilibrium, and joint stability (Hagert et al., 2009). In

TABLE 5-4

Range of Motion of the Vertebral Column

SEGMENT	FLEXION	EXTENSION	LATERAL FLEXION	ROTATION
Cervical	40 degrees	75 degrees	35 to 45 degrees	45 to 50 degrees
Thoracic	—	—	20 degrees	35 degrees
Lumbar	—	—	20 degrees	5 degrees

Adapted from Gillen, G., & Burkhardt, A. (2004). *Stroke rehabilitation: A function-based approach* (2nd ed.). Mosby.

BOX 5-3

COORDINATION OF MOVEMENTS

The coordination between head, trunk, and arm movements, such as self-feeding in children, is dependent on adequate postural control.

(Sveistrup et al., 2007)

---

sitting postures, proprioceptive input is generated at the pelvic region. The proprioceptive input to the hip helps to elicit a muscular response from the trunk extensors to improve trunk posture. Therefore, it is helpful to allow some freedom of movement for an individual who maintains a seated posture for long periods of time, such as a wheelchair user.

Postural control is an ongoing skill for infants. The development of head and trunk control begins very early in infancy and continues to develop into adolescent years (Sveistrup et al., 2007). Stabilization of the head in space is an important aspect of postural stability. Head stabilization provides a stable gravitational reference for the vestibular system and facilitates visual information (Allum et al., 1998); therefore, the position of the head can also influence functional tasks, such as swallowing, reading, and eye contact. Additionally, when individuals use a wheelchair as a means of mobility, it is essential to consider their posture and balance, recognizing the importance of head alignment as it relates to vision.

Posture is a combined activity requiring many anatomical body parts, such as the pelvis, spine, feet, head, and neck. It is helpful to understand what parts of the vertebral column move when considering posture, balance, and postural control as they relate to functional abilities. Additionally, the amount and type of motion available in each of the various sections of the vertebral column is important to note. Table 5-4 provides an outline of the ROM of each section of the vertebral column. Box 5-3 further points out the relationship between postural control and function.

Common Problems Associated With the Spine and Pelvis

Occupational performance, and all movement, requires an extensive array of movement capabilities of the trunk, pelvis, and head. When an individual experiences an orthopedic alignment problem in any aspect of the spine or pelvis, it will influence their ability to perform functional movements. An individual's ability to move the distal segments, such as the hands or LEs, is greatly influenced by pelvic and spinal alignment, stability, and mobility. This is an important consideration in wheelchair positioning. For example, if a client is unable to shift weight from one IT to the other due to a fixed posterior pelvic tilt or pelvic obliquity, they will have difficulty elongating the trunk on the weight-bearing side to allow for balance. In the occupational profile of Terrence, his ability to comb his hair, drink from a glass, and reach for items in his environment were all affected by his motion and positioning of his pelvis. Some of these issues were the result of orthopedic abnormalities. Several orthopedic abnormalities will be presented.

Scoliosis is a spinal deformity in the frontal plane characterized by a lateral S-shaped curvature of the vertebra, as illustrated in Figure 5-5. Scoliosis may result from congenital anomalies, neuromuscular disorders, neurofibromatosis, connective tissue disorders, skeletal dysplasia, or iatrogenic causes (Harrop et al., 2008). Scoliosis can be generally classified as either structural or nonstructural and is commonly

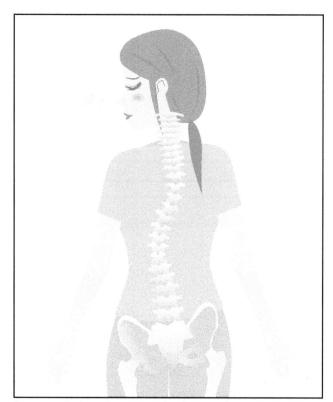

Figure 5-5. Scoliosis. (metamorworks/shutterstock.com)

associated with a variety of postural changes that affect the trunk, pelvis, and extremities. Structural or irreversible scoliosis is a lateral curve of the spine with fixed rotation and lateral curvature of two or more vertebrae, and this curve and rotation remain fixed regardless of movement or repositioning. **Structural scoliosis** is generally identified in adolescence and occurs more often in girls than boys with a prevalence of 2% to 4% of the general population (Horne et al., 2014). This spinal curvature is associated with compression of the ribs on the concave side of the curve and separation of the ribs on the convex side. The vertebral bodies will rotate toward the convex side of the curve, and the spinous processes will rotate in the opposite direction. In addition to the lateral curvature of the spine, the ribs and scapula protrude from the posterior aspect of the back when the client bends forward. This rib protrusion is known as a gibbus deformity. The severity of structural scoliosis in terms of its impact on overall health and function is highly variable depending on the degree of curvature. As the curvature and rotation increases, the internal organs decline in their ability to function normally. This occurs primarily in the thorax, affecting organs such as the lungs and heart. Scoliosis can become so severe that it impedes proper respiratory and circulatory functioning and can lead to death. The cause of structural scoliosis may be due to a specific disorder, such as spina bifida or cerebral palsy (CP), but in most cases the cause is not known (i.e., idiopathic).

Nonstructural scoliosis is a reversible lateral curve of the vertebral spine, meaning that the curve is no longer visible when the trunk is repositioned or when spinal movement such as flexion or lateral bending occurs. Nonstructural scoliosis is very common and may occur due to differences in LE limb length or imbalances of strength or flexibility in the trunk or lower limbs. Nonstructural scoliosis may be corrected if adequate support and muscle re-education are provided. Most pelvic obliquities will present with some degree of scoliosis.

Kyphosis is a convex curve of the spine, and a certain amount normally occurs in the thoracic area of the spine; however, a kyphosis of the lumbar spine is considered abnormal because the normal lumbar curvature is concave. Kyphosis can normally occur in the lumbar area with temporary posterior tilting of the pelvis or with other normal postural adjustments. As a result of long periods of immobilization in a flexed posture, such as when a person is full-time wheelchair user or is sedentary, the lumbar kyphosis can become accentuated or even fixed. Kyphosis may also be present in the lumbar spine in children with spina bifida. In the thoracic spine, kyphosis is abnormal when it is increased beyond what is considered a normal anatomic feature. When the thoracic kyphosis is excessive, the trunk flexes and the rib cage is compressed anteriorly, such that the spine forms a C-shaped bend when viewed laterally. This can impair respiratory function and balance. An increased thoracic kyphosis is commonly seen in older women as a result of osteoporosis and associated thoracic compression fractures.

Lumbar lordosis is a normal curve, however when the lordosis is exacerbated, or if it is inflexible, it is considered abnormal. When the pelvis is in an excessive anterior pelvic tilt, the spine forms an increased lumbar lordosis as part of the normal movement pattern. When this position is observed as part of the posture analysis, however, the abdomen may appear to protrude forward, and when sitting, the lumbar spine may not contact with the seat back. This posture is sometimes referred to as *sway back*.

In the occupational profile presented at the beginning of this chapter, Terrence demonstrates a sitting posture of posterior pelvic tilt, with a mild increased thoracic kyphosis, pelvic obliquity to the right side, and mild increased cervical lordosis. When sitting in a posterior pelvic tilt, the body attempts to correct this misalignment by altering the placement of the spine and attempting to place the head and center of vision in line with the horizon. This is an effort to keep vision functional. In other words, if a person sits in a posterior pelvic tilt with thoracic kyphosis, the eyes will face downward onto their lap. To correct this, a person may hyperextend the neck in order to see the environment. Again, the optimal seated posture is one of neutral pelvic tilt with normal trunk and cervical alignment.

TABLE 5-5

Definitions of Vertebral Structures

STRUCTURE	DEFINITION
Body	A cylindrical mass of cancellous bone. This is the anterior and weight-bearing portion of the vertebrae. It is not palpable on the back. C1 does not have a body.
Facet	A small, flat, smooth surface on a bone. A facet refers to the articulation of the thoracic vertebrae and the rib bone.
Facet joint	The facet joint is the articulation between the superior articular process of the vertebrae below and the corresponding inferior articular process of the vertebrae above.
Foramen	An opening.
Intervertebral foramen	The opening formed by the inferior and superior vertebral notches that allows passage of a nerve root.
Lamina	Portion of the vertebrae that connects the spinous process to the transverse process.
Neural arch	The posterior portion of the vertebrae.
Pedicle	The portion of the vertebral arch. It lies posterior to the body and anterior to the lamina.
Spinous process	The posterior projection found on the neural arch. It is also an attachment point for muscles and ligaments. The seventh cervical vertebra, also known as the *vertebrae prominens*, has an unusually long spinous process. One can easily palpate this aspect. This is where the cervical and thoracic area conjoin.
Transverse process	The union of the lamina and pedicle where the ligaments and muscle attach to the spine.
Vertebral foramen	The opening formed by the joining of the neural arch and vertebral body that contains the spinal cord.

Adapted from Lippert, L. S. (2023). *Clinical kinesiology and anatomy* (7th ed.). F. A. Davis Company.

Generally, when alignment problems occur with the vertebral column, there are also associated alignment problems of the pelvis. These problems can be either fixed or movable and can be observed with the individual either seated or standing. These pelvic alignment problems include those previously mentioned, specifically anterior and posterior pelvic tilt, lateral pelvic obliquity and forward or backward pelvic rotation. The alignment of the LEs, pelvis and trunk are dependent on one another and can change with body position. Alignment is also dependent upon available ROM and strength; therefore, it is important to address all body components together in both sitting and standing, as well as in other functional positions. Most alignment problems of the trunk and pelvis can be corrected or improved with proper seating, positioning, posture education, limb length correction, and exercise. Problems left unaddressed could contribute to the development or worsening of orthopedic problems, such as pain, muscle strain, joint sprain or disk injury.

Body Structures of the Trunk and Neck

Body Structures of the Spine and Rib Cage

The spine is formed by 33 individual bones, 23 that are movable and 10 that are fixed. These bones are called the *vertebrae*. With the exception of the first two cervical vertebrae, known as C1 and C2 (also known as the **atlas** and **axis**), the movable vertebrae all have similar structures. The vertebrae are composed of the following parts: body, facet, vertebral foramen, intervertebral foramen, lamina, neural arch, pedicle, spinous process, transverse process, and superior and inferior articular processes. The vertebral foramen is a passageway formed by the vertebral body and vertebral arch of each vertebra and houses the spinal cord. Each two vertebrae articulate with one another at the intervertebral joint (the joint between two vertebral bodies) and the facet joints (joints between the bilateral articulating facets of the superior vertebra to the one below it). These structures are defined in Table 5-5. Figure 5-6 illustrates the different parts of the vertebrae and vertebral joint.

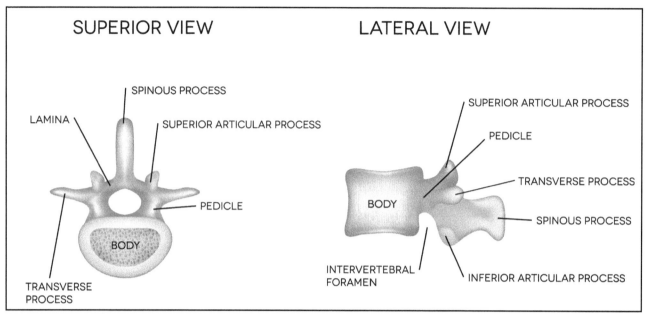

Figure 5-6. Features of a typical vertebra. (TimeLineArtist/shutterstock.com)

The combined structure of the vertebra is referred to as the *vertebral column*. The vertebral column is divided into five areas: cervical, thoracic, lumbar, sacral, and coccygeal. The purpose of the vertebral column is to maintain the longitudinal axis of the body. The vertebral column also serves as a protective covering for the spinal cord, which is composed of nerve pathways that travel between the brain and body. Additionally, the vertebral column serves to provide a pivot point for the head and neck as an anchor point onto the pelvis functioning to transmit the weight of the upper body onto the pelvis and limbs. These combined purposes allow for both the stability and mobility required for normal functional movement.

The skull, sometimes referred to as the *cranium*, sits on the most superior aspect of the vertebral column. The skull provides a covering for the brain and is composed of cranial bones. Between each of the 23 movable vertebrae is a structure known as the **intervertebral disk**. These disks function to absorb and transmit shock as well as to promote normal spinal flexibility. The disks are held in place by ligaments that allow for flexible movement yet also provide adequate strength to prevent the dislocation of the vertebrae. The external portion of the disk is made of a fibrocartilaginous ring and is called the *annulus fibrosus*, and the inner aspect is the *nucleus pulposus*. A common form of damage in the intervertebral disk is known as a slipped disk, herniated disk, or disk prolapse. Such a condition causes the soft nucleus pulposus to bulge out through a weak area of the annulus fibrosus. This may compress a spinal nerve root, causing pain, sensory loss, or muscle weakness in the arms or legs.

The Cervical Vertebrae

The neck region of the spine includes the cervical vertebrae. The seven cervical vertebrae are the smallest vertebrae in the spine. The first cervical vertebra (C1) is called the atlas and supports the cranium. Though it does not have a body, it does have a shortened spinous process and a long transverse process. The superior surface contains two large concavities that articulate with the occipital condyles of the skull. The articulation between the head and C1 is the atlanto-occipital joint. This joint allows for a small amount of flexion and extension of the head on the neck, as if nodding in agreement. Rotation does not occur at this joint.

The second cervical vertebra (C2) is the **axis**, which is characterized by a short protrusion known as the *odontoid process* or the *dens*. The dens extends into the vertebral foramen of C1 and is the pivot point of the cervical spine and head. This joint, the atlantoaxial joint, is a pivot joint and allows for rotation of the head on the neck. Eighty percent of all cervical rotation occurs at the atlantoaxial joint (Foster, 2013, p. 509).

The remaining vertebrae, C3 through C7, are capable of producing the combined motions of cervical flexion, cervical extension, cervical hyperextension, cervical rotation, and cervical lateral bending.

The combined movement of head flexion at the atlanto-occipital joint and neck extension of the joints of C2 through C7 is referred to as **cervical retraction** or axial extension. An upright posture encourages cervical retraction. This exercise is often taught as a proprioceptive activity to improve posture (Foster, 2013, p. 452).

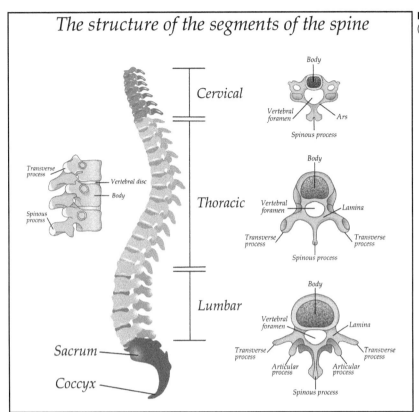

The structure of the segments of the spine

Cervical

Body

Vertebral foramen   *Ars*

Spinous process

Thoracic

Body

Vertebral foramen   *Lamina*

Transverse process   *Transverse process*

Spinous process

Transverse process

Vertebral disc

Body

Spinous process

Lumbar

Body

Vertebral foramen   *Lamina*

Transverse process   *Transverse process*

Articular process   *Articular process*

Spinous process

Sacrum

Coccyx

Figure 5-7. Unique features of the vertebrae by area. (Ellen Bronstayn/shutterstock.com)

The Thoracic Vertebrae

The thoracic vertebrae occur below, or inferior to, the cervical spine. These 12 vertebrae (T1 through T12) make up the most stable aspect of the spine. Many aspects of the thoracic vertebrae are similar to the cervical vertebrae. One significant difference, however, is the presence of costal facets. Costal joints are the areas of articulation of the thoracic vertebral bodies to the ribs. The ribs on the thoracic spine limit the ability for flexion and lateral flexion. This in turn provides for stability of the thoracic spine. The ribs also protect many internal organs. The intercostal muscles allow for the ribs to expand during respiration. Additionally, the thoracic spine differs from other vertebrae as the spinous processes point inferiorly. This characteristic in part serves to limit the thoracic spine in hyperextension.

The Lumbar Vertebrae

The lumbar vertebrae of the spine have five vertebrae, numbered L1 through L5. The lumbar vertebrae support the weight of the body; thus, they are the largest of the movable vertebrae. ROM is limited in the lumbar spine because of both the size and orientation of the articular processes. The lumbar facet joints allow for flexion and extension but limit rotation. One exception is at the largest of the lumbar vertebrae, the fifth lumbar vertebrae, which articulates with the

sacrum. The lumbar spine has more available ROM than the thoracic spine but less than the cervical spine. The lumbar spine is the most frequently injured of the spinal areas, most likely due to the fact that it supports the weight of the body and so its structures take a great deal of stress. Figure 5-7 illustrates the differences in the three types of vertebrae and Table 5-6 lists characteristics for the different types of cervical, thoracic, and lumbar vertebrae.

The Sacral Vertebrae

The sacrum represents the fusion of the five sacral vertebrae. Because these vertebrae are fused, no movement occurs. Sacral vertebrae S1 through S5 fuse together into a triangular shape and fit between the two hip bones, also known as the *pelvic bones*. The last lumbar vertebra, L5, articulates with the most superior vertebra of the sacrum at the lumbosacral joint. The most inferior vertebra in the sacrum articulates with the coccyx or the tailbone.

The Coccygeal Vertebrae

The coccyx, or tailbone, is formed of four or five fused rudimentary vertebrae. No movement occurs at these vertebrae. The most common cause of injury to the tailbone is falling on a hard surface.

TABLE 5-6

Characteristics of the Vertebrae

VERTEBRAL LOCATION	SIZE	BODY SHAPE	VERTEBRAL FORAMEN	TRANSVERSE PROCESS	SPINOUS PROCESS	SUPERIOR ARTICULAR PROCESS	VERTEBRAL NOTCHES
Cervical	Smallest	Small, oval	Large, triangular	Foramen for vertebral artery	Short, stout	Faces medially	Equal in depth
Thoracic	Intermediate	Heart-shaped, with facets that articulate with ribs	Smallest	Facets that connect with ribs, long, thick, point posterior and laterally	Long, slender, point inferiorly	Faces posterior and laterally	Deeper inferior notches
Lumbar	Largest	Large, oval	Intermediate	No foramen and no articulation	Thick, points posterior	Faces posterior	Deeper inferior notches

Adapted from Lippert, L. S. (2023). *Clinical kinesiology and anatomy* (7th ed.). F.A. Davis Company.

BOX 5-4

PRESSURE INJURY DEFINITION

A pressure injury is a localized injury to the skin and/or underlying tissue, usually over a bony prominence, as a result of pressure or pressure in combination with shear force and/or friction. A number of contributing or confounding factors are also associated with pressure injuries. The significance of these factors is yet to be elucidated.

(National Pressure Injury Advisory Panel, 2010)

Rib Cage

The rib cage is composed of the sternum, the dorsal aspect of the 12 thoracic vertebrae, and the 12 pairs of ribs. The rib cage encloses the heart and lungs. All of the ribs articulate with the vertebrae but only seven pairs attach to the sternum. These are referred to as *true ribs*, while the three pairs of ribs that attach only to the vertebra and not the sternum are called the *false ribs*. These sets of ribs all interlock with connective tissue called *costal cartilage*. The last two pairs of ribs are called the *floating ribs* and do not attach to the sternum, nor do they attach to the costal cartilage. Between the ribs are the intercostal muscles, which move the ribs up and down during respiration.

In addition to protecting the heart and lungs, the rib cage also provides support for the UEs and assists in respiration. Upon inhalation, the intercostal muscles lift the rib cage, allowing the lungs room to expand. Upon exhalation, the rib cage moves down, forcing air out of the lungs. During trunk extension, the rib cage lifts and migrates anteriorly. During spinal flexion, the rib cage moves posteriorly, depressing the ribs. Most of the available flexion occurs at the point where the rib cage ends. Thus, in a sitting position, maintaining thoracic extension is important to hold the rib cage upright, which will also allow for proper breathing. During spinal flexion while sitting, the rib cage compresses the diaphragm, making it difficult to breathe. The rib cage prohibits spinal motion from occurring in the thoracic spine to the same extent that motion occurs in the cervical or lumbar areas.

Body Structures of the Pelvic Girdle

The pelvic girdle is comprised of four bones: two hip bones, the sacrum, and the coccyx. There are three joints of the sacrum: two SI joints and the symphysis pubis. These joints will be discussed in this section. The hip bones are formed by the fusion of the pubis, ilium, and ischium. Anteriorly, the hip bones are bound together by the symphysis pubis and posteriorly by the two SI articulations known as the SI joints. The SI joint is part synovial and part **syndesmosis**. Syndesmosis indicates a fibrous joint where the ligaments provide stability. Movement at this joint is limited

because it is a nonaxial joint with ligaments that provide quite a bit of stability. In most typical individuals, the SI joint is virtually immobile.

Each of the pubic bones join anteriorly at the symphysis pubis. The symphysis pubis is a cartilaginous joint with two ligaments providing additional support. These are the superior pubic and arcuate pubic ligaments. The acetabulum is the fossa where the femoral head articulates to form the hip joint. The ITs are the prominent protuberances of the hip bones. The ITs support the weight of the body in a seated position and are particularly vulnerable to pressure injuries. A person is able to sit on these bony prominences as the gluteus maximus covers them, adding cushioning. The ITs are also covered by a fluid-filled bursa to help reduce friction as the gluteus maximus crosses over the ITs in a seated position. It is necessary to provide adequate support and cushioning for individuals who sit for long periods of time. For individuals who use wheelchairs, pressure relief cushions and repositioning are essential to prevent pressure injuries development. Box 5-4 provides a definition for pressure injuries, or decubiti.

The pelvis is the BOS for the rest of the body in sitting. "The position of the pelvis dictates body position throughout the seating arrangement" (Taylor, 1987, p. 713). The pelvis, in conjunction with the trunk, provides for a more stable support system to allow for functional movement. Therefore, proper measurement of the hips and pelvis is a key component for providing the appropriate seating. Additionally, accurate measurements for the seating system are crucial for optimal functional mobility (Pederson, 2000).

A client such as Terrence is at risk of pressure injury development. Thus, the wheelchair assessment completed by the occupational therapist must take into consideration the skin integrity of the client and ensure that proper measurements were taken for the prescribed wheelchair. Figure 5-8 shows what a pressure injury may look like.

Wheelchair research indicates that improper alignment and an inappropriate sitting surface in which the client is unable to efficiently relieve pressure are two of the main causes of pressure injuries. According to Cron and Sprigle (1993), to protect against "pressure [injuries] from a seated position, a wheelchair cushion and a properly fitted wheelchair are equally important" (p. 141). Additionally, between 36% and 50% of pressure injury formation among older adults was attributed to sitting in a wheelchair for an extended period of time (Aissaoui et al., 2001).

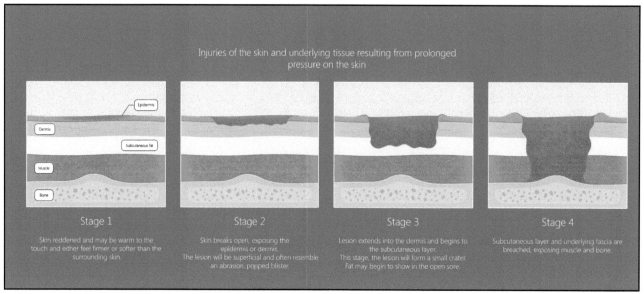

Figure 5-8. Stages of pressure injuries. (Pepermpron/shutterstock.com)

Ligaments

The stability of the trunk and neck is a result of muscular activity as well as ligamentous structures. There are two types of ligaments in the vertebral column: intrasegmental and intersegmental. The intrasegmental ligaments hold the individual vertebrae together. The intrasegmental ligaments include the ligamentum flavum, interspinous, and intertransverse ligaments.

The intersegmental ligaments span across multiple vertebrae and include the anterior longitudinal ligament, posterior longitudinal ligament, supraspinous ligament, and nuchal ligament. The anterior longitudinal ligament connects the bones of the vertebral column and attaches on the anterior surface of the vertebral bodies. This ligament helps to prevent excessive hyperextension of the spine. The posterior longitudinal ligament connects the vertebral bodies posteriorly and attaches to the vertebral bodies inside the vertebral foramen. This ligament limits excessive flexion. The supraspinous ligament extends from the seventh cervical vertebra to the sacrum and runs posteriorly over the tips of the spinous processes. The supraspinous ligament works with the posterior longitudinal ligament to limit forward flexion of the trunk. The nuchal ligament, which takes the place of the supraspinous and interspinous ligaments in the cervical region, extends from the external occipital protuberance to the spinous process of the seventh cervical vertebra. In addition to limiting flexion, this ligament serves as an attachment for the trapezius and splenius capitis muscles, which will be covered in the following section.

Muscles of the Trunk and Neck

The muscles of the neck and trunk are divided into those muscles that lie on the anterior portion and those on the posterior portion of the body. In general, anterior muscles cause flexion, whereas posterior muscles cause extension. Most muscles of the trunk are paired, one on each side of the vertebral column, or vertical axis, of the body. These pairs of muscles will cause different movements if they are contracted simultaneously, or bilaterally, as compared to a unilateral muscle contraction. For the most part, bilateral contractions cause flexion or extension, while unilateral contractions lead to rotation or lateral bending.

The two sides of the rectus abdominis span the front aspect of the trunk. They connect in the center at a point called the *linea alba*. The rectus abdominis flexes the trunk and aids in respiration. It also enables compression of the internal organs. The external oblique muscles are large, thin muscles, that, when acting together, assist in trunk flexion. When contracted bilaterally, they also compress the abdomen and aid in exhalation. When one side contracts (known as *unilateral contraction*), the muscle laterally bends the trunk to the same side while it rotates the trunk toward the opposite side of the body. In other words, the left external oblique rotates the left side of the trunk toward the midline of the body or, stated another way, toward the right. The external oblique muscle originates on the lower ribs, runs inferiorly and medially to insert on the iliac crest and at the midline onto the linea alba via an abdominal aponeurosis.

The internal oblique muscle originates on the inguinal ligament, iliac crest, and the thoracolumbar fascia. The internal oblique muscle performs two major functions. First, it acts as an antagonist to the diaphragm during exhalation. In other words, when the diaphragm contracts, it pulls the lower chest cavity down, which allows the lungs to expand.

When the internal obliques contract, they compress the abdomen and the internal organs, pushing them up into the diaphragm and forcing air out of the lungs. Second, the internal obliques rotate and laterally bend the trunk by pulling the rib cage toward the hip on the same side. Thus, they are same-side rotators, and the external obliques are opposite-side rotators. The internal obliques run deep and perpendicular to the external oblique muscles.

The internal and external obliques can work together as synergists to strengthen trunk flexion or rotation. Contracting unilaterally, the left internal oblique and the right external oblique contract as the trunk rotates to bring the right shoulder toward the left side of the body. Contracting bilaterally, these muscles work together to enhance trunk flexion and compression of the abdominal contents.

The transverse abdominis muscle is the deepest of the abdominal muscles. The fibers of this muscle run horizontally, hence the name transverse. This muscle originates from the lateral portion of the inguinal ligament, the last six ribs, the iliac crest, and the thoracolumbar fascia. It inserts on the abdominal aponeurosis and the linea alba. Because of its horizontal line of pull, it does not have any influence on trunk movement. It does, however, play a significant role in pelvic and trunk stability. Additionally, it is important in the **Valsalva maneuver**. The Valsalva maneuver is compression of the abdomen that facilitates activities such as defecation, coughing, childbirth, lifting, vomiting, and sneezing.

Muscles on the posterior aspect of the trunk include three groups of muscles: the erector spinae muscles, transversospinalis muscles, and intertransversarii muscles.

The erector spinae group lies just under the latissimus dorsi and trapezius muscles. This group includes three distinct groups that span the posterior trunk from the sacrum to the occiput. These groups include the spinalis muscle, longissimus muscle, and iliocostalis muscle. Spinalis is the most medial and occupies the gutter created by the lamina of the vertebrae; longissimus is between spinalis and iliocostalis; and iliocostalis, as the name implies, attaches on the ribs and occupies the most lateral position. These muscles collectively function in extending the spine when they act bilaterally and rotate and laterally bend the spine when they act unilaterally. Splenius capitis is an extension of erector spinae that extends the head on the neck, and splenius cervicis is an extension that extends the cervical spine. These muscles are superficial compared to the rest of the erector spinae, and, for that reason, are given individual names.

The transversospinalis muscles are the deepest muscles in the spine and include two groups of muscles that span only one vertebral segment throughout all areas of the spine. As the name implies, they travel obliquely attaching the transverse process of one vertebral segment to the spinous process of another. The two muscles are the rotatores and multifidus. One other member of the transversospinalis spans several vertebrae and is called the *semispinalis*. These muscles function to extend the spine when they act bilaterally and they rotate the spine when they act unilaterally.

The intertransversarii, the second group of the deep layer, are muscles that span one vertebral segment and connect the transverse processes of adjacent vertebra. These muscles, along with rotatores and multifidus are important segmental stabilizers of the spine and are active during maintenance of dynamic balance during most upright activities.

The quadratus lumborum muscle is a deep muscle originating from the iliac crest and inserting onto the last rib and transverse processes of the lumbar vertebrae. Its role is to balance postural distortions by stabilizing the pelvis during unilateral stance (standing on one limb). Its main function is pelvic elevation, or hip-hiking.

While the psoas and iliacus muscles are an aspect of the LE, their role in spinal stabilization is important. Research by Andersson and colleagues (1996) suggests that the psoas and iliacus muscles play an important role in the stability of the lumbar spine, pelvis, and hip in sitting as compared to standing. The psoas and iliacus muscles are often referred to as one, the *iliopsoas muscle*. Additionally, for individuals who sit in wheelchairs for extended periods of time, the iliopsoas may become shortened or contracted. This may result in a contracture of this muscle group, limiting one's ability to extend the LE.

The latissimus dorsi, although an arm mover, is also important in maintenance of trunk stability. It attaches on the axial spine from the sixth vertebrae of the thoracic spine, the dorsolumbar fascia, and crosses over the lateral aspect of the ribs and the inferior angle of the scapula. Additionally, it connects to the external oblique muscles. Its most proximal attachment is on the floor of the intertubercular groove on the anterior humerus. It traditionally acts to adduct and medially rotate the humerus on the scapula, but when the distal attachment, in this case the humerus, is fixed, such as with lifting the body using the arms while seated, the proximal segment moves instead, in this case the trunk, through an action known as reversal of muscle function. Also, if an individual is positioned in a posterior pelvic tilt, this may limit the functional excursion of the shoulder in flexion because the latissimus is already elongated at the trunk limiting full ROM of shoulder. The immobilization of the shoulder and trunk due to prolonged positioning that occurs when individuals are in a wheelchair full time may result in further limitation of shoulder movements not only due to tightness that develops in the latissimus dorsi, but tightness in the shoulder joint capsule and other muscles of the shoulder and shoulder girdle as well. Muscles of the pelvis that act on the trunk are identified in Table 5-7.

Maintaining an upright posture requires a careful balance of muscle activity around the pelvis, trunk, and abdomen. All of the muscles that support these structures work in unison to create upright trunk postures in both sitting and standing positions. When any one group of these muscles is weak, it will affect the other muscles. If the antagonist is stronger or tighter than the agonist, it will create a muscle imbalance. Such an imbalance influences the orthopedic alignment of the individual. The abnormal postural alignments previously discussed included examples such as an

TABLE 5-7

Muscles of the Pelvis That Act on the Trunk

MUSCLE	NERVE	TRUNK FLEXION	TRUNK STABILITY	PELVIC STABILITY	ANTERIOR PELVIC TILT	POSTERIOR PELVIC TILT	OTHER
Psoas major	Anterior rami, T12-L5	X	X	X			Maintains disk space
Hip flexors (rectus femoris)	Femoral nerve, L2-L4					X	
Iliacus	Femoral nerve and branches of lumbar plexus					Lifts trunk from supine	Lifts trunk from supine
Latissimus dorsi	Thoracodorsal nerve	Lateral			X		
Gluteus minimus, medius	Superior gluteal, L4, L5, and S1			X		X	

Adapted from Lippert, L. S. (2023). *Clinical kinesiology and anatomy* (7th ed.). F.A. Davis Company and Stone, R. J., & Stone, J. A. (2003). *Atlas of skeletal muscles* (4th ed.). McGraw-Hill.

TABLE 5-8

Muscles That Contribute to Pelvic Position

MUSCLE	ORIGIN	INSERTION
Neutral Pelvic Rotation		
Hip extensors (gluteus maximus)	Ilium and sacrum	Gluteal tuberosity and iliotibial band
Oblique abdominals	Lower eight ribs	ASIS, pubic crest
Hip abductors	Gluteal surface of ilium	Greater trochanter of the femur
Hip adductors	Pubis	Medial and posterior surface of the femur
Posterior Pelvic Tilt		
Hip extensors	Ilium and sacrum	Gluteal tuberosity and iliotibial band
Hip abductors (gluteus medius and minimus)	Gluteal surface of ilium	Greater trochanter of the femur
Rectus abdominis	Pubis	Costal cartilage ribs of 5 to 7, xiphoid process of sternum
Iliotibial band with hip external rotation	Supracondylar tubercle of the femur	Tibia and patella
Anterior Pelvic Tilt		
Spinal extensors: Iliocostalis, longissimus, spinalis muscles	Sacrum and vertebrae	Runs parallel to the vertebral column
Iliopsoas	Transverse process of lumbar vertebrae	Lesser trochanter of the femur
Hip adductors	Pubis	Medial and posterior surface of the femur
Rectus femoris	ASIS	Patella and tibial tuberosity
Iliotibial band with hip internal rotation	Supracondylar tubercle of the femur	Tibia and patella

increased anterior-posterior pelvic tilt vs. a neutral pelvic tilt. Orthopedic malalignment problems may lead to muscle contracture or could place strain on joints that could eventually lead to pain and, possibly, deformity, especially if the malalignment is prolonged.

Sometimes a person's tendency to stay in a specific pelvic posture is due to concomitant factors, such as increased weight or girth around the abdomen, as during pregnancy. Approximately 50% to 80% of people who are pregnant report symptoms of low back pain (Sabino & Grauer, 2008). Additionally, posterior pelvic tilt may be associated with prolonged seated postures if the seat surface is not adequate. For instance, in children with CP, the increased muscle tone around the pelvis and LE may result in posterior pelvic tilt and an unstable trunk. Lacoste et al. (2009) found that a high percentage of children with CP demonstrated increased muscle tone around the pelvis with decreased tone (hypotonicity) of the trunk. These postures contribute to pelvic obliquity, posterior pelvic tilt, and pelvic rotation.

Muscle balance around the trunk, pelvis, and abdomen contribute to a stable BOS for trunk stability and UE control. Additionally, muscular balance decreases the chance of developing an orthopedic deformity. Table 5-8 illustrates the various muscles that contribute to pelvic postures.

Muscles of the cervical spine are presented next. Muscles causing neck flexion include the sternocleidomastoid muscle, the scalene muscles, and the prevertebral muscles. The sternocleidomastoid muscle is the largest neck flexor. It has two heads. One head originates on the clavicle and is referred to as the *clavicular head*. The other head originates on the sternum and is thus referred to as the *sternal head*. Both heads insert on the mastoid process of the temporal bone. When the sternocleidomastoid muscle contracts bilaterally, it flexes the neck. When it contracts unilaterally, it laterally flexes to the same side and rotates the head toward the opposite side. That is, when you contract your left sternocleidomastoid muscle, you would be looking over your right shoulder. Of interest is the attachment on the nuchal line; this allows this muscle to extend the head on the neck if the cervical spine is hyperextended while it contracts.

Deep and lateral to the sternocleidomastoid muscle are three scalene muscles. The anterior scalene muscle originates on the transverse process of C2-C6 and inserts on the first rib. The middle scalene muscle originates on the transverse process of C2-C7 and also inserts on the first rib. The posterior scalene muscle originates on C5-C7 and inserts on the second rib. The scalene muscles as a group assist the sternocleidomastoid to perform elevation of the ribs, work bilaterally to flex the neck, and work unilaterally to perform lateral bending of the neck.

There is also a group of small muscles that are located on the anterior aspect of the cervical vertebrae called the *prevertebral muscles*. These small muscles are capable of flexion of the head, but, most importantly, they tuck the chin and help the body maintain postural control by making slight head motions. Individually, these muscles include the rectus capitis lateralis, rectus capitis anterior, longus capitis, and longus colli. Table 5-9 outlines the various muscles of the neck.

Summary

This chapter described how important pelvic positioning is to posture and function. A stable base, or pelvis, is essential for good posture as well as safe and functional movement. Proper pelvic positioning also allows for greater ROM and use of the UEs. Having good posture enables better balance and decreases the risk of falls. Common problems associated with the pelvis and spine were discussed, including pelvic tilts and scoliosis. In addition to causing pain, these deformities can impede independence. Finally, body structures of the trunk and neck were presented related to the roles they play in posture, balance, and movement.

References

Aissaoui, R., Boucher, C., Bourbonnais, D., Lacoste, M., & Dansereau, J. (2001). Effect of seat cushion on dynamic stability in sitting during a reaching task in wheelchair users with paraplegia. *Archives of Physical Medicine & Rehabilitation, 82,* 274-281.

Allum, J. H. J., Bloem, B. R., Carpenter, M. G., Hullinger, M., & Hadders-Algra, M. (1998). Proprioceptive control of posture: A review of new concepts. *Gait and Posture, 8,* 214-242.

Andersson, E. A., Oddsson, L. I. E., Grundstrom, H., Nilsson, J., & Thorstensson, A. (1996). EMG activities of the quadrates lumborum and erector spinae muscles during flexion-relaxation and other motor tasks. *Clinical Biomechanics, 11*(7), 392-400.

Arab, A. M, Abdollahi, I Joghataei, M. T, Golafshani, Z., & Kazemnaejad, A. (2009). Inter- and intra-examiner reliability of single and composites of selected motion palpation and pain provocation tests for the sacroiliac joint. *Musculoskeletal Science and Practice, 14*(2), 213-221.

Bolin, I., Bodin, P., & Kreuter, M. (2000). Sitting position: Posture and performance in C5-C6 tetraplegia. *Spinal Cord, 28,* 425-434.

Brubaker, C. E. (1986). Wheelchair prescription: An analysis of factors that affect mobility and performance. *Journal of Rehabilitation Research and Development, 23*(4), 19-26.

Cron, L., & Sprigle, S. (1993). Clinical evaluation of the hemi wheelchair cushion. *American Journal of Occupational Therapy, 47*(2), 141-144.

Davis, K. (2007, June). Seating and wheeled mobility evaluation. *National Public Website on Assistive Technology.* http://atwiki.assistivetech.net/index.php/Seating_and_wheeled_mobility_evaluation

Dean, C., Shepherd, R., & Adams, R. (1999). Sitting balance I: Trunk-arm coordination and the contribution of the lower limbs during self-paced reaching in sitting. *Gait and Posture, 10,* 135-146.

Edsberg, L. E., Black, J. M., Goldberg, M., McNichol, L., Moore, L., & Sieggreen, M. (2016). Revised National Pressure Ulcer Advisory Panel pressure injury staging system. *Journal of Wound, Ostomy, and Continence Nursing, 43*(6), 585-597. https://doi.org/10.1097/WON.0000000000000281

Foster, M. A. (2013). *Therapeutic kinesiology: Musculoskeletal systems, palpation, and body mechanics.* Prentice Hall.

Guerraz, M., Blouin, J., & Vercher, J. L. (2003). From head orientation to hand control: Evidence of both neck and vestibular involvement in hand drawing. *Experimental Brain Research, 150,* 40-49.

Hagert, E., Persson, J., Werner, M., & Ljung, B. O. (2009). Evidence of wrist proprioceptive reflexes elicited after stimulation of the scapholunate interosseous ligament. *American Society for Surgery of the Hand, 34A,* 642-651.

Harrop, J., Birknes, J., & Shaffrey, C. (2008). Noninvasive measurement and screening techniques for spinal deformities. *Neurosurgery, 63*(3), a46-a53.

Herman, J. H., & Lange, M. L. (1999). Seating and positioning to manage spasticity after brain injury. *NeuroRehabilitation, 12,* 105-117.

Horne, J. P., Flannery, R., & Saif, U. (2014) Adolescent idiopathic scoliosis diagnosis and management. *American Family Physician, 89,* 193-198.

Kyvelidou, A., Stuberg, W., Harbourne, R., Deffeyes, J., Blanke, D., & Stergiou, N. (2009). Development of upper body coordination during sitting in typically developing infants. *Pediatric Research, 65,* 553-558.

Lacoste, M., Therrien, M., & Prince, F. (2009). Stability of children with cerebral palsy in their wheelchair seating: Perceptions of parents and therapists. *Disability and Rehabilitation: Assistive Technology, 4,* 143-150.

Lauren, J., Awai, L., Bockisch, C. J., Hegemann, S., van Hedel, H. J. A., Dietz, V., & Straumann, D. (2010). Visual contribution to postural stability: Interaction between target fixation or tracking and static or dynamic large-field stimulus. *Gait and Posture, 31,* 37-41.

Lippert, L. S. (2023) *Clinical kinesiology and anatomy* (7th ed.). F. A. Davis Company.

Pederson, J. P. (2000). Functional impact of seating modifications for older adults: An occupational therapist perspective. *Wound Care and Seating, 16*(2), 73-85.

Robinson, H. S., Brox, J. I, Robinson, R., Bjelland, E., Solem, S. & Telje, T. (2007). The reliability of selected motion and pain provocation tests for the sacroiliac joint. *Manual Therapy, 12* (1), 72-79.

Sabino, J., & Grauer, J. (2008). Pregnancy and low back pain. *Current Review of Musculoskeletal Medicine, 1,* 137-141.

Sveistrup, H., Schneiberg, S., McKinley, P. A., McFadyen, B. J., & Levin, M. F. (2007). Head, arm and trunk coordination during reaching in children. *Experimental Brain Research, 188,* 237-247.

Taylor, S. J. (1987). Evaluating the client with physical disabilities for wheelchair seating. *American Journal of Occupational Therapy, 41*(11), 711-716.

Westcott, S., & Burtner, P. (2004). Postural control in children: Implications for pediatric practice. *Occupational and Physical Therapy in Pediatrics, 24*(1/2), 5-55.

Zacharkow, D. (1988). *Posture: Sitting, standing, chair design and exercise.* Charles Thomas Publisher.

TABLE 5-9

Muscles of the Neck

MUSCLE	NERVE	EXTENSION	FLEXION	LATERAL FLEXION	TILTS NECK	ROTATION	ROTATION SAME SIDE	RESPIRATION	ELEVATES RIBS
Sternocleidomastoid muscle	Cranial nerve XI, (accessory nerve), 2nd and 3rd cervical nerves		X	X		X			
Scalene muscles	Lower cervical nerves				X	X			X
Prevertebral muscles	Ventral primary rami of the cervical nerves		X						

Adapted from Lippert, L. S. (2023). *Clinical kinesiology and anatomy* (7th ed.). F.A. Davis Company and Stone, R. J., & Stone, J. A. (2003). *Atlas of skeletal muscles* (4th ed.). McGraw-Hill.

Applications

The following activities will help you apply knowledge of movements and postures of the trunk and pelvis in real-life applications. Activities can be completed individually or in a small group to enhance learning.

1. **Standing Posture**: Understanding the body structures and functions is foundational to understanding how body structures and body functions influence occupational performance. It is helpful to relate these anatomical and kinesiological principles to postures in regard to the pelvis, trunk, and head. Let's first examine a standing posture. Maintaining an upright body position over a very small BOS, like the feet, requires an intricate balance anterior to posterior and left to right. In other words, one must balance the weight of the body over the small space that the feet occupy.

   To illustrate, work with a partner. Place a plumb line with a weight on the bottom of it from the ceiling and allow it to dangle almost to the floor. Begin by standing next to the string so it is close to your shoulder and elbow beside you, rather than in front of you. Try to align your body with the plumb line, but do not touch the plumb line. It may be necessary to have cuing from your partner. Ask your partner how to position certain aspects or joints of your body to be in line with the plumb line. When you feel that you are balanced, note the location of your body in relationship to the string. Your upright and erect posture should demonstrate that the plumb line follows these points on the body when viewed laterally:
   - The mastoid process or slightly in front of your earlobe
   - A point slightly in front of the GH joint
   - A point just behind the center of the hip joints (through the greater trochanter)
   - A point just behind your patella (slightly anterior to knee joint)
   - A point slightly anterior to your lateral malleolus
   a. Can you align your body to the string as described? Why or why not?
   b. Is it possible to move your body to align to the string? Explain what you have to do.

2. **Influence of Vision on Static Standing Posture**: It is also important to note that we rely on our vision to maintain postural stability. Lauren et al. (2010) found that a stationary environment stabilizes posture and limits the amount of postural sway associated with standing postures. This may be helpful in designing treatment interventions for clients who have difficulty maintaining upright postures. That is, having a fixed-in-space stationary visual object to look at during static standing may help the client to maintain an erect posture. More will be discussed in Chapter 6.

   Try standing upright on both feet while scanning the room. You will most likely not lose your balance. Now, try scanning the room while only one foot is on the ground. Fixating on a nonmoving object should help you to maintain your balance. Try this same activity on a balance board to help accentuate this point.
   a. Was it easier to maintain your balance while fixating on an object or scanning the room?
   b. Do you think your BOS or COG has any influence? Why or why not?

3. **Sitting Posture**: In a standing posture, the BOS is small. Sitting is a more stable position because the BOS is larger than that of standing. In a sitting posture, the BOS extends from the feet to the most posterior aspect of the seated surface of the buttocks. In the case where there is a back support, an increase in stability may be noted. In fact, approximately 82% of the body weight is supported across the femurs and the remainder of the weight through the feet while sitting (Dean et al., 1999). However, if an individual is in a wheelchair and the femurs are not adequately supported, their sitting posture may be affected.

   Try this: While seated in a wheelchair, flex your knees and place them on the footplates. This positions the knees above the angle of the hips. Where do you feel the weight of your legs? You should feel more weight on the posterior aspect of the femurs. Thus, it places increased pressure on the ITs. Recall from the previous section that the ITs are bony prominences on the pelvis. Excessive pressure on the bony prominences and infrequent movement in a seated posture may contribute to increased risk of pressure injury development. Thus, when working with individuals who sit for long periods of time, it is essential to provide education on proper sitting posture and pressure redistribution.

a. Create a handout that describes proper sitting posture for a client. Include pictures or diagrams of proper positioning. Also include a section related to skin breakdown, decubiti, and distribution of pressure. Remember to write this using vocabulary your client will understand. If you are unfamiliar with this topic, a good resource is the National Pressure Injury Advisory Panel. Patient education materials may also be found on their website.

b. Modify a wheelchair for yourself or a student in the classroom. Try to achieve a neutral pelvic tilt, hips at about 90 degrees flexion, knees at about 90 degrees flexion, and ankles in a neutral position supported on the leg rests. Again, try to support the femurs on the wheelchair.

4. **Sitting Posture**: Sit in a firm chair with your feet directly under your knees and on the ground so that your knees are in 90 degrees of flexion. Flex your right shoulder 90 degrees, or so that your arm is at shoulder level outstretched to the front with your elbow fully extended. Have your partner hold the tip of a yardstick beginning at your fingertips. Now, reach out in front of you as far as you can while maintaining your trunk positioning and your hand at shoulder level. Have your partner write down how far you were able to reach.

Repeat this activity. This time, extend your legs by straightening your knee so that your feet are far out in front of you and your knees are not bent. Reach out in front of you with your trunk maintaining the same position as you did before. Have your partner record how far you were able to reach with your knees extended.

a. If these numbers varied, explain why you think this occurred?

b. Reach sideways and diagonally and complete the same measurements. Were they the same? Explain why or why not?

c. What are the implications of this to occupational performance, particularly for someone who uses wheelchair?

5. **Anatomical Considerations for Sitting**: Review the anatomical considerations for sitting. First, sit in a solid seat chair with your feet on the ground. Do not have your back resting against the seat back. Slump your back, and assume a posterior pelvic tilt posture. Think of reaching your belly button back toward your spine. Note how this posture creates an increased cervical lordosis and increased thoracic kyphosis. Also note how you must position your head in order to see in front of you. Now, raise your arms in front of you. Notice that the end range is about at your shoulder level. Holding this arm position, move your pelvis into anterior pelvic tilt. Note how your arms suddenly feel lighter and automatically move above your shoulders. You may also note that your humerus bone moves into an externally rotated position. Now place your pelvis in a neutral position and notice how your spine aligns from the pelvis upward. Think about ways you could support this posture with towel rolls, pillows, or a firmer seat in order to help you maintain this alignment in sitting.

a. How does your need to examine your world visually affect your posture in sitting and standing?

b. Can you explain how the position of the pelvis affects the alignment of the trunk and head?

6. **Body Structures of Trunk Muscles**: Work with a partner to review the origin and insertion of a few key trunk muscles. Think specifically about the latissimus dorsi, rhomboids, and trapezius muscles. When muscles are overly stretched, they cannot exert adequate strength to overcome the effects of gravity.

a. In an upright unsupported trunk posture, are the trapezius and rhomboids active?

b. What role do these muscles play in sitting?

7. **Body Structures of Cervical Trunk Muscles**: While lying supine, without lifting your shoulder, lean your head to your left shoulder.

a. What joint motion is occurring in the cervical spine?

b. What is the normal ROM for this aspect of the spine?

c. What is the name of this movement?

d. What muscles are the prime movers for this motion?

8. **Body Structures of Abdominal Muscles**: Lie supine on a mat with your knees bent and your feet firmly placed on the mat. Clasp your hands together and place them under your head. Move your right shoulder toward your left knee, as if attempting to do a sit-up.

a. What trunk motions are occurring?

b. What muscles cause these trunk motions to occur?

9. **Body Structures of Posterior Cervical and Trunk Muscles**: Lying prone on a mat with your arms extended at your sides and your face on the mat, raise your trunk off the mat. Be sure to keep your head in neutral alignment, and do not rotate or laterally flex to either side. As you raise yourself off the mat, determine how far you can move.

   a. What aspects of the spine are moving (cervical, thoracic, or lumbar)? It may vary depending on how far you can raise yourself up off the mat.

   b. What muscle groups are involved in this activity?

   c. What structures prevent you from moving further off the mat?

10. **OTPF-4: Occupation and Activity Demands**: Occupation and activity demands include all aspects of the actual activity, which also include relevance and importance, the objects being used and their properties, space and social demands, and sequencing. Underlying required actions, performance skills, body functions, and body structures are also considered. The purpose of this activity is to be more mindful of the life demands that impact what appears to be a simple activity. This activity should raise your awareness of what is really involved in completing an activity. It is important to realize that you have control over many of these demands and can modify or change them to enhance your overall success in performing the activity. Identify an activity and area of occupation that is relevant in your life. Table 5-10 can help to identify activity demands. Place this item in the left-hand column of Table 5-10. Next, list the associated activity demands. An example has been done for you.

   a. Are there activity demands that interfere with your completion of an activity? Identify these with a negative sign (–). Identify activity demands that might promote your activity with a positive sign (+).

   b. Is there an example in class where one student identified a negative activity demand and another student identified that same activity demand as positive? Discuss why this might have occurred.

   c. What activity demands do you feel are out of your ability to control? How can you change any of the activity demands with a negative sign to enable your engagement in the activity?

TABLE 5-10

Occupational Therapy Practice Framework: Domain and Process, Fourth Edition—Occupation and Activity Demands

ACTIVITY AND AREAS OF OCCUPATION	RELEVANCE AND IMPORTANCE	OBJECTS USED AND THEIR PROPERTIES	SPACE DEMANDS	SOCIAL DEMANDS	SEQUENCING AND TIMING DEMANDS	REQUIRED ACTIONS AND PERFORMANCE SKILLS	REQUIRED BODY FUNCTIONS	REQUIRED BODY STRUCTURES
Reaching items in the refrigerator; area of occupation is instrumental self-care	Nutrition, fulfilling role, leisure activity	Refrigerator, wheelchair	18 inches to the side of the refrigerator to allow door to open	Food preferences for all, including food traditions	Move self to side of door, open door, retrieve item, close door, carry item to a table	Trunk extension with shoulder movement to reach item in refrigerator, ability to weight shift and maintain trunk extension	Cognitive, motor, sensory	Nerves, muscles, skeletal alignment
Your example here								
Your example here								
Your example here								

CHAPTER 6

Function and Movement of the Lower Extremity

Maribeth P. Vowell, PT, MPH, EdD and Carolyn L. Roller, OTR/L

Key Terms

ambulation

circumduction

double support

equilibrium

foot drop

gait

gait cycle

gait patterns

hypertonic

pronation

single support

spasticity

supination

Chapter Outline

Introduction

Occupational Profile

Body Functions of the Lower Extremity

    Role of Occupational Therapy and the Lower Extremity

    Motions of the Lower Extremity

    Occupation-Based Mobility: The Visual Observation of Gait

    Common Problems of the Lower Extremity

Body Structures of the Lower Extremity

    Body Structures of the Hip

    Body Structures of the Knee

    Body Structures of the Ankle and Foot

Summary

References

Applications

Sain, S. J., & Roller, C. L. *Kinesiology for the Occupational Therapy Assistant: Essential Components of Function and Movement, Third Edition* (pp. 123-147).
© 2024 Taylor & Francis Group.

Chapter Objectives

After completion of this chapter, students should be able to:

1. Define key terminology.
2. Explain common functional relationships between the lower extremity, trunk, and upper extremity.
3. Analyze the provided client information to identify specific client problems and impairments of the lower extremities.
4. Predict how specific impairments of the lower extremities can affect functional movements, such as transfers, gait, and activities of daily living involving the upper extremities.
5. Identify potential corrections of impairments as a mechanism for improving a patient's functional movements.

Introduction

This chapter describes the movement and function of the lower extremities (LEs), specifically how it relates to the trunk and upper extremity (UE) function. The primary purpose of the LEs is to enable an individual to have an upright posture in standing, which increases a person's ability to engage in the environment. The LEs also participate in maintaining sitting and standing balance and **equilibrium** and support the weight of the body. The LEs enable movement through **gait**, or the way a person ambulates or walks. This chapter will also explore, with examples, the role of occupational therapy and the LEs. Movements of the LEs include motions of the pelvic girdle, hip, knee, ankle, and foot. The occupational therapist and the occupational therapy assistant need to be able to observe **gait patterns** as they relate to occupations of daily life activities. This observation of gait analysis can be used to prevent injury, ensure safety, reinforce carryover of physical therapy treatment, and facilitate progress toward occupational therapy goals. Two LE problems seen in occupational therapy are **foot drop** and cerebrovascular accident (CVA). Foot drop is a common neurological condition where a person cannot pick up the foot or dorsiflex the ankle. The damage can either be to the central nervous system (CNS) or peripheral nervous system. This disorder causes an unsafe and nonfunctional gait. Often, an ankle-foot orthosis (AFO) is used to maintain ankle position. The occupational therapy assistant can incorporate the donning and doffing of the AFO in LE dressing and functional mobility. A CVA, or stroke, is commonly seen in both occupational therapy and physical therapy. Sometimes the two disciplines will work together on functional mobility issues involved in gait and ADL skills. Lastly, the reader will learn all the structures of the LEs and their influence on occupational performance.

Occupational Profile

The following occupational profile is provided to demonstrate how body functions and body structures are related to function and movement of the LE. Through the client, Betty, this occupational profile will show how occupational therapy incorporates knowledge of function and movement in the LE. References to Betty will be made throughout this chapter.

Betty is a 68-year-old widow and retired Certified Nursing Assistant (CNA) who is receiving skilled occupational therapy at a long-term care facility. Betty was diagnosed with a right CVA with left hemiparesis 1.5 months ago.

During the occupational therapy evaluation, the following data were gathered.

Subjective: Betty reports living in a two-bedroom, one-level home with five steps to enter. She has lived alone during the past year following her husband passing away. Betty has no children but has a good support system of neighbors and friends from church. Betty belongs to a ladies' golf league and enjoys bridge and watching talk shows. Betty states that she was driving and was able to complete all activities of daily living (ADLs) and instrumental activities of daily living (IADLs) independently with no adaptive equipment prior to onset. Betty enjoys going to church when she can and volunteering 2 or 3 days per week at the long-term care facility where she previously worked. Betty expressed that her goals are to eventually drive again, increase the functional ability of her left dominant UE, return home within the next couple of months, and return to independent living. Betty states that she is thankful that the doctor said she only had a mild stroke.

Objective: Upon admission to the inpatient rehabilitation facility, Betty demonstrated the following ADL abilities:
- Self-feeding: Independent
- Grooming: Independent
- UE bathing: Set-up assistance
- LE bathing: Moderate assistance

BOX 6-1

GENERAL CATEGORIES OF AN ACTIVITIES OF DAILY LIVING SCALE

Independence: Client completes 100% of task typically by self.

Modified independence: Client completes ADL task with adaptations.

Supervision: Client requires assistance of someone present to complete a task. This may include standby assistance or standing next to the person.

Minimum assistance: Client requires less than 20% assistance. Contact guard assistance may also be included in this category.

Moderate assistance: Client requires between 20% to 50% assistance for ADL tasks.

Maximum assistance: Client requires between 50% to 80% assistance for ADL tasks.

Dependent assistance: Client requires between 80% to 100% assistance for ADL tasks.

(Foti & Kanazawa, 2006)

- UE dressing: Supervision for static sitting balance and set-up assistance
- LE dressing: Moderate assistance
- Toileting: Dependent assistance
- Toilet transfer: Moderate assistance
- Tub transfer: Moderate assistance

Box 6-1 identifies the general categories of an ADL scale that identify a client's performance in self-care tasks.

UE Observations: Betty is left-hand dominant and displays left UE weakness. Betty cannot use her left UE alone to complete functional tasks due to weakness and impaired initiation of muscle activation for controlled movement. She can use her left UE as a secondary assist in functional activities. Betty displays slight, increased **spasticity** (variable increased tone that restricts normal movement) in her left UE during functional tasks, which further increases the difficulty of regaining use of the arm. She demonstrates left UE active range of motion (AROM) grossly within functional limits (WFL) except for having only 0 to 60 degrees of shoulder flexion. Manual muscle testing (MMT) strength of the left UE is grossly 3+/5, except for shoulder MMT strength, which is grossly 2/5. Left UE shoulder strength was identified by observation of functional movement because of the inability to separate when voluntary movement becomes involuntary due to spasticity. Betty has full AROM and passive range of motion (PROM) with her right UE and 4/5 MMT strength grossly.

LE Observations: Betty displays foot drop impairment with the affected left LE and no increased tone during left LE AROM movements. During standing and stand pivot transfers, Betty is observed hyperextending her left knee and displays difficulty transferring her weight onto the affected left LE in standing. Betty initially used a rolling walker for stand pivot functional transfers and gait as recorded in the physical therapy evaluation, and the physical therapist recommended an assistive mobility device for improved safety and balance. Betty was later advanced to a quad cane for functional mobility by physical therapy. Betty can also use grab bars for UE support with transferring to the commode. As per the physical therapy evaluation, Betty displays AROM left LE grossly WFL except for less than half of normal active left ankle dorsiflexion. She also displays MMT strength of the left LE to include trace left ankle, 3+/5 left knee, and 3+/5 left hip muscles grossly. AROM and MMT strength of the intact right LE are grossly WFL and 4+/5 MMT strength.

Sensory/Perception/Cognition: Betty reports no visual or sensory impairments. She demonstrates intact proprioception and sensation bilaterally. Betty is alert and oriented x4 (person/place/date/situation) and can follow three-step commands.

Occupational therapy goals were established by the occupational therapist in collaboration with Betty and the interdisciplinary team and are presented in the following sections.

Short-Term Goals:

1. Client will be educated in and demonstrate independence with a home exercise program for increased left UE functional ability within 1 week.

2. Client will demonstrate supervision with stand pivot transfers using adaptive equipment appropriately by 2 weeks.

3. Client will demonstrate supervision with standing balance to sweep floors by 2 weeks.

4. Client will demonstrate modified independence to supervision with all ADL tasks by 2 weeks.

Long-Term Goals:

1. Client will demonstrate modified independence with all functional stand pivot transfers by discharge.

2. Client will demonstrate modified independence with self-care tasks using bilateral UEs by discharge.

3. Client will demonstrate MMT and grip pinch strength WFL in the left UE by discharge.

4. Client will demonstrate modified independence with simple home management tasks by discharge.

The outcome of Betty's occupational therapy intervention along with treatment techniques and goals achieved can be found in Appendix C.

Body Functions of the Lower Extremity

The LE has many functional purposes. Primarily, the LE enables an upright posture in standing, which increases a person's ability to engage in the environment. The LE also significantly participates in maintaining sitting and standing balance and equilibrium and supports the weight of the body (Greene & Roberts, 2005). Whenever the body leans away from the center of gravity (COG), the LE adjusts to help maintain balance. Equilibrium is maintained through sensory receptors throughout the body, including the LE. The LE provides support for the weight of the body in standing and shock absorption as the foot meets the ground. It is also involved with pushing up off the ground during walking. The LE enables movement through gait or **ambulation** for mobility. Gait is defined as the way a person walks. There are multiple types of gait patterns, both functional and impaired (O'Sullivan et al., 2014). Ambulation is defined as the process of moving from place to place by walking. For this text, gait and ambulation will be used interchangeably. *Functional mobility in the home* is often referred to when a client can ambulate distances greater than 50 feet with or without assistive devices. An example might include the client being able to walk from one side of the home to the other. *Functional mobility in the community* is achieved when a client can ambulate distances greater than 150 feet with or without assistive devices. An example might include a client's ability to walk from a car in a parking lot to a grocery store entrance. A greater review of gait will be provided later in this chapter.

Role of Occupational Therapy and the Lower Extremity

Occupational therapy is not defined as or constrained to the treatment of the UE as may be inaccurately perceived. Typically, however, occupational therapy is not the primary treatment for LE injuries and impairments. Physical therapy is often prescribed for LE injuries and impairments due to the emphasis on gait and LE function. As occupational therapy treats the whole body, therapists cannot ignore the trunk and LE because they significantly influence function. Specifically, occupational therapy practitioners may collaborate with physical therapists to reinforce physical therapy intervention in standing balance and safety; functional mobility using appropriate adaptive equipment; functional transfer techniques; range of motion (ROM); and observation of clinical factors, precautions, and contraindications. It is important to recognize that these approaches should also support and target occupational therapy treatment plans and goals, ideally incorporating the client and interdisciplinary team.

Examples of occupational therapy incorporating the LE in treatment include, but are not limited to, the following:

- An occupational therapy assistant walking a client using a rolling walker to the commode during ADL retraining. The occupational therapy assistant ensures safe use of the walker and avoidance of knee hyperextension and ankle injury by proper foot placement. Betty could use a rolling walker to transfer to the commode during toileting self-care retraining. The occupational therapy assistant would ensure that Betty always keeps her rolling walker to her front, her body remains within the frame of the walker, all four legs of the walker are kept in contact with the ground, and that she makes small turns with the walker.

- An occupational therapy assistant collaborating with physical therapy and reinforcing functional safe transfer techniques by the client. The occupational therapy assistant may aid in the progression of transfer training, such as knowing when to move from a sliding board transfer to a lateral pivot transfer, or even a stand pivot transfer. Additionally, the occupational therapy assistant may need to educate the client on proper transfer techniques, as well as ensure that proper transitional movements are being used. Refer to Box 6-2 for a definition of transitional movements. For Betty in the occupational profile, the occupational therapy assistant can collaborate with physical therapy for when to advance Betty from the rolling walker to a quad cane or standard cane. Additionally, the proper sequence of sit-to-stand can be reinforced by ensuring that Betty pushes up from the arm rests on the wheelchair vs. pulling herself up by the handholds on the walker.

- An occupational therapy assistant adapting and grading static or dynamic standing and sitting balance while looking at the base of support (BOS); muscle activation; and sequence of LE movement, trunk posture, and weight shifting as they influence UE functional reaching. Refer to Box 6-2 for a definition of static and dynamic balance. In the case of Betty, the occupational therapy assistant can monitor sitting balance at the edge of the bed when reaching during upper or lower body dressing. Another example may include standing to complete IADL tasks.

- An occupational therapy assistant treatment session where the patient is reaching into a kitchen cabinet for a plate using appropriate adaptive equipment and safety while static and dynamic standing balance are monitored. An example would include Betty using a quad cane to help maintain her balance while reaching into a cabinet or standing at the kitchen counter. Figure 6-1 illustrates Betty reaching into a kitchen cabinet.

- Aiding a patient diagnosed with spinal cord injury to perform circle sitting for the self-care task of dressing. In the example of Betty, she most likely would not need to learn to circle sit due to her intact trunk and LE function. Adaptive approaches, PROM, and impaired balance response may be appropriate for a client with a spinal cord injury who could benefit from circle sitting to increase independence.

BOX 6-2

Dynamic balance: Balance with movement occurring or to move or function within a position; can describe movement in sitting or standing. Opposite of static balance. The ability to maintain a controlled position of the head and body during movement in relation to gravity.

Static balance: Balance where no movement is occurring; can describe a position in sitting or standing. The ability to maintain a steady position of the head and body in relation to gravity.

Transitional movements: Change of posture or movement from one position to another.

(Kisner & Colby, 2023)

Occupational therapy is not limited to these examples. A common factor in all these examples include the use of therapeutic activities and engagement in occupations. It is important to note that a client is not standing for the sake of standing, a client is standing to participate in an occupational role. Standing can be used in occupation-based interventions, purposeful activities, and preparatory methods in occupational therapy treatment. Transitional movements are also important to consider. Transitional movements occur between different positions or postures. Examples may include rolling from supine to prone, moving from sitting to standing, or moving from supine to sitting. Transitional movements are obviously very important during functional transfers. Quite often, the occupational therapy assistant is not selecting or initiating LE adaptive equipment, and certainly the occupational therapy assistant is not duplicating treatment performed by physical therapy. No one, though, should inaccurately describe occupational therapy as just treating the UE.

Occupational therapy assistants should also be familiar with adaptive equipment used to increase the safety and efficiency of gait or standing as well as adaptive equipment used to correct and prevent deformity or impairment. Equipment used to increase the safety or efficiency of gait or standing may include, but is not limited to, crutches, canes, quad canes, hemi-walkers, standard walkers, and rolling walkers. Usually, physical therapy practitioners determine which equipment is most advantageous for the client. A standard wheelchair or powered mobility device may also be used to enable functional mobility. Depending on the facility, training, and role expectations within the facility, occupational therapy or physical therapy practitioners may assume the primary responsibility for determining wheelchair and seating client needs. This responsibility may also be a shared expectation between occupational therapy and physical therapy practitioners. Some information is provided in Chapter 5; however, due to the complexity involved with wheelchair seating and positioning, in-depth discussion is outside the scope of this book and will be covered in other treatment courses.

Equipment used to correct or prevent deformity or impairments may include AFOs, casts, air splints, and various types and sizes of ankle and knee braces. Again, physical therapy practitioners often assess and issue this equipment.

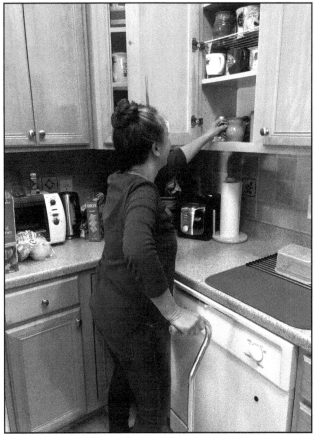

Figure 6-1. Betty with a quad cane reaching into the cabinets.

Service competency should be achieved as the occupational therapy assistant learns to appropriately don and doff splints and orthotic devices with clients. The occupational therapy assistant may need to instruct a client or educate caregivers on how to don and doff a splint or orthotic device as part of LE dressing. As in the occupational profile with Betty, a physical therapy practitioner may decide that an AFO or ankle air cast is appropriate due to the decreased ability to produce ankle dorsiflexion. In certain cases, physical therapy may recommend knee braces to prevent hyperextension or uncontrolled knee flexion. Part of lower body dressing may include independently donning or doffing these devices to enable a return to safe independent living at home.

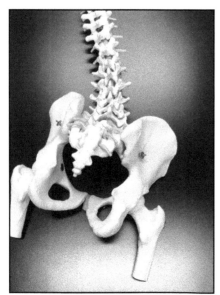

Figure 6-2. Movement of the pelvis: left lateral tilt.

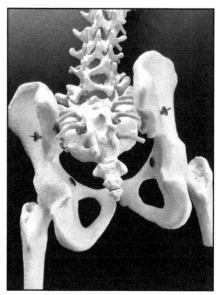

Figure 6-3. Movement of the pelvis: right lateral tilt.

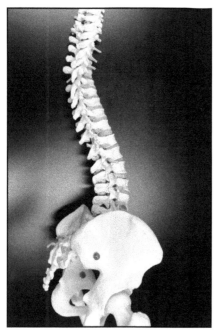

Figure 6-4. Movement of the pelvis: anterior pelvic tilt.

Motions of the Lower Extremity

The motions of the LE include motions of the pelvic girdle, hip, knee, ankle, and foot. Typically, movements of the LE are generally described by these joint motions; however, variations at each joint increase the complexity and specificity for describing the specific movement at each joint. It is important for the occupational therapy assistant to be able to identify the most common joint movements of the LE

and how each joint influences function. The pelvic girdle is a good place to start because it is the most proximal body structure and connects the appendicular skeleton to the axial skeleton.

The pelvic girdle may appear to be part of the trunk due to its location proximal to the hip joint; however, the pelvic girdle is considered part of the appendicular skeleton. As presented in Chapter 5, the pelvic girdle is important because it influences posture and sitting balance and establishes stability for reaching with the UE. The pelvic girdle is also important to the LE because it influences posture and curvature of the spine in standing, provides stabilization needed for standing balance, and enables mobility to allow for movement of the LE as in gait. Movements of the pelvic girdle often occur in combination with movements in the LE to achieve functional goals. For example, all movements of the pelvic girdle occur during walking. The movements of the pelvic girdle include left lateral tilt (Figure 6-2), right lateral tilt (Figure 6-3), anterior pelvic tilt (Figure 6-4), posterior pelvic tilt (Figure 6-5), and forward/backward rotation in the transverse plane (Figure 6-6).

The reference points for pelvic girdle motions are the anterior superior iliac spine (ASIS) landmarks, which are located on each pelvic bone.

The hip joint has three degrees of freedom and thus can move in three planes of movement, which is typical for a triaxial joint. Structurally, the hip joint provides for greater stability as compared to the glenohumeral joint, but with this greater stability comes lesser mobility. The motions of the hip joint include flexion (Figure 6-7), extension (Figure 6-8), abduction (Figure 6-9), adduction (Figure 6-10), internal rotation (Figure 6-11), and external rotation (Figure 6-12).

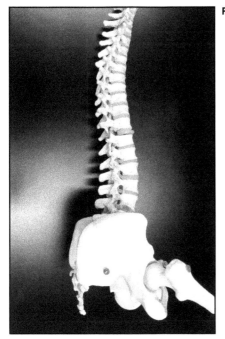

Figure 6-5. Movement of the pelvis: posterior pelvic tilt.

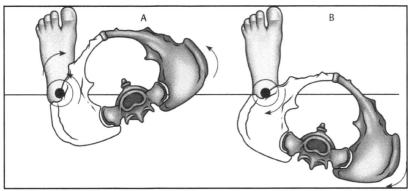

Figure 6-6. Rotation movements of the pelvis. (A) Right forward rotation. (B) Left forward rotation.

The knee and ankle are the next joints following the appendicular skeleton. The primary motion of the knee joint is flexion and extension. The knee is a combination of three articulations that enable movement. Due to the three articulations of the knee, a rotary movement also occurs to a lesser degree. The occupational therapy assistant is primarily concerned with the main joint motions of knee flexion (Figure 6-13) and extension (Figure 6-14).

The ankle joint also includes multiple articulations. The motions of the ankle can be referred to by different terms depending on the source. For this text, the primary motions of the ankle will be referred to as *plantarflexion* (Figure 6-15), *dorsiflexion* (Figure 6-16), *eversion* (Figure 6-17), and *inversion* (Figure 6-18). Greene and Roberts (2005) identify inversion and eversion as important because these movements are used when the body shifts weight. They also provide better balance when on uneven ground. Plantarflexion and dorsiflexion are important movements as they allow the

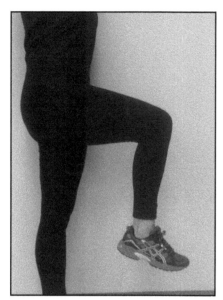

Figure 6-7. Movement of the hip joint: flexion.

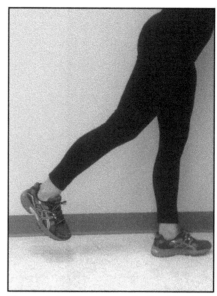

Figure 6-8. Movement of the hip joint: extension.

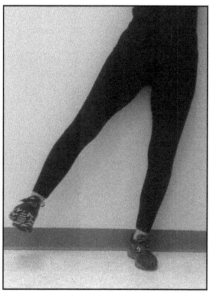

Figure 6-9. Movement of the hip joint: abduction.

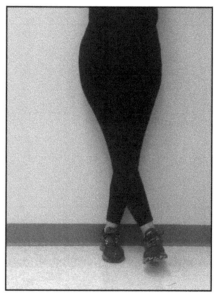

Figure 6-10. Movement of the hip joint: adduction.

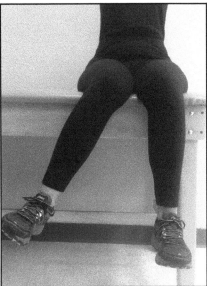

Figure 6-11. Movement of the hip joint: internal rotation.

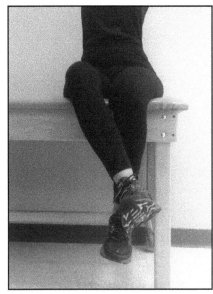

Figure 6-12. Movement of the hip joint: external rotation.

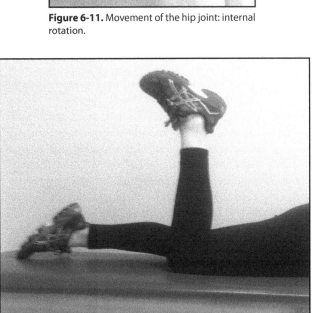

Figure 6-13. Movement of the knee joint: flexion.

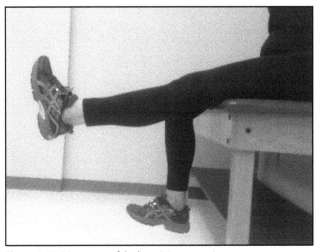

Figure 6-14. Movement of the knee joint: extension.

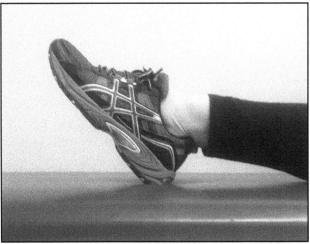

Figure 6-15. Movement of the ankle joint: plantarflexion.

foot to clear the ground during walking and enable proper foot placement when the foot comes back in touch with the ground.

In addition to the motions already mentioned for the LE, there are joints and motions that occur distal to the ankle joint. ROM and strength of the toes influence standing balance and push off during gait when the foot lifts off the ground. The occupational therapy assistant primarily will need to be aware of the motions at the pelvic girdle, hip, knee, and ankle as they are involved in functional tasks during sitting or standing. Table 6-1 identifies the joint, motion, landmark for joint measurement, and available ROM for each joint of the LE. Complicating the analysis of the LE is that most or all joints will be simultaneously involved in

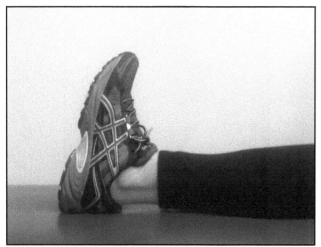

Figure 6-16. Movement of the ankle joint: dorsiflexion.

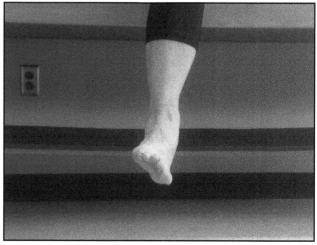

Figure 6-17. Movement of the ankle joint: eversion.

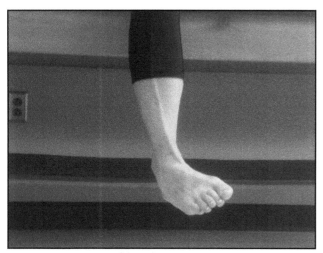

Figure 6-18. Movement of the ankle joint: inversion.

a functional activity and require observation of their movement. Consultation with physical therapy should be performed if more specific analysis of movement is needed or if variations to typical joint movement exist.

Occupation-Based Mobility: The Visual Observation of Gait

The *Occupational Therapy Practice Framework: Domain and Process, Fourth Edition* (OTPF-4), as displayed in Box 6-3, identifies gait patterns (also called *walking patterns*), as a body function commonly considered by occupational therapy practitioners (American Occupational Therapy Association [AOTA], 2020). Traditionally, physical therapy can analyze and detail the strengths and weaknesses associated with LE function and ambulation. While physical therapy may provide an in-depth evaluation of gait, occupational therapy assistants need to be able to provide observational gait analysis during treatment and occupational roles. Observational gait analysis can reflect distance traveled and the absence or presence of common characteristics of gait. This observational analysis can be used to ensure safety, prevent injury, reinforce carryover of physical therapy treatment, and facilitate progress toward occupational therapy goals. The occupational therapy assistant should also be able to communicate what they see with physical therapy practitioners. Knowledge of gait and walking patterns as well as common terminology are needed to enable this communication with physical therapy and the rehabilitation team.

While every person may have slightly different gait patterns, gait patterns have been broken down into common components within what is called the **gait cycle** (Figure 6-19). The gait cycle describes the events that occur between the initial contact with the heel of one LE to the initial contact of the same LE on the ground. The gait cycle must be able to accommodate changes in the level of the ground, dodging obstacles, and various speeds and distances. The gait cycle may also be referred to as *stride*. The distance traveled for one stride is called the *stride length*. Each stride length has two step lengths, meaning one stride contains a step with the right LE and a step with the left LE. Figure 6-19A illustrates a client at the start of the gait cycle taking a step with her right LE. Figure 6-19C illustrates the client halfway through

TABLE 6-1

Joints, Motions, Landmarks, and Normal Range of Motion of the Lower Extremity

JOINT AND MOTION	LANDMARK*	AVAILABLE ROM**
Hip flexion	Lateral aspect of greater trochanter	0 to 100 degrees
Hip extension		0 to 30 degrees*
Hip abduction	Over ASIS	0 to 25 degrees
Hip adduction		Adduction is the return to 0 degrees
Hip internal rotation	Over midpoint of the patella	0 to 20 degrees
Hip external rotation		0 to 30 degrees
Knee flexion	Over the lateral epicondyle of the femur	0 to 110 degrees
Knee extension		Extension is the return to 0 degrees
Ankle plantarflexion	Lateral aspect of the lateral malleolus	0 to 50 degrees
Ankle dorsiflexion		0 to 10 degrees
Ankle eversion	Over the anterior aspect of the ankle midway between malleoli	0 to 10 degrees
Ankle inversion		0 to 20 degrees

*Data source: Latella, D., & Meriano, C. (2003). *Occupational therapy manual for evaluation of range of motion and muscle strength.* Delmar Cengage Learning.

**Data source: Rondinelli, R. D., Genoverse, E., Katz, R. T., Mayer, T. G., Mueller, K., & Ranavaya, M. (2008). *Guides to the evaluation of permanent impairment* (6th ed.). American Medical Association..

BOX 6-3

The OTPF-4 identifies **gait patterns** as neuromusculoskeletal and movement-related functions, as a body function commonly considered by occupational therapy practitioners as it relates to occupations of daily life activities.

(AOTA, 2020, p. 53)

---

the gait cycle as the left LE advances forward. Lastly, Figure 6-19H illustrates the client at the end of the gait cycle as the right foot again touches the ground.

The gait cycle can be broken down into two phases: the stance phase and the swing phase. Figure 6-19 illustrates the individual phases and the events that occur in those phases. Box 6-4 identifies the ROM needed in the LE for gait. The stance phase occurs when the LE is in contact with the ground and is about 60% of the gait cycle. Skinner et al. (1985) identify that the limb must demonstrate weight bearing, stability, progressional mobility, and shock absorption during the stance phase. The traditional terminology for describing the events of gait is provided in the following list in parentheses; however, the Rancho Los Amigos terminology is the most widely accepted. Using the Rancho Los Amigos terminology, the following terms describe the events of the stance and swing phases:

1. Initial contact (heel strike)
2. Loading response (foot flat)
3. Midstance
4. Terminal stance (heel off)
5. Preswing (toe off)

Initial contact identifies when the heel comes in contact with the ground. Loading response describes when the weight is shifted onto the stance leg. Midstance occurs when the body passes directly over the foot that is in contact with the ground. Terminal stance explains when the heel begins to lift off the ground, and preswing portrays when weight has shifted to the opposite leg and the toes push off the ground to propel the foot forward (Lippert, 2022).

The swing phase occurs when the foot leaves the ground, but before it comes in contact with the ground again, and accounts for 40% of the gait cycle. The traditional phases of the swing phase include the following:

1. Initial swing (acceleration)
2. Midswing
3. Terminal swing (deceleration)

Initial swing occurs when the foot lifts off the ground, is behind the body, and is moving forward. Midswing describes the phase when the toes pass over the ground and the

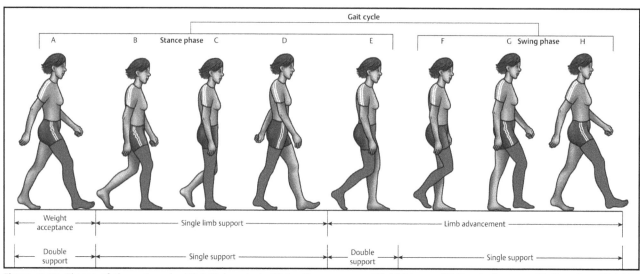

Figure 6-19. Phases of the gait cycle. (A) Initial contact. (B) Loading response. (C) Midstance. (D) Terminal stance. (E) Preswing. (F) Initial swing. (G) Midswing. (H) Terminal swing.

BOX 6-4

RANGE OF MOTION NEEDED DURING GAIT

Joint and Motion	Stance Phase	Swing Phase
Hip flexion	0 to 30 degrees	0 to 30 degrees
Hip extension	0 to 20 degrees	0 to 20 degrees
Knee flexion	0 to 40 degrees	0 to 60 degrees
Knee extension	0 degrees	0 degrees
Plantarflexion	0 to 20 degrees	0 to 10 degrees
Dorsiflexion	0 to 10 degrees	0 degrees
Subtalar joint inversion	0 to 35 degrees	0 degrees
Subtalar joint eversion	0 to 15 degrees	0 degrees

(Loudon et al., 2008)

foot moves ahead of the weight-bearing leg. Finally, terminal swing occurs when the toes point upward and the leg advances just prior to initial contact with the ground (Lippert, 2022).

There are additional aspects that can be highlighted to describe ambulation. First is the number of feet in contact with the ground. **Single support** describes the part of the gait cycle when only one leg is in contact with the ground. **Double support** describes when both legs are in contact with the ground. During ambulation, the gait cycle is in either single support or double support, unless the person is running, in which case there is a period of non-support. In addition to the number of legs in contact with the ground, the distance between both feet is called the *step width*. Typically, people

do not step directly in front of each foot. Lippert (2022) identifies that step width may range from 2 to 4 inches during ambulation; however, this distance may increase when there is balance impairment.

Functional ambulation can be identified by several different factors. As mentioned previously, distance traversed is quite often used to identify independence with ambulation. The use of adaptive equipment may also be important to identify functional ambulation. Adaptive equipment may increase the speed of walking as well as improve weight bearing on the targeted LE. The goal may be to maximize safe independence with mobility using the least amount of restrictive device. Overall quality of movement should be important to meet individual goals.

Another consideration for functional ambulation is the excursion of the COG during gait. *Excursion* refers to the wandering from usual course of the COG during gait. All three planes of pelvic movement are needed for typical excursion of the line of progression (Yavuzer & Süreyya, 2002). During ambulation, the COG displaces up to 2 inches vertically and 2 inches horizontally as the body and pelvis move (Lippert, 2022). This vertical and horizontal displacement is called the *line of progression* and should typically be constant with stable variables. Increasing the excursion of the line of progression will increase energy expenditure and decrease stability and efficiency of walking.

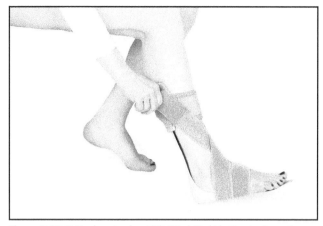

Figure 6-20. Betty donning her AFO. (Med_Ved/shutterstock.com)

Common Problems of the Lower Extremity

Foot Drop

Foot drop is a common disorder in neurological conditions where a person has an inability to or difficulty in creating ankle dorsiflexion. The foot, toes, and ankle have difficulty pointing up in the air, procuring the name foot drop. Reduced knee function, hip flexion, and ankle dorsiflexion all may complicate toe clearance during swing phase. While neurological damage, either of the CNS or peripheral nervous system, is most often associated with this disorder, muscle damage, anatomical deviations, diabetes mellitus, tumors, motor neuron disease, multiple sclerosis, and adverse reactions to drugs and alcohol can also lead to foot drop (Hayes, 2004; Pritchett & Porembski, 2010).

In foot drop, the common fibular nerve is often affected as it innervates the anterior tibialis muscle, which is the main muscle associated with picking up the foot, also called *dorsiflexion*. The common fibular nerve branches off the sciatic nerve, lumbosacral plexus, and the L5 nerve root proximally. Functionally, foot drop can significantly and negatively affect function. Foot drop does not allow for the normal dorsiflexion that should occur when the heel contacts the ground. As a result, the forefoot makes initial contact before the heel. Foot drop is most problematic during the swing phase of gait because clients may have trouble clearing the foot and toes from the ground as they advance the foot forward. If untreated, the client can incorporate nonfunctional gait patterns that limit functional mobility and recovery. Most importantly, the client can also be at risk for increased falls and further functional decline.

An example of a nonfunctional gait pattern used by clients with foot drop is a circumducted gait (also known as **circumduction**), when during the swing phase the pelvis hikes while the hip abducts on the unsupported side. The leg then advances in a circular motion out to the side, swinging forward toward midline where the foot strikes the ground.

This type of gait pattern can decrease safety, increase energy expenditure, and decrease movement options for the development of more functional gait patterns.

Treatment approaches will depend on the source of injury. Quite often, an AFO can be used to maintain the position of the ankle through compensation, which allows improved function. Remedial approaches by physical therapy may include the use of neuromuscular electrical stimulation (NMES) or exercises to strengthen the tibialis anterior. The occupational therapy practitioner does not typically provide the direct treatment for foot drop. Betty in the occupational profile presents with foot drop. In Betty's case, the physical therapy practitioner is using both electrical stimulation and exercises to strengthen and improve coordination of the affected LE. Physical therapy practitioners may use an AFO during gait training to prevent injury, increase safety, decrease risk for falls, and increase functional mobility. The occupational therapy assistant ensures that the AFO is donned correctly whenever the client is up out of bed and incorporates treatment of donning and doffing the AFO in lower body dressing training. By ensuring that the AFO is donned correctly, the occupational therapy assistant is also helping to prevent further injury and deformity, facilitating the recovery process. Figure 6-20 illustrates Betty as she dons her AFO.

Cerebrovascular Accident

A CVA, also called a *stroke*, is one of the most common medical/health conditions among clients being treated by occupational therapy. A CVA frequently involves a blockage in the supply of blood to the brain, resulting in wide array of impairments, activity limitations, and participation restrictions depending on the severity of the injury. While a CVA affects the brain, it is also a condition that affects the CNS. Although the whole body may be affected by a CVA, impairments and activity limitations of the LE will be the focus in this chapter.

Foot drop, as mentioned earlier, can be an impairment caused by a CVA. Specifically, Cruz and Dhaher (2008) identified that reduced knee flexion, hip flexion, and ankle dorsiflexion can affect toe clearance during the swing phase of walking. As a result, the client can compensate by hiking the hip or circumducting gait to allow the clearance needed to advance the foot forward. Lippert (2022) identifies circumducted gait as the leg swinging out to the side during the swing phase and returning toward the midline for the heel strike. Hemiplegic gait more readily describes the full movement synergy of a client who has been diagnosed with a CVA.

Hemiplegic gait typically describes the involved LE gait pattern of a client who has experienced a stroke. Lippert (2022) describes this synergy of movement or pattern as hip adduction, hip extension, hip medial rotation, knee extension, ankle plantarflexion, and ankle inversion. Yavuzer and Süreyya (2002) described characteristics of hemiplegic gait, including slow speed, short stance phase, poorly coordinated movements, and decreased weight bearing on the affected extremity.

Additional kinematic characteristics have been identified in the gait cycle. Moseley et al. (1993) identified common stance phase kinematic deviations to include the following:

- Decreased peak hip extension in late stance phase
- Decreased peak lateral pelvic displacement in stance phase
- Increased peak lateral pelvic displacement in stance phase
- Decreased knee flexion (or hyperextension) in stance phase
- Increased knee flexion in stance phase
- Decreased ankle plantarflexion at terminal swing

In addition, Moore et al. (1993) identified common swing phase kinematic deviations to include the following:

- Decreased peak hip flexion in swing phase
- Decreased peak knee flexion in early swing phase
- Decreased knee extension prior to initial contact
- Decreased dorsiflexion in swing phase

The UE and trunk also affect gait in a client who has experienced a stroke. The client may not be able to produce a reciprocal arm swing due to weakness in the involved UE. A client may not swing the uninvolved limb to maintain balance, which will affect a typical LE gait cycle. Due to compensatory movements and weakness, the trunk also may not be able to maintain the alignment of the shoulders with the pelvis, as well as eliminate all unnecessary or excessive movements to maintain the body over the BOS. Interestingly, holding onto an object or even slightly touching an object with a fingertip can decrease postural sway (Jeka, 1997). Postural sway is the natural anterior/posterior movement of the body in standing caused by movement at the ankles (Lippert, 2022). The trunk muscles may be **hypertonic**, restricting normal pelvic forward rotation during gait.

Hypertonicity is similar to spasticity and refers to increased tone in muscles that prevents normal movement. As can be seen, multiple factors in the trunk, LE, and UE combine to influence functional mobility.

Unfortunately, the characteristics of neurological gait patterns can increase energy expenditure and prevent functional progress. These movement patterns can also limit functional recovery and movement potential. Clients may dislike their new movement repertoire for walking because it differs from their prior ability, while others may be able to visually perceive this difference during walking. Ultimately, deviations from normal gait following a stroke can be caused by multiple factors important to both occupational and physical therapy practitioners.

Body Structures of the Lower Extremity

Body Structures of the Hip

The hip joint is a ball-and-socket joint. Unlike the shoulder joint, the hip joint sacrifices some ROM to attain more stability. The hip joint is a triaxial joint, which means that it has movement in three planes. Logically, location of muscle groups can identify its function. Muscles on the anterior side can be associated with hip flexion, while muscles on the posterior side are associated with extension. Muscles located on the lateral side of the hip can be associated with muscles that create hip abduction.

Table 6-2 presents the muscles, nerves, spinal root levels, and actions of muscles of the hip joint.

The ligaments of the hip increase stability and limit mobility. The ligaments of the hip include the following:

- **Iliofemoral ligament**: Anterior ligament that resists loss of balance posteriorly, limiting hyperextension.
- **Pubofemoral ligament**: Limits hyperextension and limits abduction.
- **Ischiofemoral ligament**: Limits hyperextension and medial rotation.
- **Ligamentum teres**: Helps to stabilize the head of the femur to the acetabulum and may provide some blood supply to the head of the femur.

Body Structures of the Knee

The knee, also called the *tibiofemoral joint*, is made up of the distal end of the femur, the patella, and the proximal end of the tibia. The knee is a synovial hinge joint, the largest joint in the body, and the joint most prone to injury. The fibula is not specifically included in consideration with the knee joint as it does not come in contact with the femur. The

Function and Movement of the Lower Extremity   137

TABLE 6-2

Muscles, Nerves, Spinal Root Level, and Actions of Muscles of the Hip Joint

MUSCLE	NERVE	L2	L3	L4	L5	S1	S2	S3	HIP FLEXION	HIP EXTENSION	HIP ABDUCTION	HIP ADDUCTION	HIP INTERNAL ROTATION	HIP EXTERNAL ROTATION
		SPINAL NERVE ROOT												
Tensor fasciae latae	Superior gluteal nerve			X	X	X			X		X			
Rectus femoris	Femoral nerve	X	X	X					X					
Biceps femoris: long head	Sciatic nerve				X	X	X	X		X				
short head						X	X							
Pectineus	Femoral nerve	X	X	X					X			X		
Gracilis	Obturator nerve		X	X								X		
Adductor longus	Obturator nerve		X	X					X			X		
Adductor brevis	Obturator nerve		X	X								X		
Adductor magnus	Obturator nerve		X	X								X		
Semitendinosus	Sciatic nerve				X	X	X			X				
Semimembranosus	Sciatic nerve				X	X	X			X				

Adapted from Lippert, L. S. (2022). *Clinical kinesiology and anatomy* (7th ed.). F. A. Davis Company; Stone, R. J., and Stone, J. A. (2003). *Atlas of skeletal muscles* (4th ed.). McGraw-Hill.

patella sits over the anterior surface of the knee in the quadriceps muscle tendon. This is called the *patellofemoral joint*. The patella provides a mechanical advantage for improved quadriceps function.

The knee muscles primarily produce knee extension or knee flexion. The knee also produces slight medial and lateral rotation. The knee flexors can be grouped together, called the *hamstring group*, and the knee extensors can be grouped together, called the *quadriceps group*. Quite often, treatment may focus more on strengthening the quadriceps group to decrease contracture formation and counter the powerful hamstring group. Table 6-3 identifies the muscles, nerves, spinal root levels, and actions for the muscles of the knee.

The ligaments of the knee increase stability, limit mobility, and protect the articular capsule. The ligaments of the knee include the following:

- **Medial collateral ligament**: Contributes to knee stability, specifically medial stability.
- **Lateral collateral ligament**: Contributes to knee stability, specifically lateral stability.
- **Anterior cruciate ligament**: Prevents anterior displacement of the tibia in relation to the femur. It is commonly injured in sports during twisting and bending of the knee.
- **Posterior cruciate ligament**: Prevents posterior displacement of the tibia in relation to the femur. The posterior cruciate ligament is not commonly injured.
- **Transverse ligament**: Attaches to the anterior horns of the medial and lateral menisci.
- **Patellar ligament**: Helps the patella to create its mechanical advantage.

Body Structures of the Ankle and Foot

The primary joint of the ankle is called the *talocrural joint*, or sometimes the *talotibial* or *true ankle joint*. This synovial hinge joint is responsible for the movements of plantarflexion and dorsiflexion. This joint is the articulation between the fibula and tibia proximally and with the talus distally. The subtalar joint, alternatively called the *talocalcaneal joint*, is the articulation between the talus proximally and the calcaneus distally. This joint is responsible for the motions of inversion and eversion. The transverse tarsal joint is distal to the subtalar joint, and, while there is no specific action motion associated with the transverse tarsal joint, during weight bearing this joint allows adduction and abduction of the forefoot, enabling the foot to adapt to uneven surfaces, and, therefore, it is important to the maintenance of standing and balance during gait.

Ankle muscles can be grouped by the motions they create. The ankle muscles primarily produce movements of plantarflexion, dorsiflexion, inversion, and eversion. **Supination** is a combined active motion of plantarflexion, inversion, and adduction, and **pronation** is a combined active motion of dorsiflexion, eversion, and abduction. Additional ways that the ankle muscles can be grouped include those muscles that act on the ankle alone and those muscles that act on the ankle and joints distal to the ankle. Just like the hand, there are intrinsic and extrinsic muscles of the foot that enable functional movement. For the purpose of this text, only muscles of the ankle will be illustrated. Table 6-4 presents the muscles, nerves, spinal root level, and actions of muscles of the ankle joint.

The ligaments of the ankle increase stability and limit mobility. The ligaments of the ankle include the following:

- **Deltoid ligament**: Supports the medial side of the ankle joint and helps to maintain the medial longitudinal arch of the foot.
- Three lateral ligaments: (1) **Anterior talofibular ligament**, (2) **posterior talofibular ligament**, (3) **calcaneofibular ligament**—Support the lateral side of the ankle joint.

Quite often, physical therapy will focus on strengthening the dorsiflexion muscles due to the easier tendency to plantarflex the ankle. Interestingly, the ankle is also more stable in dorsiflexion. The anterior talofibular ligament is the weakest of the three lateral ligaments and is most often associated with a sprained ankle. There are additional ligaments, bones, and joints of the foot distal to the ankle that will not be addressed in this text.

TABLE 6-3
Muscles, Nerves, Spinal Root Level, and Actions of the Knee

GROUP	MUSCLE	NERVE	SPINAL NERVE ROOT							KNEE FLEXION	KNEE EXTENSION
			L2	L3	L4	L5	S1	S2	S3		
Quadriceps group	Rectus femoris	Femoral nerve	X	X	X						X
	Vastus lateralis	Femoral nerve	X	X	X						X
	Vastus intermedialis	Femoral nerve	X	X	X						X
	Vastus medialis	Femoral nerve	X	X	X						X
	Popliteus	Tibial nerve			X	X	X			X	
Hamstring group	Semitendinosus	Sciatic nerve				X	X	X		X	
	Semimembranosus	Sciatic nerve				X	X	X		X	
	Biceps femoris: long head	Sciatic nerve				X	X	X	X	X	
	short head	Common peroneal nerve					X	X			
	Gastrocnemius	Tibial nerve					X	X		X	

Adapted from Lippert, L. S. (2022). *Clinical kinesiology and anatomy* (7th ed.). F. A. Davis Company and Stone, R. J., & Stone, J. A. (2003). *Atlas of skeletal muscles* (4th ed.). McGraw-Hill.

TABLE 6-4
Muscles, Nerves, Spinal Root Level, and Actions of Muscles of the Ankle

MUSCLE	NERVE	SPINAL NERVE ROOT				ANKLE PLANTARFLEXION	ANKLE DORSIFLEXION	ANKLE INVERSION	ANKLE EVERSION
		L4	L5	S1	S2				
Gastrocnemius	Tibial nerve			X	X	X			
Soleus	Tibial nerve			X	X	X			
Plantaris	Tibial nerve	X	X	X		X			
Tibialis anterior	Deep peroneal nerve	X	X	X			X	X	
Extensor hallucis longus	Deep peroneal nerve	X	X	X			X	X	
Extensor digitorum longus	Deep peroneal nerve	X	X	X			X		X
Peroneus longus	Superficial peroneal nerve	X	X	X		X			X

(continued)

TABLE 6-4 (CONTINUED)
Muscles, Nerves, Spinal Root Level, and Actions of Muscles of the Ankle

MUSCLE	NERVE	SPINAL NERVE ROOT				ANKLE PLANTARFLEXION	ANKLE DORSIFLEXION	ANKLE INVERSION	ANKLE EVERSION
		L4	L5	S1	S2				
Peroneus brevis	Superficial peroneal nerve	X	X	X		X			X
Peroneus tertius	Superficial peroneal nerve	X	X	X			X		X
Tibialis posterior	Tibial nerve		X	X		X		X	
Flexor digitorum longus	Tibial nerve		X	X		X		X	
Flexor hallucis longus	Tibial nerve		X	X	X	X		X	

Adapted from Lippert, L. S. (2022). *Clinical kinesiology and anatomy* (7th ed.). F. A. Davis Company and Stone, R. J., & Stone, J. A. (2003). *Atlas of skeletal muscles* (4th ed.). McGraw-Hill.

Summary

Through Betty in the occupational profile, this chapter has shown how the LEs function. The LEs can affect whole-body function and movement in ADL skills. If an individual does not have functional mobility in the home and community, it is difficult to be independent. A knowledge of normal balance and gait are required to understand the disease process that can affect mobility. Even though occupational therapists rarely treat LEs, it is important to understand how the trunk and LEs influence function. When occupational therapists treat a patient with LE dysfunction, it is helpful to understand how and why the patient requires an assistive device for ambulation or an AFO to prevent foot drop after stroke. Injuries and diseases treated in occupational therapy often affect the LEs as well as the UEs. The reader has learned how the pelvic girdle and LEs influence posture and sitting balance to reach with the UEs. The knowledge gained in this chapter will aid the occupational therapy practitioner in helping to return their clients to a healthy and more independent lifestyle.

References

American Occupational Therapy Association. (2020). Occupational therapy practice framework: Domain and process (4th ed.). *American Journal of Occupational Therapy, 74*(Suppl. 2), Article 7412410010. https://doi.org/10.5014/ajot.2020.74S2001

Cruz, T. H., & Dhaher, Y. Y. (2008). *Compensatory gait movements post stroke: The influence of synergies.* North American Congress in Biomechanics.

Foti, D., & Kanazawa, L. M. (2006). Activities of daily living. In H. M. Pendleton & W. Schultz-Krohn (Eds.), *Pedretti's occupational therapy: Practice skills for physical dysfunction* (6th ed.). Mosby-Elsevier.

Greene, D. P., & Roberts, S. L. (2005). *Kinesiology: Movement in the context of activity* (2nd ed.). Elsevier-Mosby.

Hayes, S. M. (2004). Gait awareness. In G. Gillen & A. Burkhardt (Eds.), *Stroke rehabilitation: A function-based approach* (2nd ed., pp. 312-337). Mosby.

Jeka, J. (1997). Light contact as a balance aid. *Physical Therapy, 77*(5), 476-487.

Kisner, C., & Colby, L. (2023). *Therapeutic exercises: Foundations and techniques* (8th ed.). F. A. Davis Company.

Latella, D., & Meriano, C. (2003). *Occupational therapy manual for evaluation of range of motion and muscle strength.* Delmar Cengage Learning.

Lippert, L. S. (2022). *Clinical kinesiology and anatomy* (7th ed.). F. A. Davis Company.

Loudon, J., Swift, M., & Bell, S. (Eds.). (2008). *The clinical orthopedic assessment guide* (2nd ed.). Human Kinetics.

Moore, S., Schurr, K., Wales, A., Moseley, A., & Herbert, R. (1993). Observation and analysis of hemiplegic gait: Swing phase. *Australian Journal of Physiotherapy, 39*(4), 271-278.

Moseley, A., Wales, A., Herbert, R., Schurr, K., & Moore, S. (1993). Observation and analysis of hemiplegic gait: Stance phase. *Australian Journal of Physiotherapy, 39*(4), 259-267.

O'Sullivan, S., Schmitz, T., & Fulk, G. (2014). *Physical rehabilitation.* F. A. Davis Company.

Pritchett, J. W., & Porembski, M. A. (2010). Foot drop. *Medscape.* http://emedicine.medscape.com/article/1234607-print

Skinner, S. R., Antonelli, D., Perry, J., & Lester, K. (1985). Functional demands on the stance limb in walking. *Orthopedics, 8*, 355-361.

Stone, R. J., & Stone, J. A. (2003). *Atlas of skeletal muscles* (4th ed.). McGraw-Hill.

Yavuzer, G., & Süreyya, E. (2002). Effect of an arm sling on gait patterns in patients with hemiplegia. *Archives of Physical Medicine and Rehabilitation, 83*, 960-963.

Applications

The following activities will help you apply knowledge of the LE in real-life applications. Activities can be completed individually or in a small group to enhance learning.

1. **Transitional Movements—Sitting to Standing**: Transitional movements refer to changes of body position. Quite often, occupational therapy assistants reinforce certain transitional movements as part of transfer training and ADL retraining. Frequent transitional movements of concern to occupational therapy include moving from supine to sitting, sitting to supine, sitting to standing, and standing to sitting. This application is designed to increase your awareness of the sequence of movements required to complete these transitional movements. Select one of the transitional movements listed and identify the sequence of movements that occur. Practicing the transitional movement yourself may give you insight into what muscles and joints are activated during the movement. Movements of the UE and trunk also occur during transitional movements; however, for this application, the focus will be on LE movement. Focus on the movements at the pelvic girdle, hip, knee, and ankle. Select from the following transitional movements, and fill in the answers in the space below.

   a. Supine to sitting

   b. Sitting to supine

   c. Sitting to standing

   d. Standing to sitting

Lower Extremity Movement Sequence

TRANSITIONAL MOVEMENT SELECTED

Joint Movement	Muscles Involved	Identify ROM Needed
1.		
2.		
3.		
4.		
5.		
6.		
7.		

2. **The Pelvic Girdle**: The pelvic girdle is very important due to its influence on the trunk and LE in sitting and standing. This activity will help you identify the different motions of the pelvic girdle. First, with a partner or on your own, identify the location of the ASIS, which is a bony landmark located on the pelvic bone on the front side of the body. The ASIS bony landmark provides a reference point to identify the motions of the pelvic girdle. Palpate the ASIS on each pelvic bone to identify if they are roughly symmetrical or if one ASIS is not a mirror image of the other ASIS on the contralateral (opposite) side of the body. Standing upright, both ASIS landmarks should be level. Anterior tilt occurs if the ASIS landmarks are more anterior than the pubic symphysis. Posterior tilt occurs if the ASIS landmarks are more posterior than the pubic symphysis. In lateral tilt, one ASIS landmark is more superior than the contralateral side ASIS. The more superior ASIS landmark is the reference point. If the left ASIS is more inferior to the right ASIS, then the pelvic girdle is in left lateral tilt.

   a. While facing another student, place your thumbs over the ASIS landmarks. Spread your hands out to cover the sides of the hip with fingers abducted, as if you were going to catch a basketball. By moving your wrists in ulnar and radial deviation, try to palpate the movement of anterior and posterior pelvic tilt. Sit on the edge of a mat. Is your pelvic girdle in anterior or posterior pelvic tilt?

   b. Hopefully, the pelvic girdle is in anterior pelvic tilt. Carefully, so as not to fall off the mat, try to make your pelvic girdle go into posterior pelvic tilt. Does it feel like you could easily slide off the mat? Why? Note the movement of the lumbar spine that occurs with pelvic rotation. Quite often, occupational therapy practitioners treat clients sitting on the edge of a mat. Anterior pelvic tilt is important to enable an active trunk that supports reaching and decreases the risk for falls.

   c. Observe the movements of the pelvis in the transverse plane during normal gait. Palpate the ASIS landmarks during gait and observe how they move forward and backward relative to each other. In what phase of gait is the left ASIS most forward when compared to the right?

3. **LE PROM**: In some settings it may be necessary for the occupational therapy assistant to perform PROM on the LE as a preparatory treatment. With another student, either sitting or supine on a mat, practice moving each joint of the LE through its available ROM. Remember, in PROM the therapist provides the force to create joint movement. The hand placement proximal to the joint supports and isolates the joint through stabilization. The hand placement distal to the joint provides the force needed to move the joint and create PROM. Try to move each joint through its available ROM.

   Joint Motions:
   - Hip flexion
   - Hip extension
   - Hip internal rotation
   - Hip external rotation
   - Hip abduction
   - Hip adduction
   - Knee flexion
   - Knee extension
   - Ankle plantarflexion
   - Ankle dorsiflexion
   - Ankle inversion
   - Ankle eversion

4. **LE AROM**: In some settings it may be necessary for the occupational therapy assistant to measure the available joint ROM for the LE. For this application, measure the available AROM of the LE with a partner. Use Table 6-5 for this application.

TABLE 6-5
Lower Extremity Active Range of Motion Application

POSITION	JOINT AND MOTION	LANDMARK	STABLE ARM	MOVING ARM	RECORDED ROM
Supine	Hip flexion	Lateral aspect of greater trochanter	Parallel to the midaxillary line of the trunk	Parallel to the lateral aspect of the femur	
Prone	Hip extension				
Supine	Hip abduction	Over ASIS	Horizontal between the right and left ASIS	Parallel to the anterior midline of the femur	
Supine	Hip adduction				
Sitting	Hip internal rotation	Over midpoint of the patella	Perpendicular to the floor	Parallel to the anterior midline of the tibial midway between the two malleoli	
Sitting	Hip external rotation				
Sitting or supine	Knee flexion	Over the lateral epicondyle of the femur	Parallel to the lateral midline of the femur	Parallel to the lateral midline of the fibula	
Sitting or supine	Knee extension				
Sitting	Ankle plantarflexion	Lateral aspect of the lateral malleolus	Parallel to the lateral midline of the fibula	Parallel to the lateral midline of the fifth metatarsal	
Sitting	Ankle dorsiflexion				
Sitting	Ankle eversion	Over the anterior aspect of the ankle midway between malleoli	Parallel to the anterior midline of the lower leg	Parallel to the anterior midline of the second metatarsal	
Sitting	Ankle inversion				

Adapted from Latella, D., & Meriano, C. (2003). *Occupational therapy manual for evaluation of range of motion and muscle strength.* Delmar Cengage Learning.

5. **LE Adaptive Equipment for Mobility**: Occupational therapy assistants frequently need to educate and reinforce safety and proper use of adaptive equipment for safe mobility during engagement in occupations. Examples of adaptive equipment related to enhancing mobility include rolling walkers, standard walkers, wheelchairs, and various types of canes. Using a standard or rolling walker, answer the following questions.

   a. Describe the BOS without the adaptive equipment.

   b. Describe the BOS with the adaptive equipment.

   c. If the client is sitting down and tries to stand by pulling on the walker handholds, is this safe? What happens to the BOS? Is there a better alternative method to stand?

   d. When the client stands and holds the walker by the handholds as far to the front as possible, is this safe? Is the BOS larger or smaller? Where is the COG? How could you make this safer for the client to stand with a walker?

   e. Is it safe for the client to stand and turn with a walker by only twisting the trunk, not changing foot placement, so that the front of the walker is more toward the side of the person during turning? How is the BOS affected? Where is the COG? How could you make this safer for the client to stand with a walker?

6. **Stride Length**: This application will help you comprehend that while components of gait are similar for each person, everyone has their own individualized characteristics. Anatomical characteristics, environmental adaptations, and contextual factors all influence gait and stride length. Individuals can have different leg lengths or body structure components that affect gait. A person walking downhill may have a greater stride length than when walking uphill. A person may also have a different stride length when walking on a level surface vs. an unlevel surface. Knowing your stride length is useful in determining distances traveled for functional mobility. As stated previously, stride length is the distance traveled during the gait cycle or from one initial contact to the same initial contact on the ground. You can measure one stride length to find the distance traveled; however, it may be inaccurate due to the conscious effort to take a step. A more accurate method may be to walk a premeasured distance of 50 or 100 feet and count the number of strides for that distance. For this application, identify the following:

    a. What is the step length for your right leg? What is the step length for your left leg? Are they the same or different? Why?

    b. What is your number of stride lengths for 50 feet? Is it the same or different than a friend or classmate? Why?

    c. Identify five factors that influenced the stride length that was recorded.

7. **OTPF-4 Areas of Occupation**: The OTPF-4, specifically areas of occupation, was introduced in Chapter 1. Remember, areas of occupation include life activities in which a person engages (AOTA, 2020). This application will build on the use of the OTPF-4 by using Betty's occupational profile. Identify areas of occupation that may apply to Betty by using the occupational profile and Table 6-6. If you cannot identify an area of occupation from the occupational profile, identify what may be appropriate for Betty considering her age and the information provided.

TABLE 6-6

Occupational Therapy Practice Framework: Domain and Process, Fourth Edition Domain Aspect: Areas of Occupation

AREAS OF OCCUPATION

Activities of Daily Living	Instrumental Activities of Daily Living	Health Management	Rest and Sleep	Education	Work	Play	Leisure	Social Participation
Upper and lower body dressing	Sweep floor	Balance training	Sleep at night	Sunday school at church	Retired CNA	Golf league	*The Ellen DeGeneres Show*	Volunteers at a long-term care facility
Your example here								
Your example here								
Your example here								
Your example here								
Your example here								
Your example here								
Your example here								
Your example here								

8. **OTPF-4 Occupation and Activity Demands**: This application will build on the use of the OTPF-4 by using Betty's occupational profile. Identify an activity and its area of occupation in the first column of Table 6-7. Then, identify the activity demands for this activity that apply to Betty to be able to complete that activity. Remember, some activities may need to be adapted in order for Betty to complete the activity due to her impairments. Record your examples in Table 6-7.

TABLE 6-7

Occupational Therapy Practice Framework: Domain and Process, Fourth Edition Process Aspect: Evaluation Analysis of Occupational Performance—Activity Demands

ACTIVITY AND AREAS OF OCCUPATION	RELEVANCE AND IMPORTANCE	OBJECTS USED AND THEIR PROPERTIES	SPACE DEMANDS	SOCIAL DEMANDS	TIME DEMANDS	REQUIRED ACTIONS AND PERFORMANCE SKILLS	REQUIRED BODY FUNCTIONS	REQUIRED BODY STRUCTURES
Toileting: Self-care ability; area of occupation is ADLs	Regularity	Bedside commode, bedpan, grab bars, toilet paper	Lighting needs, area for a wheelchair, reaching for toilet paper	Appropriate hygiene for community engagement	Typical time needed to complete toileting task Needed items present, safe multistep processing, timeliness with toilet hygiene	Transfer to commode, lower pants, peri hygiene, stand balance	Level of arousal, impulse control, sensory functions, urinary and bowel functions	Nerves, muscles, eyes, ears, sensory receptors
Your example here								
Your example here								
Your example here								
Your example here								

CHAPTER 7

Function and Movement of the Shoulder and Scapula

Carolyn L. Roller, OTR/L

Key Terms

antagonists

Erb's palsy

force couple

glenohumeral joint

hemiplegia

humeral positioners

humeral propellers

primary adhesive capsulitis

rotator cuff

rotator cuff tendinitis

scaption

scapular pivoters

scapulohumeral rhythm

shoulder complex

shoulder dystocia

shoulder girdle

shoulder impingement

shoulder protectors

shoulder subluxation

synergists

winging of the scapula

Chapter Outline

Sain, S. J., & Roller, C. L. *Kinesiology for the Occupational Therapy Assistant: Essential Components of Function and Movement, Third Edition* (pp. 149-178).
© 2024 Taylor & Francis Group.

Introduction

This chapter discusses the **shoulder complex** and how it relates to function during occupation. The shoulder complex, which is a portion of the **shoulder girdle**, provides movement at the **glenohumeral (GH) joint**, scapula, and clavicle. The term shoulder girdle includes all muscles that provide motion when using the shoulder. The way the shoulder is designed allows more movement than any other joint in the body. **Scapulohumeral rhythm** is the term used to describe the motion of the clavicle, scapula, and humerus working together to bring the arm overhead. Discussion will include all movements of the shoulder girdle and how they relate to occupation. Muscles of the shoulder complex that work together to strengthen a movement or provide stability are called **synergists**. **Antagonists** are muscles that work against each other to form a cocontraction, which also provides stability. Throughout the chapter the goals and activities of the client in the occupational profile demonstrate how body functions and structures are related to the shoulder complex and how occupational therapy intervention can help individuals with shoulder impairments. Four problems seen in occupational therapy relating to the shoulder complex are also presented, including adhesive capsulitis (or frozen shoulder), **shoulder subluxation** after stroke, **Erb's palsy** (a brachial plexus injury occasionally found in newborns after a difficult birth), and **rotator cuff** tendinitis, which can cause shoulder pain, stiffness, and weakness. Finally, the reader will learn structures of the shoulder girdle, including muscles, ligaments, tendons and nerve innervations, their influence on occupational performance.

Occupational Profile

The following occupational profile is provided to demonstrate how body functions and body structure are related to the shoulder complex and tie into occupational therapy intervention of shoulder impairments. Linda, the client in the following occupational profile, will be referred to throughout the chapter.

Linda is a 77-year-old grandmother who is participating in occupational therapy with a physician's referral to improve right dominant shoulder function.

During the evaluation, the following data were gathered.

Subjective: Linda reports decreased function in her right shoulder for approximately 3 months with an increase in her symptoms of right shoulder pain and stiffness over the past month. Her main complaints include an inability to properly care for her grandchildren and difficulty with grooming, toileting, bathing, and sleeping. Her occupational roles include caring for her two grandchildren since her daughter returned to part-time employment. Linda has a grandson who is 3 years old and a granddaughter who is 6 months old.

Linda states her biggest problem occurs when she is providing care for her grandchildren, especially when getting them in and out of their car seats. She also reports that it is difficult to change diapers on her 6-month-old granddaughter safely and without increased pain. The client denies any injury to her right shoulder; however, she slipped while gardening about 6 months ago and broke her fall with her right arm. She stated that she had some "achy"-type pain in her whole arm occasionally, but especially at night after this incident. She reported an inability to sleep on her right side, which has always been her most comfortable position. The client reports a medical history of type 2 diabetes, hypertension, and high cholesterol. She reports that she does not have a pacemaker. Besides insulin, she takes medication to control her blood pressure and cholesterol. She denies any other health problems and affirms that "I feel healthy and get around quite well for my age."

Objective: The client rates her pain on a 0 to 10 scale, 0 being no pain and 10 being "emergency room" pain. She rates her pain as a 3/10 when at rest and an overall rating of 8/10 at her worst. She reports her worst pain is with right shoulder movement during resistive functional activities. Examples of these functional activities include lifting her grandchildren out of their car seats and donning and doffing her bra.

Active range of motion (AROM) is within functional limits in both upper extremities (UEs) except the right dominant shoulder. Formal measurements follow:

- GH joint flexion:
  Right: 75 degrees   Left: 170 degrees
- GH joint abduction:
  Right: 60 degrees   Left: 165 degrees
- GH joint external rotation:
  Right: 25 degrees   Left: 75 degrees
- GH joint internal rotation:
  Right: 35 degrees   Left: 70 degrees

The client reports pain at the end of AROM in the right shoulder during strength measurements. Grip strength is tested bilaterally with the right grip averaging 45 pounds and the left grip averaging 50 pounds. Linda denies any numbness or tingling in her UEs. There was no edema observed in the UEs at the time of the evaluation.

Goals were established by the occupational therapist in collaboration with Linda and are presented in the following sections.

Short-Term Goals:

1. Client will be instructed in and comply with a home exercise program within 2 weeks.
2. Client will decrease pain from 3/10 to 0/10 at rest and will be able to sleep through the night within 4 weeks by sleeping on her left side or back and using a pillow under her right shoulder.
3. Client will decrease pain from 8/10 to 4/10 at worst with transferring grandchildren out of car seats within 4 weeks by using modified lifting techniques.
4. Client will increase AROM in all limited planes of right shoulder range of motion (ROM) by 10 degrees within 3 weeks.
5. Client will increase right grip strength by 5 pounds within 4 weeks.
6. Client will be able to perform donning/doffing of bra using right UE independently and with fewer complaints of pain within 4 weeks.

Long-Term Goals:

1. Client will demonstrate compliance and independence in home exercise program at discharge.
2. Client will be independent with use of right UE in self-care and occupational roles with only minimal complaints of discomfort within 3 months.
3. Client will demonstrate AROM in right shoulder and right grip strength to within functional limits within 3 months.

The outcome of Linda's occupational intervention along with treatment techniques and goals achieved can be found in Appendix C.

Body Functions of the Shoulder Complex

Joint motions, as well as the strength characteristics, of the GH joint and scapula will be identified in the following sections as they relate to function. Scapulohumeral rhythm will also be defined and explained. Additionally, four shoulder problems seen in occupational therapy treatment will be identified and discussed. Throughout this chapter, references will be made to the occupational profile of Linda.

The shoulder complex includes all of the body structures that provide motion at the GH joint and scapula. The shoulder complex includes in one part the motions of the scapula and clavicle, which can also be referred to as the shoulder girdle. Additionally, motions of the scapula and humerus are often referred to as the *shoulder joint* as well as the *glenohumeral (GH) joint*. Overall, the shoulder complex consists of four joints that function in a coordinated and rhythmic manner. Changes in the position of the UE involve movements of the clavicle, scapula, and humerus (Peat, 1986). This is accomplished by the sternoclavicular joint, acromioclavicular joint, GH joint, and the scapulothoracic gliding mechanism (Oatis, 2004).

The design of the shoulder complex is related to overall function of the UE. For example, the shoulder complex controls placement of the hand in its occupational space in front of and to the side of the body. The shoulder complex provides the UE with a ROM that is greater than any other joint in the body. This ROM is more than what is required for most activities of daily living (ADLs; Peat, 1986). Linda, in the occupational profile, may not need to regain all of her right shoulder movement to resume care of her grandchildren, although that may be a treatment goal. She may be able to compensate with the other joints of her right arm and left UE to safely lift her grandchildren from the car seat. Even though she may not regain full ROM, she may have functional movement of a very mobile body part, the shoulder complex.

Motions of the Shoulder Girdle and Glenohumeral Joint

Movements of the shoulder complex rely on the motion of all components. Specifically, the humerus, which moves in synchronization with the scapula at the GH joint. The scapula moves while in contact with the clavicle at the acromioclavicular joint, while the clavicle attaches to the sternum at the sternoclavicular joint. Movement at all of these joints must occur for the arm to reach 180 degrees of GH joint flexion or abduction (Schenkman & Rugo de Cartaya, 1987). The ability to achieve full AROM of the UE, however, depends more heavily on certain joints, namely the GH and scapulothoracic joints.

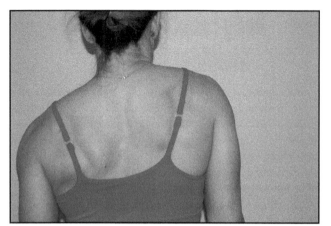

Figure 7-1. Scapular elevation.

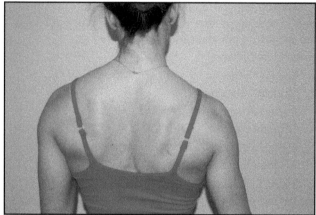

Figure 7-2. Scapular depression.

Motions of the scapula are identified as scapular elevation, scapular depression, scapular adduction or retraction, scapular abduction or protraction, scapular upward rotation, and scapular downward rotation. Scapular elevation is achieved when the client elevates their shoulder complex as in shrugging the shoulders. Scapular depression is achieved when the client attempts to depress the shoulder complex as in reaching toward the ground. Scapular adduction, also called *retraction*, is when the client moves their scapula closer to the vertebrae. This can be achieved by sticking the chest out and pulling the shoulder complex toward the rear of the person. The opposite is scapular abduction, also referred to as *protraction*. Scapular abduction is achieved when the client moves the shoulder complex toward the front of the person as when reaching forward, resulting in an increase in distance between the scapula and vertebrae. Scapular upward rotation is achieved with either GH joint flexion or GH joint abduction. This occurs when the inferior angle of the scapula moves upward and away from the spinal column. Downward rotation occurs when the arm returns to the neutral or anatomical position. Of importance, scapular upward rotation is important and necessary to achieve full GH joint AROM. Each scapular motion is labeled in Figures 7-1 through 7-6.

Motions of the GH joint are identified as GH joint flexion, extension, abduction, adduction, internal rotation, external rotation, horizontal adduction, and horizontal abduction. GH joint flexion is achieved when the client raises their arm overhead in front of the body, such as placing an item in a cupboard above the head. **Scaption**, short for scapular plane elevation, is a commonly used term in shoulder rehabilitation.

Scaption is a functional movement of the GH joint that occurs about midway between shoulder flexion and abduction. Please refer to Chapter 2 and Table 2-8 in this text for a more detailed description of scaption. GH joint extension (sometimes called *hyperextension*) is when the client moves their arm straight back from the neutral or anatomical position at the side of the body. This movement could be used to place an object in the back seat of the car with the right arm while seated in the driver's seat. GH joint abduction occurs when the client moves their arm away from the body out to the side, away from the anatomical position. This movement may be seen functionally when the client reaches up and out to the side to turn on a light switch. GH joint adduction is the movement of the client's arm returning to the side of the body from GH joint abduction. GH joint internal rotation is achieved when the greater tubercle of the humerus rotates toward the midline in front of the body. Functionally, during this motion, the client would be reaching behind the small of their back as though they were tucking in a shirt or placing the palm of the hand on their stomach. GH joint external rotation is seen when the client rotates the greater tubercle of the humerus away from the midline. This movement can be seen when a client is reaching with their left arm for the seat belt prior to driving the car or placing the palm of the hand on the back of the head. GH joint horizontal adduction is shown when the client moves the arm in a horizontal or transverse plane toward and across the chest, such as reaching across the body to bathe the left shoulder with the right hand. Finally, GH joint horizontal abduction is achieved when the person moves the arm in a horizontal or transverse plane away from the chest. Each motion is identified in Figures 7-7 through 7-14.

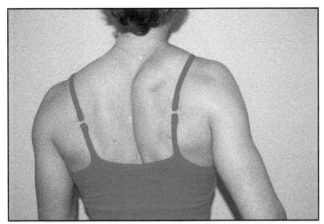

Figure 7-3. Scapular retraction (also called adduction).

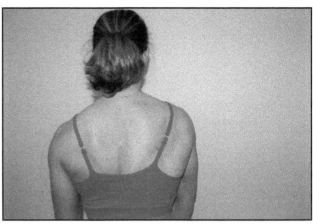

Figure 7-4. Scapular protraction (also called abduction).

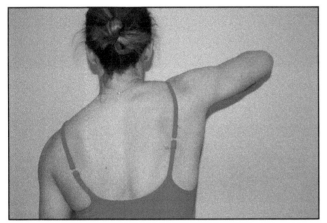

Figure 7-5. Scapular upward rotation.

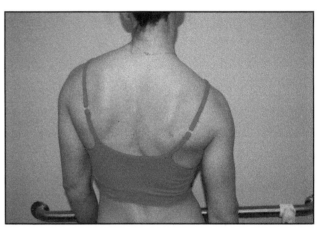

Figure 7-6. Scapular downward rotation.

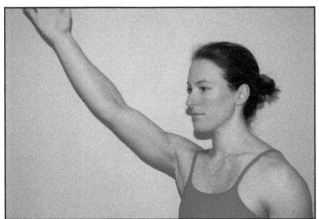

Figure 7-7. GH joint flexion.

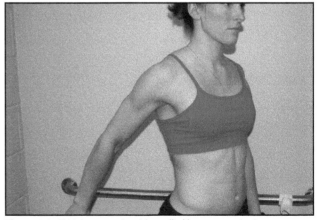

Figure 7-8. GH joint extension (also called hyperextension).

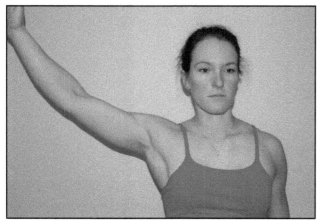

Figure 7-9. GH joint abduction.

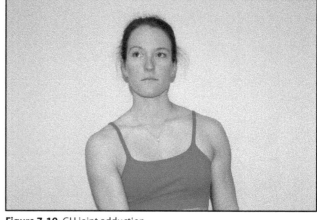

Figure 7-10. GH joint adduction.

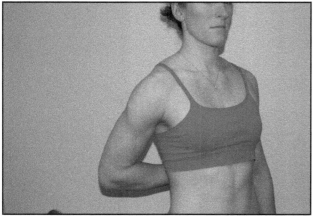

Figure 7-11. GH joint internal rotation.

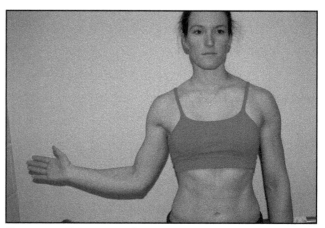

Figure 7-12. GH joint external rotation.

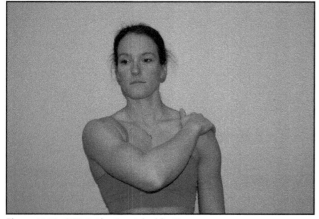

Figure 7-13. GH joint horizontal adduction.

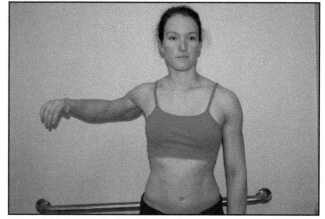

Figure 7-14. GH joint horizontal abduction.

Scapulohumeral Rhythm

Understanding the concept of scapulohumeral rhythm may be enhanced by multiple definitions. According to Lippert (2000), scapulohumeral rhythm describes the movement relationship between the scapula in the shoulder girdle and the GH joint. This movement can be described as a synchronization of combined movements that occur between the scapula and humerus during GH joint flexion or abduction (Dutton, 2004). Scapulohumeral rhythm can also be defined as motions of the clavicle, scapula, and humerus all working together to achieve full elevation of the arm (Hunter et al., 2002). Due to the importance of scapulohumeral rhythm, its definition is provided in Box 7-1.

The first 30 degrees of GH joint flexion or abduction is called the *setting phase* of scapulohumeral rhythm. During this phase, scapulothoracic movement is very small and

BOX 7-1

Scapulohumeral rhythm: The motion of the clavicle, scapula, and humerus working together to achieve full elevation of the arm. This movement relationship exists between the scapula in the shoulder girdle and the GH joint.

(Dutton, 2004; Hunter et al., 2002)

inconsistent (Schenkman & Rugo de Cartaya, 1987). During the second phase, the scapula abducts and upwardly rotates 1 degree of motion for every 2 degrees of GH joint flexion or abduction. The second phase occurs between 30 and 90 degrees of GH joint flexion or abduction (Glinn, 2008). This 2:1 ratio is the measurement of scapulohumeral rhythm. After 90 degrees of GH joint movement, 60 degrees of motion occurs at the GH joint with the remaining 30 degrees consisting of scapular movement. In this final phase of scapulohumeral rhythm, this 2:1 ratio is not consistent throughout the ROM. Early movement as in the first phase involves more GH joint motion, while end-range movement involves more scapular movement (Dutton, 2004).

Scapulohumeral rhythm serves two purposes. First, scapular upward rotation allows the GH joint muscles to maintain the length–tension relationship. This allows the muscles to sustain their force through a larger portion of the available ROM and effectively limits active insufficiency. Second, simultaneous movement of the humerus and scapula during GH joint flexion or abduction prevents impingement between the greater tubercle of the humerus and the acromion process (Hunter et al., 2002).

Strength Characteristics of the Shoulder Girdle and Glenohumeral Joint

Most muscles of the shoulder complex perform a variety of movements. Additionally, most muscles work together to either strengthen a movement or provide stability. Synergists are muscles that work together to increase the strength of a desired movement as they work in unison. If stability is the goal, rather than increased strength, then muscles will work in unison to counter each other, thus stabilizing a joint. Antagonists are muscles that work against each other to equal or cancel out the movement and therefore gain stability. This is also called a *cocontraction*.

Synergists are muscles whose fibers (line of force) lie approximately in the same direction. Muscles that act as synergists to one another provide a stronger action on the joint resulting in stronger functional movement for the client. A **force couple**, as seen in upward and downward rotation, is a special type of synergy. The muscles in the force couple still act together to provide a stronger functional movement; however, they do so in a different manner. To be classified as a force couple, two basic requirements must be met. First, the resulting movement must be rotary in nature. Second, the line of force and the pull or angle of muscle fibers of all muscles involved must be in opposing directions. One muscle's line of force might be vertical, another lateral, and still another medial. A common example of a force couple is the motion used to turn a steering wheel when the power steering goes out. One hand pushes or turns the steering wheel upward while the other hand pushes or turns the steering wheel in a downward direction. The forces are in opposite directions but work together to strengthen the rotary movement of the steering wheel.

Table 7-1 can be used to identify muscles that act as synergists for scapular motions. Synergists can be found by selecting a movement and then looking in the column beneath it for the muscles marked with an X. To discuss specific movements required during selected daily activities, refer back to the client, Linda. Looking at the table, we see that scapular protraction, which Linda uses when she reaches forward to get her grandchild out of the car seat, is performed by the serratus anterior and pectoralis minor muscles working as synergists. In a similar manner, this table can also be used to find antagonists for each movement. Retraction is the motion that is opposite to, or antagonist to, protraction. Therefore, the muscles that cause retraction are antagonists to the muscles that cause protraction. Using the table as a reference, one sees that the middle trapezius and rhomboid muscles cause scapular retraction; thus, they are antagonists to the serratus anterior and pectoralis minor for the motion of scapular protraction.

Some muscles of the shoulder girdle are so large that the muscle fibers in different portions of the muscle are oriented in different directions, meaning that their line of pull will be different. In this case, the different portions of the same muscle may work as synergists to each other or as antagonists, depending on the motion desired at a given joint. The trapezius and deltoid muscles both fit this description and are both divided into three parts. The trapezius muscle is divided into upper, middle, and lower sections while the deltoid muscle is divided into anterior, middle, and posterior sections. Again, refer to Table 7-1 to observe the upper portion of the trapezius functions as a synergist with the lower portion of the trapezius for scapular upward rotation. The upper portion of the trapezius also functions as an antagonist to the lower portion of the trapezius for the movement of scapular depression.

TABLE 7-1

Motions of the Scapula

MUSCLE	NERVE	NERVE ROOT						DEPRESSION	ELEVATION	PROTRACTION	RETRACTION	UPWARD ROTATION*	DOWNWARD ROTATION*
		C3	C4	C5	C6	C7	C8						
Trapezius (upper)	Spinal accessory	X	X						X			X	
Trapezius (middle)	Spinal accessory	X	X								X		
Trapezius (lower)	Spinal accessory	X	X					X				X	
Levator scapulae	Dorsal scapular	X	X						X				X
Rhomboids	Dorsal scapular			X							X		X
Serratus anterior	Long thoracic			X	X	X				X		X	
Pectoralis minor	Pectoral				X	X	X	X		X			X

*Indicates force couple.

Adapted from Kendall, F. P., McCreary, E. K., Provance, P. G., Rodgers, M. M., & Romani, W. A. (2005). *Muscle testing and function with posture and pain* (5th ed.). Lippincott Williams & Wilkins.

TABLE 7-2
Shampooing Hair: Movements, Muscles, and Innervations

MUSCLE	NERVE	NERVE ROOTS
Scapular Elevation		
Trapezius (upper)	Spinal accessory	C3, C4
Levator scapulae	Dorsal scapular	C3, C4
Scapular Upward Rotation		
Trapezius (upper)	Spinal accessory	C3, C4
Trapezius (lower)	Spinal accessory	C3, C4
Serratus anterior	Long thoracic	C5, C6, C7
Glenohumeral Joint Flexion		
Deltoid (anterior)	Axillary	C5, C6
Biceps brachii	Musculocutaneous	C5, C6
Pectoralis major (clavicle)	Medial pectoral	C8, T1
Coracobrachialis	Musculocutaneous	C5, C6
Glenohumeral Abduction		
Deltoid	Axillary	C5, C6
Supraspinatus	Suprascapular	C5, C6
Glenohumeral External Rotation		
Deltoid (posterior)	Axillary	C5, C6
Infraspinatus	Suprascapular	C5, C6
Teres minor	Axillary	C5, C6

To determine which motions are necessary at the shoulder complex to complete specific daily activities, refer again to Linda in the occupational profile. The interrelatedness of joint actions, muscular control, and innervations can be seen in reference to an activity important to Linda. One of Linda's ADLs, shampooing her hair, requires many movements to include scapular elevation and upward rotation, GH joint flexion and abduction, and GH joint external rotation. Examples of motions, muscles, nerves, and innervations that may be needed to shampoo hair are provided in Table 7-2.

An instrumental activity of daily living for Linda, caring for her grandchildren, includes diapering and getting the children into and out of car seats. For these actions Linda uses scapular protraction and GH joint internal rotation in reaching forward and holding the child, GH joint extension and scapular retraction in lifting the child toward herself, and GH joint horizontal abduction and adduction in reaching for and placing a diaper on the baby. Scapular depression and downward rotation accompany GH joint extension. As you can see, all of the motions of the shoulder girdle listed earlier in this chapter are necessary for our client to engage in her chosen occupations. Typically, in order for most people to accomplish their daily chosen activities, they will need to be able to perform all the motions of the shoulder girdle. The ability to perform these motions will require an intricate and detailed coordination of muscle, nerve, and joint motion.

Four Problems of the Shoulder Girdle and Glenohumeral Joint

There are many injuries and diseases that can affect the scapula and GH joint, requiring occupational therapy intervention. Four of the most common shoulder injuries and diseases seen in occupational therapy will be presented in the following section. While reading about these injuries and diseases, consider Linda in the occupational profile. Think about Linda's signs and symptoms and the functional tasks that are limited. Appendix C will provide further information on Linda's treatment plan and the outcome of her interventions.

Primary Adhesive Capsulitis (Frozen Shoulder)

Most clients report a history of progressive shoulder stiffness with **primary adhesive capsulitis**, or frozen shoulder. The stiffness is usually preceded by diffuse pain with no prior obvious shoulder problem. This may last from 2 weeks to several months. In some cases, there may have been a period of immobilization or minor trauma to the extremity. According to Hunter and colleagues (2002), women over the age of 40 appear to be more commonly affected with adhesive capsulitis. Clients with type 1 diabetes, degenerative disk disease of the cervical spine, and those with a history of stroke involving shoulder **hemiplegia** are also more likely to experience adhesive capsulitis (Boyle-Walker et al., 1997).

Frozen shoulder typically develops slowly and in three stages. In the freezing stage, the client often complains of limited ROM and pain with movement. In the second stage, called the *frozen stage*, the client may report less pain, but the shoulder is stiffer and using it becomes more difficult. The thawing stage is the last stage when the shoulder movement begins to return. Each stage can last anywhere from 2 to 9 months (Mayo Clinic, 2015).

Shoulder Hemiplegia and Subluxation After a Stroke

Hemiplegia is the paralysis of one side of the body after a cerebrovascular accident or stroke. A stroke can occur when a clot reduces or blocks blood flow through an artery supplying blood to the brain. When the brain is without blood or oxygen for even a short period of time, damage occurs (American Stroke Association, 2017). The rehabilitation of clients after stroke is very complex; however, an overview of treatment applications will be focused on shoulder subluxation in this chapter. Shoulder subluxation is the misalignment of the humeral head in the glenoid fossa after stroke (Mahle & Ward, 2019). When the shoulder complex is affected by weakness or paralysis after a stroke, subluxation of the GH joint can occur. The shoulder, in particular, is vulnerable to stretch, especially when the arm is hanging unsupported by the side of the body and there is less stability at the GH joint (Ryerson & Levit, 1987).

GH joint integrity and rhythm are important for typical and pain-free shoulder movement. Even after recovery from stroke is achieved, pain and stiffness can lead to limitations in movement and function (Vliet et al., 1995). Another example of pain-limiting movement is in the previous condition of adhesive capsulitis.

It is important to protect the affected arm from injury and to keep the affected extremity in a supported position early in the treatment of clients with shoulder hemiplegia after stroke to prevent shoulder subluxation. Pillows can be used in bed or a lap board can be used in the wheelchair to support the arm while positioned to help keep the shoulder joint intact and prevent shoulder subluxation. According to Zorowitz et al. (1996), the client should be educated in movement techniques to maximize functional recovery with AROM and active assist range of motion. Additionally, occupational therapy techniques may also include neuromuscular re-education, modalities, shoulder cuffs or adaptive therapeutic equipment, taping protocols, and forced use or constraint-induced movement programs. Ideally, the therapist will focus on functional tasks to achieve rehabilitation of the affected UE.

Erb's Palsy or Upper Obstetric Brachial Plexus Palsy

Erb's palsy is often seen in newborns after a difficult delivery. The difficult birth can cause an injury to the baby's brachial plexus, which is an interconnected group of nerves passing through the shoulder. The brachial plexus includes the nerves that control movement and sensation to the arm, hand, and fingers. Erb's palsy is characterized by weakness or paralysis of the arm by affecting nerve roots C5, C6, and C7. Typically, the paralyzed limb is positioned in internal rotation, elbow extension, forearm pronation, and wrist and finger flexion. Approximately 1 to 2 babies per 1000 births are affected with this impairment.

Erb's palsy can result from several causes connected to a difficult delivery. Breech birth and larger-than-average baby weight (greater than 8 pounds 13 ounces), present an increased risk. During breech birth, which is feet first, the baby's arms are usually raised, and excess pressure can cause a stretching injury to the brachial plexus. In births where the baby is larger than average, a condition called **shoulder dystocia** occurs more frequently. In shoulder dystocia, the infant's head is delivered normally, but one shoulder becomes stuck under a portion of the mother's pelvic bones. The doctor's use of manipulations, such as forceps or a vacuum extractor, to free the baby can then increase the risk of a brachial plexus injury. People who are short, have gestational diabetes, pelvic abnormalities, or have experienced prolonged labor, are more at risk for a birth involving shoulder dystocia. A Cesarean birth may be scheduled for people at greater risk of shoulder dystocia (Brain and Spinal Cord. org, 2009).

Most cases of Erb's palsy are due to stretching of the brachial plexus and will heal within 6 to 12 months. Sometimes, total recovery is not possible due to scar tissue that forms around healthy nerves after the stretching injury. Only 10% of brachial plexus birth injuries result in permanent paralysis or impairment. Erb's palsy is almost always apparent immediately because it is caused by an injury at birth. The extent of the injury may not be known for months to years due to the slow rate of nerve healing. Signs and symptoms that parents may notice are limited spontaneous arm movement of the baby's affected side and decreased grip or fisting in the affected hand. Infants with Erb's palsy may lack a Moro reflex on the injured side. The Moro reflex, which is present

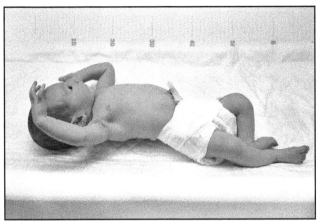

Figure 7-15. Infant with a normal Moro reflex. (Zhuravlev Andrey/shutterstock.com)

in healthy newborns, occurs when the infant is startled. A healthy infant, when startled, will throw out the arms to the side with the palms up and the thumbs flexed. Figure 7-15 illustrates a baby with a Moro reflex.

Occupational therapy treatment for infants with Erb's palsy may include gentle massage and passive range of motion to improve circulation and prevent joint contractures while the injured nerves are healing. Neoprene serpentine splinting, which promotes supination, or splinting to bring the affected hand to midline near the chin may also be incorporated.

Rotator Cuff Tendinitis and Shoulder Impingement

The rotator cuff is a tendon connecting four muscles that cover the head of the humerus. The muscles are the supraspinatus, infraspinatus, teres minor, and subscapularis. Box 7-2 provides an easy acronym to memorize these muscles. The rotator cuff muscles work together to lift and rotate the humerus and maintain the head of the humerus in the glenoid fossa. **Rotator cuff tendinitis** and **shoulder impingement** are some of the most common causes shoulder pain adults. Impingement happens when there is pressure on the surface of the rotator cuff from the acromion process as the arm is lifted.

Impingement can cause local swelling and soreness in the front of the shoulder. Pain and stiffness may occur when raising the arm and sometimes when the arm is lowered from an elevated position. As the condition progresses, there may also be pain at night and difficulty sleeping. Over time strength and movement may continue to vanish, and functional movements requiring placement of the arm behind the back may also become difficult and painful. Figure 7-16 illustrates the difference between a normal shoulder and a shoulder with impingement.

BOX 7-2

ROTATOR CUFF MUSCLES: USE THE ACRONYM SITS

S = Supraspinatus
I = Infraspinatus
T = Teres minor
S = Subscapularis

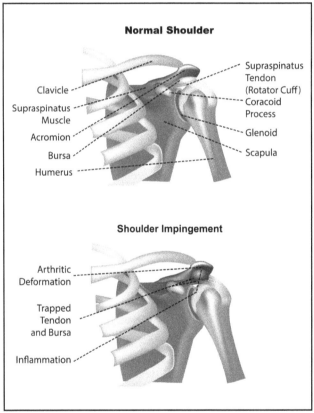

Figure 7-16. Shoulder impingement. The inflamed rotator cuff tendons become impinged between the humeral head, the swollen bursa and the acromion process. (La vector/shutterstock.com)

A history of forward-head posture with rounded shoulders, clinically called *thoracic kyphosis*, is especially seen in clients 45 years and older with shoulder impingement. Clients may also report a history of overuse of the UEs. Other signs and symptoms may include pain after activity, pain at night, and a "catching" sensation in the shoulder with overhead activities. Clients may report arm fatigue during and after functional activities as well. The symptom of night pain, which often involves sleeplessness, is usually the main reason an individual seeks medical attention (Glinn, 2008).

Risk factors that can lead to shoulder impingement are categorized as structural or functional. Structural risk factors include degenerative spurring of the acromion process, inflammation of the bursa, calcification or thickening of the rotator cuff tendon, or tears of the rotator cuff. Additionally, there are three types of acromion shapes (Figure 7-17). Type 1 is flat, type 2 is curved, and type 3 is hooked. Individuals with a type 2– or type 3–shaped acromion process are also at greater structural risk for shoulder impingement.

Unfortunately, most individuals have either type 2 or type 3 acromion process shapes, which are more often associated with impingement. The hook or curved shape can lead to degeneration and eventual tearing of the rotator cuff (Weiss & Falkenstein, 2005). Functional risk factors include abnormal scapular and GH joint positioning during functional use from thoracic kyphosis, depression of the humeral head in the glenoid fossa due to rotator cuff weakness or tear, and tightness of the posterior capsule. Over time these conditions can lead to decreased blood flow, inflammation, and rotator tendon tears or rupture (American Academy of Orthopaedic Surgeons, 2007). Supraspinatus tendinitis accounts for 80% to 90% of rotator cuff tendinitis, possibly because of this tendon's location at the GH joint. There is constant pressure on the supraspinatus tendon from the humeral head that impinges against the coracoacromial arch during normal joint movements (Weiss & Falkenstein, 2005).

Occupational therapy treatment may focus on decreasing pain and inflammation, which will promote the healing process and assist in regaining normal GH joint motion required for typical shoulder function. Treatment approaches may also include education on positioning of the shoulder to decrease pain and inflammation, activity modification, and protective positions for the shoulder during sleeping, sitting, and walking. Ideally, rotator cuff tears, as well as subsequent surgical intervention, can be prevented (Burke et al., 2006).

Body Structures of the Shoulder Complex

Muscle Actions of the Shoulder Complex

A significant number of muscles control movement of the shoulder complex. The movements of the shoulder complex will be discussed in terms of their kinetic functional roles. These functional roles include **scapular pivoters**, **humeral positioners**, **humeral propellers**, and **shoulder protectors** (Glinn, 2008). The functional roles are identified in Box 7-3. An overview of the shoulder complex muscles and their functional roles are presented in Table 7-3.

The scapular pivoters include the trapezius, serratus anterior, levator scapulae, pectoralis minor, and rhomboid major and minor muscles. Together, these muscles are involved with movement at the scapulothoracic joint. The trapezius muscle is divided into upper, middle, and lower portions because of its different actions.

The upper portion of the trapezius is a prime mover in scapular elevation and upward rotation. The middle trapezius muscle is effective at scapular retraction. The lower portion of the trapezius depresses and upwardly rotates the scapula (Lippert, 2000). One of the main functions of the trapezius is to provide shoulder girdle elevation on the fixed cervical spine. For the trapezius to perform its job well, the cervical spine must be stabilized by anterior neck flexors, which will prevent forward head posture if stable and strong. The trapezius muscle is used strenuously when using the hands to hold a heavy object overhead or when moving a heavy wheelbarrow, for example (Floyd & Thompson, 2001). Downward rotation of the scapulothoracic joint is performed by the rhomboid, pectoralis minor, and levator scapula muscles.

The serratus anterior muscle is a prime mover in scapular protraction. It works with the upper and lower trapezius muscles in rotating the scapula upward. Another function of the serratus anterior muscle is to hold the vertebral border of the scapula against the ribs, preventing **winging of the scapula**. Winging of the scapula occurs when the inferior angle of the scapula sticks out from the body. Figure 7-18 illustrates winging of the scapula.

The action of the serratus anterior muscle is commonly seen in functional movements used to throw a baseball, tackle in football, or shoot a gun while hunting (Floyd & Thompson, 2001). According to Lippert (2000), an individual could not raise their arm overhead without the action of the serratus anterior.

The levator scapula muscle elevates the scapula and allows us to shrug our shoulders. It is also a prime mover in downward rotation. The rhomboid muscles retract and elevate the scapula. Along with the levator scapula, they assist in downward rotation of the scapula as well. The proper function of these scapular pivoters is important to normal movement of the entire shoulder complex and functional tasks involving the UE (Van Dyck, 2000).

Humeral positioners are muscles that position the humerus in space during or after actions of the scapular pivoters. The humeral positioner muscles include the anterior, middle, and posterior deltoid. The different sections of the deltoid are separated by their different origins and functions. All sections have a common insertion, the deltoid tuberosity of the lateral humerus. The anterior fibers of the deltoid muscle originate on the clavicle and perform actions of shoulder GH joint abduction, flexion, horizontal adduction, and internal rotation. The middle fibers of the deltoid originate on the acromion process of the scapula and perform shoulder GH abduction. The posterior fibers originate on the spine of the scapula. The posterior deltoid performs abduction, extension, horizontal abduction, and external rotation of the GH joint.

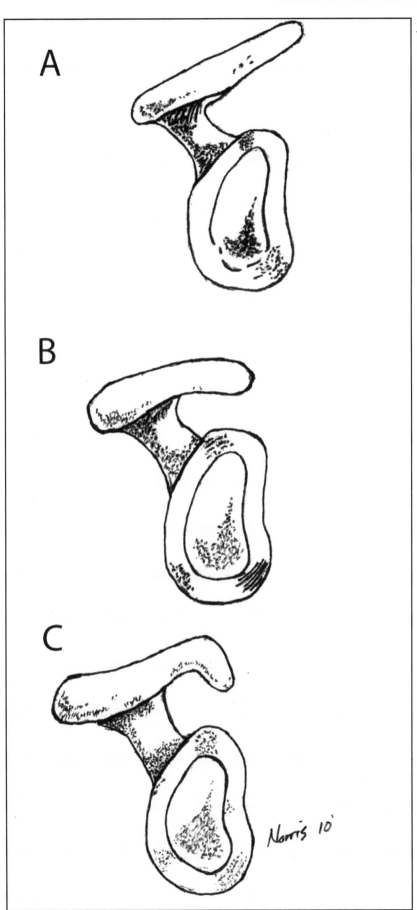

Figure 7-17. Acromion types. (A) Type 1, flat. (B) Type 2, curved. (C) Type 3, hooked. (Reproduced with permission from Kevin Norris.)

BOX 7-3

KINETIC FUNCTIONAL ROLES OF THE SHOULDER COMPLEX

Humeral positioners: Muscles that position the humerus in space during or after actions of the scapular pivoters.
Humeral propellers: Muscles that propel the humerus.
Scapular pivoters: Muscles that are involved with motion at the scapulothoracic joint.
Shoulder protectors: Muscles that work with the humeral positioners to keep the structures of the shoulder complex safe. These include the rotator cuff muscles.

(Glinn, 2008)

TABLE 7-3
Functional Roles of Shoulder Complex Muscles

SCAPULAR PIVOTERS	HUMERAL POSITIONERS	HUMERAL PROPELLERS	SHOULDER PROTECTORS (ROTATOR CUFF)	MUSCLES OF THE SHOULDER COMPLEX
• Trapezius • Serratus anterior • Levator scapulae • Rhomboids • Pectoralis minor	• Deltoid, anterior fibers • Deltoid, middle fibers • Deltoid, posterior fibers	• Latissimus dorsi • Pectoralis major • Teres major	• Supraspinatus • Infraspinatus • Teres minor • Subscapularis	• Biceps brachii • Coracobrachialis • Triceps brachii (long head only) • Subclavius • Pectoralis minor

Adapted from Dutton, M. (2004). *Orthopaedic examination, evaluation, and intervention*. McGraw-Hill.

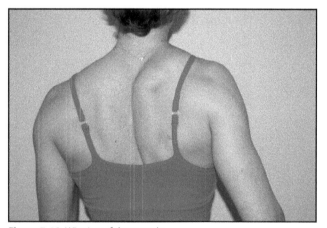

Figure 7-18. Winging of the scapula.

The deltoid muscle is commonly used in lifting movements with the arms at the side. Floyd and Thompson (2001) identify that the trapezius muscle stabilizes the scapula as the deltoid pulls on the humerus. Any movement of the humerus on the scapula will involve all or a portion of the deltoid muscle.

Humeral propellers are muscles that propel the humerus and include the latissimus dorsi, pectoralis major, and teres major. These muscles have been shown to have a positive impact on pitching speed and the propulsive phase of the swim stroke in athletes (Dutton, 2004). The latissimus dorsi muscle functions include GH extension, adduction, and internal rotation. It also assists with scapular depression, retraction, and downward rotation. If the arms are stabilized, the latissimus dorsi will elevate the pelvis. This is an example of reversal of muscle function described in earlier chapters of this text. Examples of this reversal action could be seen in walking with crutches or while performing a sitting push-up.

The pectoralis major and teres major are other muscles that serve as humeral propellers. The pectoralis major has different lines of pull depending on its attachments. It is a large chest muscle originating on the clavicle and sternum and inserts on the lateral lip of the bicipital groove of the humerus. The clavicular portion of the pectoralis major has a vertical line of pull and assists in GH joint flexion during the first part or to approximately 90 degrees. The sternal portion of the pectoralis major, named due to its origin on the sternum, assists in GH joint extension from 180 degrees to

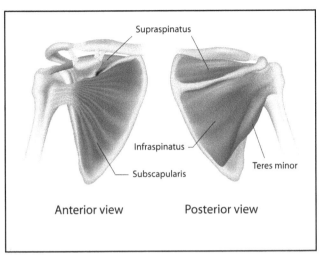

Figure 7-19. Rotator cuff muscles. (Alila Medical Media/shutterstock.com)

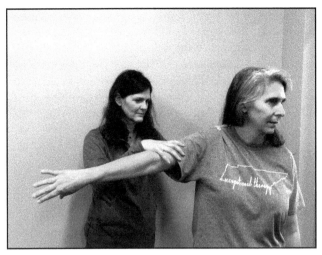

Figure 7-20. Client performing empty can exercise.

approximately 90 degrees. Both the clavicular and sternal portions provide GH joint adduction, internal rotation, and horizontal adduction (Glinn, 2008).

Even though the pectoralis major muscle does not insert on the scapula, it acts on the scapulothoracic joint through its insertion on the humerus (Dutton, 2004). The pectoralis major muscle works closely with the anterior deltoid muscle while performing push-ups and pull-ups and during tennis serves. The teres major muscle is the last of the humeral propeller muscles discussed. It assists the latissimus dorsi and the pectoralis major muscles in adduction, internal rotation, and extension of the humerus along with one of the rotator cuff muscles, the subscapularis. According to Floyd and Thompson (2001), it is commonly called the *latissimus dorsi's little helper*.

The shoulder protectors act as a force couple with the humeral positioners (the anterior, middle, and posterior deltoid) to keep the structures of the shoulder complex safe. It also works to fine tune the humeral head position during arm elevation. This allows for a greater surface area of the head of the humerus to remain in contact with the smaller glenoid fossa. The shoulder protectors also serve as decelerators to prevent subluxation and dislocation during repetitive motions, such as pitching, or in heavy lifting. The shoulder protectors are known as the rotator cuff muscles and consist of the supraspinatus, infraspinatus, teres minor, and subscapularis muscles. These four muscles have different origins on the scapula and they all insert on the humerus as displayed in Figure 7-19. The rotator cuff acts as a dynamic unit, playing an important role in movements of the GH joint (Peat, 1986).

The muscles of the rotator cuff assist in rotation of the GH joint. They also stabilize the humeral head in the glenoid cavity during functional tasks of the UEs, especially when the arms are abducted to 45 degrees and externally rotated (Dutton, 2004).

The supraspinatus is the most superior muscle of the rotator cuff group. It acts in GH joint abduction along with the middle deltoid, as well as in GH joint extension. This muscle

stabilizes the humeral head in the glenoid fossa (mainly inferiorly). The empty can exercise can be used to show supraspinatus action, according to Floyd and Thompson (2001). During empty can exercises, the client is asked to position their arm at approximately 90 degrees of GH joint flexion with the elbow extended as they move into full GH joint internal rotation, as in emptying a can. Figure 7-20 shows a client performing an empty can exercise.

The infraspinatus and the teres minor muscles act together to provide external rotation, horizontal abduction, and extension of the GH joint. These two muscles also work with the other rotator cuff muscles to stabilize the humeral head in the glenoid fossa. The infraspinatus muscle is important in maintaining posterior stability of the GH joint with the help of the teres minor muscle. The infraspinatus is the strongest external rotator of the shoulder complex and is the second most commonly injured of the rotator cuff group (Floyd & Thompson, 2001).

The subscapularis muscle is the largest muscle of the rotator cuff muscles. It has the prefix "sub" because it lies under, or on the anterior surface of, the scapula. It lies between the scapula and rib cage; therefore, it is so deep that it cannot be palpated. It acts to internally rotate, adduct, and extend the GH joint in unison with the latissimus dorsi and teres major muscles. Oatis (2004) states that it has the most anterior attachment of the four rotator cuff muscles, which allows it to stabilize the head of the humerus in front and below. It is rare for the subscapularis to receive an isolated tear. Partial ruptures have been reported occasionally, associated only with anterior dislocation of the GH joint (Weiss & Falkenstein, 2005).

There are additional muscles that play a lesser role in functional movement of the shoulder complex. They will be briefly discussed here along with their motions at the scapula and GH joint.

The biceps brachii muscle is better known as an elbow flexor and a forearm supinator; however, due to the origin of its two heads on the scapula, it does act as a weak flexor of the shoulder joint. It also assists in anterior stabilization of the humeral head of the glenoid fossa (Floyd & Thompson, 2001). It has been called the fifth tendon of the rotator cuff group (Weiss & Falkenstein, 2005).

The coracobrachialis muscle is not a strong muscle, but it assists in flexion and adduction of the GH joint. It is most functional in moving the arm across the chest during horizontal adduction of the shoulder (Dutton, 2004).

The subclavius muscle pulls the clavicle toward the sternum or assists in depressing the clavicle and the shoulder girdle. Its significant function is protecting and stabilizing the sternoclavicular joint during UE movements (Floyd & Thompson, 2001).

The pectoralis minor muscle produces scapular downward rotation and is used with the serratus anterior muscle in scapular abduction or protraction. This is seen in movements like performing push-ups. These muscles work together in most movements requiring pushing with the hands.

The long head of the triceps brachii muscle originates on the glenoid fossa of the scapula and inserts on the olecranon process of the ulna. Its main action is to extend the elbow; however, the long head is also an important GH joint extensor (Lippert, 2000). The long head of the triceps brachii also aids in shoulder adduction. It is always used in any pushing movement of the UE (Floyd & Thompson, 2001). The sternocleidomastoid muscle is a strong flexor of the neck. It is mentioned here because of its origin on the shoulder girdle, specifically on the sternum and clavicle (Lippert, 2000).

In summarizing the motions and muscles of the shoulder and scapula, it is important to remember that the incredible movement and consequent function available in the shoulder complex cannot be achieved by independent muscles and joints. As each structure works together to provide mobility and stability to the shoulder and scapula, each muscle group relies on the other to provide functional motion in the UEs. For example, the rotator cuff muscles cannot work together to move and protect the shoulder if the scapular pivoters, such as the rhomboids, are not stabilizing and rotating the scapula.

To demonstrate how integrated the shoulder complex movements are during functional roles, let's return to Linda. One of the problems that Linda reported was pain in her right shoulder while unhooking her bra with a back clasp. For Linda, this functional task requires the following movements from the shoulder complex: scapular elevation, depression, retraction, downward rotation, and GH joint horizontal adduction, abduction, extension, and internal rotation. Performing just this one task during undressing requires 13 muscles of the shoulder complex working together to stabilize and move the structures to complete this functional role.

Muscles, Nerves, and Spinal Cord Levels

Most of the muscles in the shoulder complex are innervated by nerve roots C3 through C6 with C7, C8, and T1 playing a lesser role. All of the nerve branches, except the long thoracic nerve and the spinal accessory nerve, are considered part of the brachial plexus. The long thoracic nerve and the spinal accessory nerve originate prior to the formation of the plexus, from the nerve roots themselves (Gench et al., 1999). The fact that most of the innervations in shoulder girdle movement emerge from the brachial plexus indicates a certain protection for these motions. Injury or damage to one nerve or nerve root will most likely only weaken a given movement, not render it completely unusable.

In general, the muscles that act on the scapula originate on the trunk and insert on the scapula. Muscles that act at the GH joint also originate on the trunk, as well as on the scapula, but insert on the humerus. The muscles needed for each movement and the innervation required for these movements will be discussed in relation to Linda's daily activities. Given that upward rotation of the scapula must accompany GH flexion or abduction, strengthening these muscles and, therefore, the associated movements, would have a positive impact on Linda's ability to raise her arms above her shoulders, thus allowing her to complete her daily activity of shampooing her hair.

Again, the muscles for these movements, and their respective innervations, can be found in Table 7-2. One sees that the upper and lower sections of the trapezius muscle, in addition to the serratus anterior, act together to cause the movement of scapular upward rotation. Other information found on the table indicates that the spinal accessory nerve, from roots C3 and C4, innervates the trapezius muscle and the long thoracic nerve, roots C5, C6, and C7, innervates the serratus anterior muscle. In other words, all of the nerve roots from C3 through C7 contribute to scapular upward rotation.

What other scapular movements might Linda need to use to shampoo her hair? Think of how you perform this activity. The actual movements may vary from person to person. Identify the movements you use and then determine, by referencing Tables 7-1 and 7-2 which muscles you are using.

In addition to scapular movements, GH movements must be used to raise the arms above shoulder level for shampooing hair. Table 7-4 can be used in the same manner as Table 7-1 to determine synergists or antagonists for a given GH joint movement. Information on innervation and normative ROM is also included. The normative ROM for GH flexion is between 150 and 180 degrees, depending on the source. This amount of motion, however, is not necessary to perform most daily activities. A more functional ROM for GH flexion is 100 to 110 degrees.

TABLE 7-4

Motions of the Glenohumeral Joint

MUSCLE	NERVE	C5	C6	C7	C8	T1	FLEXION 0 to 180 degrees	EXTENSION 0 to 50 degrees	ABDUCTION 0 to 180 degrees	ADDUCTION 180 to 0 degrees	INTERNAL ROTATION 0 to 90 degrees	EXTERNAL ROTATION 0 to 90 degrees	HORIZONTAL ABDUCTION 0 to 45 degrees	HORIZONTAL ADDUCTION 0 to 135 degrees
Deltoid (anterior)	Axillary	X	X				X		X		X			X
Deltoid (middle)	Axillary	X	X						X					
Deltoid (posterior)	Axillary	X	X					X	X			X	X	
Coracobrachialis	Musculocutaneous	X	X				X							
Biceps brachii	Musculocutaneous	X	X				X							
Pectoralis major (clavicular)	Medial pectoral				X	X	X			X				X
Pectoralis major (sternal)	Lateral pectoral	X	X	X				X 180–90						X
Latissimus dorsi	Thoracodorsal		X	X	X			X		X	X			
Teres major	Lower subscapular	X	X					X		X	X			
Triceps brachii	Radial			X	X			X						

(continued)

TABLE 7-4 (CONTINUED)

Motions of the Glenohumeral Joint

MUSCLE	NERVE	NERVE ROOT					FLEXION 0 to 180 degrees	EXTENSION 0 to 50 degrees	ABDUCTION 0 to 180 degrees	ADDUCTION 180 to 0 degrees	INTERNAL ROTATION 0 to 90 degrees	EXTERNAL ROTATION 0 to 90 degrees	HORIZONTAL ABDUCTION 0 to 45 degrees	HORIZONTAL ADDUCTION 0 to 135 degrees
		C5	C6	C7	C8	T1								
Rotator Cuff Muscles														
Supraspinatus	Suprascapular	X	X						X					
Infraspinatus	Suprascapular	X	X									X	X	
Teres minor	Axillary	X	X									X	X	
Subscapularis	Subscapular	X	X								X			

Adapted from Kendall, F. P., McCreary, E. K., Provance, P. G., Rodgers, M. M., & Romani, W. A. (2005). *Muscle testing and function with posture and pain* (5th ed.). Lippincott Williams & Wilkins.

Another use of these tables is to determine what effects certain nerve damage might have on the client's movements. Considering the movement of scapular protraction in Table 7-1, injury to the spinal accessory or dorsal scapular nerves would have no effect, nor would damage to nerve roots C3 or C4. On the other hand, injury to the long thoracic nerve would cause weakened protraction just as injury to any nerve root C5 through C8 would also weaken this movement. Consider the movements you identified, in relation to performing your own ADL tasks. Consult the tables to determine the innervations needed for these motions. Consider what would happen if you had an injury to nerve root C5.

Reviewing the tables will give a clear picture of the muscles that Linda uses and necessary innervations for successful completion of this one ADL. Would Linda be able to wash her own hair if she sustained an injury to nerve roots C5 and C6? Defend your answer. Select a daily activity that is important to you. Determine the scapular and GH motions necessary to complete this activity. Create a table similar to the one created for Linda. What do you learn about yourself and your movement needs for this activity from analyzing this table?

Tendons and Ligaments

The shoulder complex and its associated joints allow more ROM than any other joint in the body, but in so doing lose much of their stability. The skeletal structure allows movement in all planes but these bony structures do not provide needed stability. In the GH joint, the relatively lateral position of the glenoid fossa, along with its small size and shallow depth, allow the potential for the head of the humerus to easily slip out of the glenoid fossa. Additionally, the looseness of the joint capsule, necessary to allow full movement, provides little stability. Were it not for other structures, such as tendons and ligaments, this joint would not be able to sustain the weight of the arm, or the resistance needed during daily activities. Tendons, via contraction of the attached muscles, cause joint movement, while ligaments provide stability for the skeletal system. However, in addition to providing movement, the tendons around the GH joint provide stability as well. One of the primary functions of the rotator cuff muscles is to hold the head of the humerus in the glenoid fossa to provide joint stability. The tendons of these muscles combine with a variety of ligaments to strengthen and stabilize this joint. Additional stability is provided by the glenoid labrum, which deepens the shallow glenoid fossa, especially inferiorly.

Stability is not provided by the skeletal structure of the other joints of the shoulder complex either. Laterally, at the acromioclavicular joint, the relatively flat acromion process could slide over the clavicle. Medially, at the sternoclavicular joint, the clavicle and sternum present with flat surfaces that could glide past one another. The sternoclavicular joint needs added support as it is the only structural or bony attachment of the scapula, clavicle, and UE to the axial skeleton. Along with ligaments, the sternoclavicular joint has a thick articular disk that aids in stability and, perhaps more importantly, absorbs forces from falling or leaning on the UE.

The strength and stability of these joints is provided by ligaments. The ligaments of all of the joints of the shoulder complex are named for their locations. Each ligament performs a unique function in counteracting dislocation in a certain direction. Together they allow the GH joint to move safely in any plane, or in a combination of planes, allowing us to perform any activity of our choosing. Trauma or stress to the GH joint can occur from any direction and is more common than one would initially think. Falling and catching yourself with your hand, performing closed-chain actions with the UE, such as pull-ups or push-ups, carrying heavy objects, or even carrying a heavy backpack or purse over one shoulder, can lead to trauma of the GH joint. Refer to Table 7-5 for a listing of shoulder complex ligaments and their respective functions.

Summary

Through Linda in the occupational profile, the reader has explored how the shoulder complex moves and functions. Scapulohumeral rhythm describes how the movement of the clavicle, scapula, and humerus work together to bring a healthy arm overhead. In this chapter, we learned the shoulder is extremely flexible, placing the hand where needed to complete functional tasks. When a joint has more ROM it is more susceptible to injury, especially as the client ages. Learning about several pathologies of the shoulder complex treated in occupational therapy may be helpful with treatment strategies. Learning the muscles, nerves, tendons, and ligaments that support the shoulder complex will help the occupational therapy practitioner know how to help clients return to a more independent lifestyle as they age.

References

American Academy of Orthopaedic Surgeons. (2007). Shoulder impingement. http://orthoinfo.aaos.org/topic.cfm?topic=a00032

American Stroke Association. (2017) About Stroke. https://www.stroke.org/en/about-stroke

Boyle-Walker, K. L., Gabard, D. L., Bietsch, E., Masek-Van Arsdale, D. M., & Robinson, B. L. (1997). A profile of patients with adhesive capsulitis. *Journal of Hand Therapy, 10*(3), 222-227.

Brain and Spinal Cord.org. (2009). Erb's palsy. http://www.brain-andspinalcord.org/erbs-palsy/

Burke, S. L., Higgins, J. P., McClinton, M. A., Saunders, R., & Valdata, L. (2006). *Hand and upper extremity rehabilitation: A practical guide* (3rd ed.). Elsevier-Mosby.

Dutton, M. (2004). *Orthopaedic examination, evaluation and intervention.* McGraw-Hill.

TABLE 7-5
Ligaments and Their Functions

JOINT	LIGAMENT	FUNCTION
Glenohumeral	Coracohumeral	Major structure to prevent downward or upward displacement; limits lateral rotation and extension of humeral head; supports weight of UE.
	Superior GH	Prevents downward displacement of humeral head; limits lateral rotation; provides anterior stability.
	Middle GH	Provides anterior stability; limits lateral rotation of humeral head.
	Inferior GH	Prevents anterior displacement; limits lateral rotation; supports GH abduction.
Sternoclavicular	Costoclavicular	Major stabilizing structure, especially in GH elevation or scapular protraction; supports weight of UE.
	Anterior sternoclavicular	Limits excessive retraction; supports weight of UE.
	Posterior sternoclavicular	Limits excessive protraction; supports weight of UE.
	Interclavicular	Provides stability on superior aspect of joint; supports weight of UE; protects brachial plexus via limiting clavicular depression.
Acromioclavicular	Supra-acromioclavicular	Strengthens upper portion of joint; prevents clavicle overriding acromion process; controls anterior-posterior joint stability.
	Coracoclavicular	Major stabilizer; maintains clavicle in contact with acromion process; prevents dislocation here; limits upward rotation of scapula.
	Coracoacromial	With acromion and coracoid process forms protective arch over GH joint; prevents superior displacement.

Adapted from Peat, M. (1986). Functional anatomy of the shoulder complex. *Physical Therapy, 66*(12), 1855-1865; Schenkman, M., & Rugo de Cartaya, V. (1987). Kinesiology of the shoulder complex. *Journal of Orthopaedic and Sports Physical Therapy, 8*(9), 438-450; and Levangie, P., & Norkin, C. (2005). *Joint structure and function: A comprehensive analysis* (4th ed.). F. A. Davis Company.

Floyd, R. T., & Thompson, C. W. (2001). *Manual of structural kinesiology* (14th ed.). McGraw-Hill.

Gench, B., Hinson, M., & Harvey, P. (1999). *Anatomical kinesiology* (2nd ed.). Eddie Bowers Publishing.

Glinn, J. E., Jr. (2008). Shoulder biomechanics. *Physical Therapy Clinical Educator*, 49-53.

Hislop, H. J., & Montgomery, J. (2002). *Daniel's and Worthingham's muscle testing: Techniques of manual examinations* (7th ed.). Saunders.

Hunter, J. M., Macklin, E. J., Callahan, H. D., Skirven, T. M., Schneider, L. H., & Osterman, A. E. (2002). *Rehabilitation of the hand and upper extremity* (5th ed.). Mosby.

Latella, D., & Meriano, C. (2003). *Occupational therapy manual for the evaluation of range of motion and muscle strength*. Delmar Carnage Learning.

Lippert, L. S. (2000). *Clinical kinesiology for physical therapist assistants* (3rd ed.). F. A. Davis Company.

Mahle, A. J., & Ward, A. L. (2019), *Adult physical conditions: Intervention strategies for occupational therapy assistants*. F. A. Davis Company.

Mayo Clinic. (2015) Frozen shoulder. http://www.mayoclinic. org/diseases-conditions/frozen-shoulder/basics/symptoms/ con-20022510

Oatis, C. A. (2004). *Kinesiology: The mechanics and pathomechanics of human movement*. Lippincott Williams & Wilkins.

Peat, M. (1986). Functional anatomy of the shoulder complex. *Physical Therapy, 66*(12), 1855-1865.

Rondinelli, R. D., Genoverse, E., Katz, R. T., Mayer, T. G., Mueller, K., & Ranavaya, M. (2008). *Guides to the evaluation of permanent impairment* (6th ed.). American Medical Association..

Ryerson, S., & Levit, K. (1987). The shoulder in hemiplegia. In R. Donatelli (Ed.), *Physical therapy of the shoulder* (pp. 105-129). Churchill Livingstone.

Schenkman, M., & Rugo de Cartaya, V. (1987). Kinesiology of the shoulder complex. *Journal of Orthopaedic and Sports Physical Therapy, 8*(9), 438-450.

Van Dyck, W. R. (2000). The trunk–upper extremity connection: Understanding the origins of scapula control. *AOTA's Physical Disabilities SI Section Quarterly, 23*(2), 1-4.

Vliet, P., Sheidan, M., Kerwin, D., & Fenton, P. (1995). The influence of functional goals on the kinematics of reaching following stroke. *Neurology Report, 9*(1), 111-116.

Weiss, S., & Falkenstein, N. (2005). *Hand rehabilitation: A quick reference guide and review*. Elsevier-Mosby.

Zorowitz, R., Hughes, M., Idank, D., Idai, T., & Johnston, M. (1996). Shoulder pain and subluxation after stroke: Correlation or coincidence. *American Journal of Occupational Therapy, 50*(3), 194-201.

Applications

The following activities will help you apply knowledge of the shoulder girdle and GH joint in real-life applications. Activities can be completed individually or in small groups to enhance learning.

1. **The Shoulder Girdle/Scapula**: The shoulder girdle is another term to describe the movement of the scapula. The shoulder joint is more accurately referred to as the *glenohumeral joint*. Scapular motion and GH joint motion combine to allow for stability, mobility of the arm, and placement of the arm in numerous positions in space. Limitations in scapular motion may affect GH joint motion. Likewise, limitations in GH joint motion may affect scapular motion. As such, ROM of the GH joint cannot be fully appreciated without first considering the influence of the scapula on movement. With a partner, complete the following activities to increase your familiarity with aspects and movements of the scapula.

   a. Palpate the scapula and identify the bony landmarks of the scapula. Identify the inferior angle and superior angle, and trace your fingers along the vertebral border and axillary border. Also trace your fingers along the spine of the scapula ending at the acromion process. Follow the acromion process around to the top of the GH joint all the way to the acromioclavicular joint. Then, follow the clavicle to the sternum and palpate the sternoclavicular joint. Of importance, the acromion process is a reference point for a goniometer in measuring multiple GH joint motions. Additionally, the sternoclavicular and acromioclavicular joints minimally influence the movement of the GH joint. It may be easier to palpate these joints if the client moves their GH joint at the same time.

   b. Observe the position of the scapula on the back of your partner. Are both scapulas relatively mirrored on the left and right sides of the body? If not, what seems different? Look at the vertebral border of the scapula. Is it equally distant from the spinal column? Look at the height of both shoulders at rest. Are they equal or is one shoulder slightly higher than the other? Developed shoulder musculature, as in the pitching arm of a pitcher or the dominant arm of a client, may present slightly depressed as compared to the other arm.

   c. Lastly, refer to the movements and pictures of the scapula earlier in this chapter. As your partner moves their scapula, palpate it: Palpate the scapular movements of retraction, protraction, elevation, depression, upward rotation, and downward rotation. You are not trying to move the scapula, but feeling the scapula move under your hand. *Scapular mobilization* refers to a therapeutic treatment technique whereby the therapist assists with the movement of the scapula. Due to the complexity of scapular mobilization, additional training may be necessary to incorporate this treatment technique into occupational therapy practice.

   d. Identify the position of the scapula during the following functional movements:
      i. Brushing the hair on the back of your head:
      ii. Bringing your arm back to throw a ball:
      iii. Standing, reaching down to scratch your knee:
      iv. Doing a push-up when arms are extended:
      v. Reaching up to touch the ceiling:

   e. Identify the position of the GH joint during the following functional movements:
      i. Brushing the hair on the back of your head:
      ii. Bringing your arm back to throw a ball:
      iii. Standing, reaching down to scratch your knee:
      iv. Doing a push-up when arms are extended:
      v. Reaching up to touch the ceiling:

2. **ROM Chart**: Proceed through each joint motion with your partner and record the available ROM in Table 7-6.

TABLE 7-6
Range of Motion Application Table

JOINT	MOTIONS	AVAILABLE RANGE OF MOTION (Degrees)	RANGE OF MOTION OF PARTNER
Glenohumeral	Flexion	0 to 180	
	Extension (also called hyperextension)	0 to 50	
	Abduction	0 to 180	
	Adduction	180 to 0	
	Internal rotation	0 to 90	
	External rotation	0 to 90	
	Horizontal abduction	0 to 45	
	Horizontal adduction	0 to 135	

3. **ROM of the GH Joint**: Motions of the GH joint and ROM norms are identified in Table 7-7. ROM norms can vary depending on the reference source. One norm is provided for each motion within this text to increase ease of applications. Additionally, while multiple muscles may influence a particular motion, only the main muscles responsible for a joint motion are included. References for the following information can be found in Box 7-4. With your partner, practice using a goniometer to measure each motion available at the GH joint.

TABLE 7-7
Range of Motion of the Shoulder—Glenohumeral Joint

GLENOHUMERAL JOINT/ SHOULDER MOTION	RANGE OF MOTION (Degrees)	ASSOCIATED SHOULDER GIRDLE MOTIONS**
Flexion	0 to 180	Abduction, upward rotation, slight elevation
Extension (also referred to as hyperextension)	0 to 50	Depression, adduction
Abduction	0 to 180	Elevation and upward rotation
Adduction	180 to 0	Depression, downward rotation, and adduction
Internal rotation	0 to 90	Abduction
External rotation	0 to 90	Adduction
Horizontal abduction	0 to 45*	Abduction
Horizontal adduction	0 to 135*	Adduction

*Identified from Latella, D., & Meriano, C. (2003). *Occupational therapy manual for the evaluation of range of motion and muscle strength.* Delmar Carnage Learning.

**Identified from Killingsworth, A., & Pedretti, L. (2006). Joint range of motion. In: H. M. Pendleton & W. Schultz-Krohn (Eds.), *Pedretti's occupational therapy: Practice skills for physical dysfunction* (6th ed., pp. 437-468). Mosby-Elsevier.

BOX 7-4

REFERENCED WORKS FOR RANGE OF MOTION

Sections Referenced (a to e)	Reference
Goniometric landmark, end feel, and start and end positions	Latella & Meriano, 2003
Muscles responsible	Hislop & Montgomery, 2002
Available ROM	Rondinelli et al., 2008

a. GH joint flexion
   i. Goniometric landmark: Lateral surface of the acromion process
      Moving arm: Midline of the humerus
      Stable arm: Mid axilla/thorax
   ii. Available ROM: 0 to 180 degrees
   iii. End feel: Firm
   iv. Muscles responsible: Anterior deltoid
   v. Start and end position: Figure 7-21 displays the start position. The arm is positioned at the side of the body with the arm in the functional position. Raise the arm up straight to the front with the thumb up, while maintaining elbow extension. Figure 7-22 displays the end position. The arm is raised to full length reaching up.

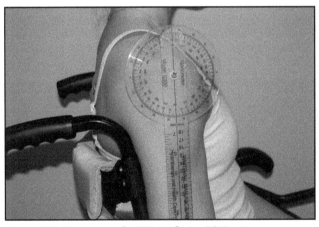

Figure 7-21. Start position for GH joint flexion ROM testing.

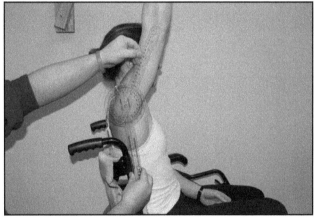

Figure 7-22. End position for GH joint flexion ROM testing.

b. GH joint extension (also called hyperextension)
   i. Goniometric landmark: Lateral surface of the acromion process
      Moving arm: Midline of the humerus
      Stable arm: Mid axilla/thorax
   ii. Available ROM: 0 to 50 degrees
   iii. End feel: Firm
   iv. Muscles responsible: Latissimus dorsi, posterior deltoid, and teres major
   v. Start and end position: Figure 7-23 displays the start position. During GH joint extension, the arm returns to the side of the body after GH joint flexion to return the hand to the side of the body. With GH joint extension, the start position is the hand at the side of the body and the arm moves posteriorly to the furthest position available. Figure 7-24 displays the end position.

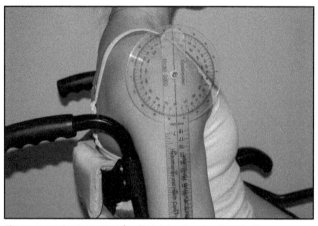

Figure 7-23. Start position for GH joint extension ROM testing.

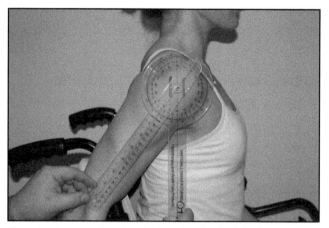

Figure 7-24. End position for GH joint extension ROM testing.

c. Anterior GH joint abduction
  i. Goniometric landmark: Anterior surface of the acromion process
     Moving arm: Medial aspect of the humerus
     Stable arm: Parallel to the spine
  ii. Available ROM: 0 to 180 degrees
  iii. End feel: Firm
  iv. Muscles responsible: Middle deltoid and supraspinatus
  v. Start and end position: Figure 7-25 displays the start position. The arm is by the side of the body in the anatomical position (GH joint adduction). The client raises their arm to the side at the shoulder with shoulder abduction maintaining the position of all other joints of the arm. The arm is raised to full height. The end position is pictured in Figure 7-26. Remember, the thumb should remain facing up when raising the arm. (This could be performed with client in supine position.)

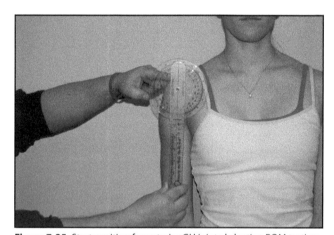

Figure 7-25. Start position for anterior GH joint abduction ROM testing.

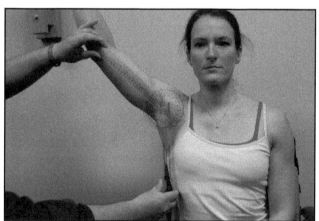

Figure 7-26. End position for anterior GH joint abduction ROM testing.

d. Posterior GH joint abduction
  i. Goniometric landmark: Posterior surface of the acromion process
     Moving arm: Medial aspect of the humerus
     Stable arm: Parallel to the spine
  ii. Available ROM: 180 to 0 degrees
  iii. End feel: Firm
  iv. Muscles responsible: Middle deltoid and supraspinatus
  v. Start and end position: Figure 7-27 displays the start position. The arm is by the side of the body in the anatomical position (GH joint adduction). The client raises their arm to the side at the shoulder with shoulder abduction maintaining the position of all other joints of the arm. The arm is raised to full height. Figure 7-28 displays the end position. (GH joint adduction is not addressed here as it is rarely measured.)

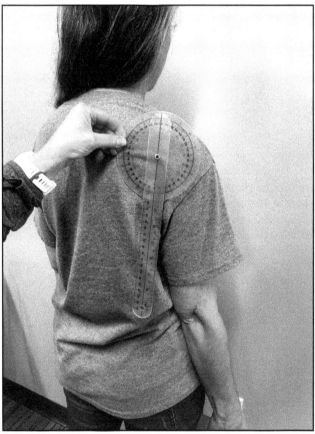
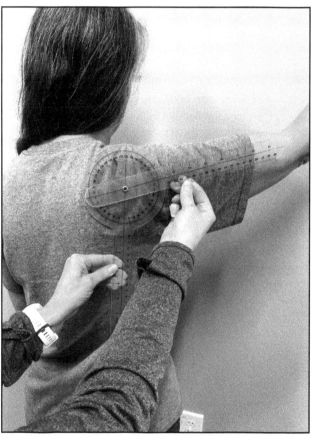

Figure 7-27. Start position for posterior GH joint abduction ROM testing.   **Figure 7-28.** End position for posterior GH joint abduction ROM testing.

e. GH joint internal rotation
  i. Goniometric landmark: Middle of the olecranon process
     Moving arm: Parallel to the midline of the ulna
     Stable arm: Maintains parallel to the forearm at the start position
  ii. Available ROM: 0 to 90 degrees
  iii. End feel: Firm
  iv. Muscles responsible: Subscapularis
  v. Start and end position: Figure 7-29 displays the start position. The client's GH joint is adducted with the upper arm positioned by the side of the body. The client's elbow is bent at 90 degrees to the front with the forearm at neutral, wrist extended. The client keeps the elbow positioned at the side of the body and rotates the hand and forearm in an arc around to the front side of the body. Figure 7-30 displays the end position.

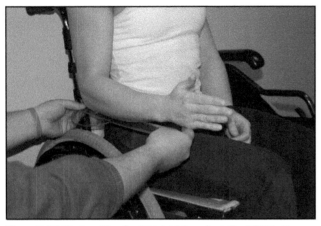

Figure 7-29. Start position for GH joint internal rotation ROM testing.

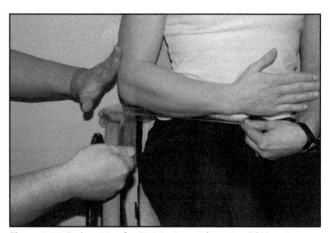

Figure 7-30. End position for GH joint internal rotation ROM testing.

f. GH joint external rotation

   i. Goniometric landmark: Middle of the olecranon process

      Moving arm: Parallel to the midline of the ulna

      Stable arm: Parallel to the forearm at the start position

   ii. Available ROM: 0 to 90 degrees

   iii. End feel: Firm

   iv. Muscles responsible: Infraspinatus, teres minor

   v. Start and end position: Figure 7-31 displays the start position. The client's GH joint is adducted with the upper arm positioned by the side of the body. The client's elbow is bent at 90 degrees to the front with the forearm at neutral, wrist extended. The client keeps the elbow positioned at the side of the body and rotates the hand and forearm in an arc away from the midline of the body. Figure 7-32 displays the end position.

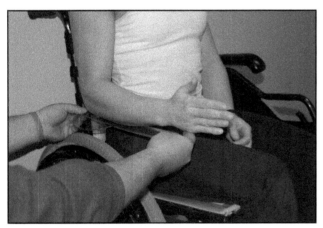

Figure 7-31. Start position for GH joint external rotation ROM testing.

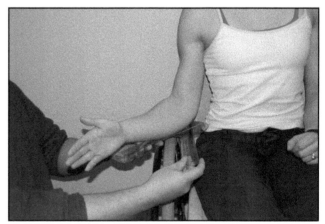

Figure 7-32. End position for GH joint external rotation ROM testing.

g. GH joint horizontal adduction

   i. Goniometric landmark: Superior aspect of the acromion process

      Moving arm: Remains parallel to the humerus position during motion

      Stable arm: Remains parallel to the humerus position prior to motion

   ii. Available ROM: 0 to 135 degrees

   iii. End feel: Firm/soft

   iv. Muscles responsible: Pectoralis major

   v. Start and end position: Figure 7-33 displays the start position. The GH joint is positioned at 90 degrees shoulder abduction and the elbow can be flexed at 90 degrees or extended. The thumb is facing up. The client moves the arm horizontally above the ground with the arm moving across the front of the body. Figure 7-34 displays the end position.

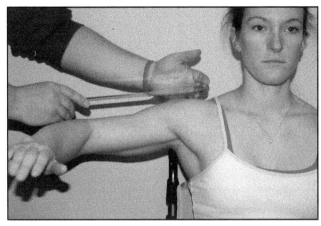

Figure 7-33. Start position for GH joint horizontal adduction ROM testing.

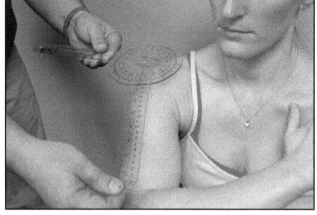

Figure 7-34. End position for GH joint horizontal adduction ROM testing.

h. GH joint horizontal abduction

    i. Goniometric landmark: Superior aspect of the acromion process

       Moving arm: Remains parallel to the humerus position during motion

       Stable arm: Remains parallel to the humerus position prior to motion

    ii. Available ROM: 0 to 45 degrees

    iii. End feel: Firm

    iv. Muscles responsible: Posterior deltoid

    v. Start and end position: Figure 7-35 displays the start position. The GH joint is positioned at 90 degrees shoulder abduction and the elbow can be flexed at 90 degrees or extended. The thumb is facing up. The client moves the arm horizontally above the ground with the elbow moving posteriorly. Figure 7-36 displays the end position.

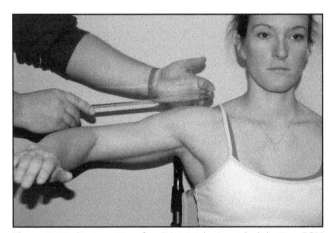

Figure 7-35. Start position for GH joint horizontal abduction ROM testing.

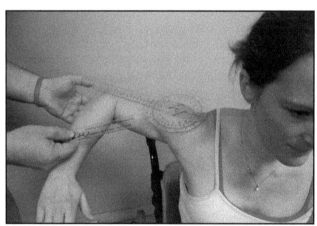

Figure 7-36. End position for GH joint horizontal abduction ROM testing.

4. **Manual Muscle Testing (MMT)**: Complete gross MMT for motions of the GH joint using Table 7-8.

TABLE 7-8
Manual Muscle Testing Application Table

JOINT	MOTIONS	PALPATE MUSCLE GROUPS/ MUSCLES	GROSS MANUAL MUSCLE TESTING SCORE
Glenohumeral	Flexion		
	Extension		
	Hyperextension		
	Abduction		
	Adduction		
	Internal rotation		
	External rotation		
	Horizontal abduction		
	Horizontal adduction		

5. **MMT of the GH Joint**: With your partner, practice the standardized procedure for identifying gross MMT for each GH joint motion.

   a. GH joint flexion and extension: Testing procedure: Figure 7-37 displays the start position for GH joint flexion. The client moves their arm halfway into GH joint flexion, or to about 90 degrees of flexion. The therapist stabilizes just proximal to the GH joint to avoid compensation. Resistance is applied just distal to the GH joint, half the distance to the elbow. The client is asked to maintain their arm position as resistance is provided on the humerus in the opposite direction to GH joint flexion. Figure 7-38 displays the testing position. GH joint extension is tested similarly. The arm is positioned at the side of the body. The client moves their GH joint posteriorly to about 25 degrees. Some books identify this motion as hyperextension. The therapist stabilizes just proximal to the GH joint to avoid compensation. Resistance is applied just distal to the GH joint, half the distance to the elbow. The client is asked to maintain their arm position while resistance is provided on the humerus in the opposite direction to GH joint extension.

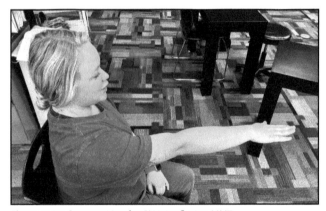

Figure 7-37. Start position for GH joint flexion MMT.

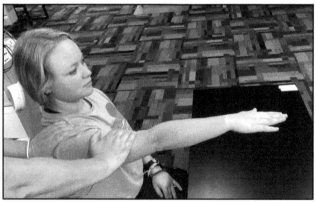

Figure 7-38. Test position for GH joint flexion MMT.

b. GH joint abduction and adduction: Testing procedure: Figure 7-39 displays the start position for GH joint abduction. The arm is positioned at 90 degrees shoulder abduction. The therapist stabilizes just proximal to the GH joint to avoid compensation. Resistance is applied just distal to the GH joint, half the distance to the elbow. The client is asked to maintain this position as resistance is provided on the humerus in the opposite direction to GH joint abduction. Figure 7-40 displays the testing position. GH joint adduction is tested similarly. The arm is positioned at 90 degrees shoulder abduction. The client is asked to maintain their arm position while resistance is provided on the humerus in the opposite direction to GH joint adduction.

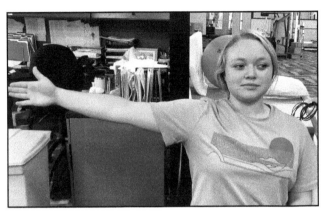

Figure 7-39. Start position for GH joint abduction MMT.

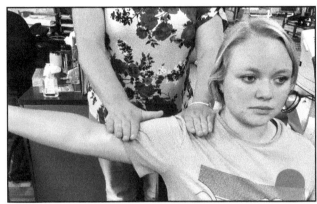

Figure 7-40. Test position for GH joint abduction MMT.

c. GH joint internal rotation and external rotation: Testing procedure: Figure 7-41 displays the start position for GH joint internal rotation. The arm is positioned at the side of the body with the elbow bent at 90 degrees to the front with the thumb facing up. The forearm is positioned at 45 degrees internal rotation. The therapist stabilizes the arm at the elbow against the body to avoid compensation. Resistance is applied just distal to the elbow. The client is asked to maintain their position of the arm while resistance is provided on the side of the forearm in the opposite direction to GH joint internal rotation. Figure 7-42 displays the testing position. GH joint external rotation is tested similarly, except the arm is positioned in 45 degrees of external rotation. Again, the client is asked to maintain their arm position as resistance is provided on the humerus in the opposite direction to GH joint external rotation.

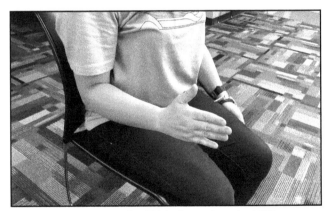

Figure 7-41. Start position for GH joint internal rotation MMT.

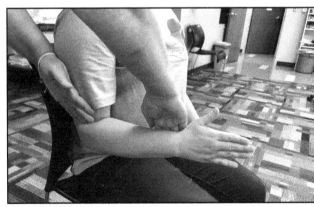

Figure 7-42. Test position for GH joint internal rotation MMT.

d. GH joint horizontal adduction and horizontal abduction: Testing procedure: Figure 7-43 displays the start position for GH joint horizontal adduction. The arm is positioned at 90 degrees shoulder abduction and 90 degrees elbow flexion with the palm facing the ground. The arm is then positioned about 70 degrees GH joint horizontal adduction. The therapist stabilizes the arm distal to the GH joint to avoid compensation. Resistance is applied just distal to the shoulder, against the humerus, halfway to the elbow. The client is asked to maintain the arm position as resistance is provided on the side of the humerus in the opposite direction to GH joint horizontal adduction. Figure 7-44 displays the testing position. GH joint horizontal abduction is tested similarly. The arm is positioned at about 20 degrees GH joint horizontal abduction. Again, the client is asked to maintain their arm position as resistance is provided on the humerus in the opposite direction to GH joint horizontal abduction.

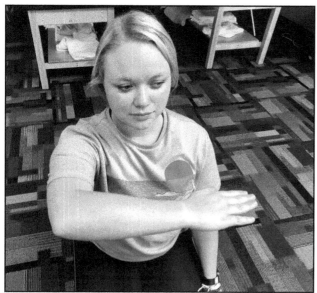

Figure 7-43. Start position for GH joint horizontal adduction MMT.

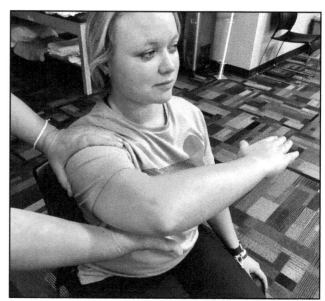

Figure 7-44. Test position for GH joint horizontal adduction MMT.

CHAPTER 8

Function and Movement of the Elbow Complex

Carolyn L. Roller, OTR/L

Key Terms

carrying angle

cubital tunnel syndrome

distal biceps tendon rupture

elbow complex

ergonomics

force couple

lateral epicondylitis

nursemaid's elbow

palpation

repetitive stress injuries

ulnar collateral ligament

Chapter Outline

Introduction

Occupational Profile

Body Functions of the Elbow Complex

    Motions of the Elbow Complex

    Strength Characteristics of the Elbow Complex

    Four Problems of the Elbow Complex

Body Structures of the Elbow Complex

    Muscle Actions of the Elbow Complex

    Muscles, Nerves, and Spinal Cord Levels

    Tendons and Ligaments

Summary

References

Applications

Sain, S. J., & Roller, C. L. *Kinesiology for the Occupational Therapy Assistant:
Essential Components of Function and Movement, Third Edition* (pp. 179-202).
© 2024 Taylor & Francis Group.

Chapter Objectives

After completion of this chapter, students should be able to:

1. Define key terminology.
2. Justify how the movement and strength of the elbow complex affects occupational performance of the upper extremity.
3. Describe four problems of the elbow complex treated in occupational therapy.
4. Analyze how body structures of the elbow complex combine to allow occupational roles.
5. Organize the muscles of the elbow and forearm and their actions and innervations.
6. List the strength characteristics of the elbow complex.

Introduction

This chapter describes the movement and function of the **elbow complex**, which consists of body structures that provide motion at the elbow and forearm. The interrelated joints of the elbow are the humeroradial and the humeroulnar joints. The forearm consists of the proximal radioulnar joint. The elbow complex provides strength and stability with its primary role positioning the hand for functional activities. The tightly fitting bony articulations of the elbow joint limits certain movements to provide the strength and stability to withstand forces one to three times the body weight when the arm is extended during weight-bearing activities. Because of this, the elbow complex is prone to **repetitive stress injuries**, which are addressed through repeated references to the client in the occupational profile and when describing common problems treated by occupational therapists. Three of the four problems presented in this chapter are introduced here. **Cubital tunnel syndrome** or ulnar nerve entrapment can be caused by pressure over the superficial ulnar nerve at the medial elbow, frequent positioning of the elbow in extreme flexion, and/or repetitive motion. Symptoms may include tingling and numbness in the ring and small fingers. **Lateral epicondylitis** or tennis elbow presents with pain and inflammation in the lateral elbow caused by repetitive use. An **ulnar collateral ligament** (UCL) tear is seen more frequently in college and professional baseball pitchers. Throwers will complain of pain and instability on the medial side of the elbow. Finally, readers will learn all body structures of the elbow complex as they relate to function.

Occupational Profile

The following occupational profile is provided to demonstrate how body functions and body structures are related to the elbow complex. Through the client, David, this profile will show how occupational therapy intervention can affect elbow complex impairment. References to David will be made throughout this chapter.

David is a 47-year-old carpenter working in construction and receiving occupational therapy with a physician's referral to improve right dominant elbow function with less pain.

During the occupational therapy evaluation, the following data were gathered.

Subjective: David states that he has experienced pain in his right lateral elbow for about 8 months. The pain has worsened over the past month, negatively affecting his function. He reports that he was referred to occupational therapy and placed on a 10-pound weightlifting restriction at work for the right upper extremity (UE) after seeing the doctor last week. David reports his signs and symptoms have included pain in the right elbow, which is exacerbated when gripping with the elbow extended and palm facing down. He states that his grip has weakened, causing him to drop items at times while working. David has been using his carpentry skills at home, remodeling his kitchen on the weekends for the past 6 months. He says that he has been unable to work on his remodeling project over the past month due to right elbow pain and weakness. He has not been able to enjoy his favorite leisure activity of fishing and has not been able to play catch with his son, who is a star pitcher for the high school baseball team.

David denies any history of past medical problems. He reports occasionally taking over-the-counter medicine for his elbow pain.

Objective: David rates the pain in his right elbow as 2/10 when he is at rest and 7/10 at its worst during active range of motion (AROM). He reports his worst pain is with resistive gripping, such as using a hammer at work, casting a fishing line and reeling it in, or throwing the baseball back to his son during practice. He states, "It hurts my arm when I start the truck or shift it into gear, and I even have pain when I brush my teeth!"

AROM is within normal limits in the bilateral UEs; however, the client reports pain in the lateral epicondyle at the end range of motion (ROM) of elbow extension, full wrist extension, and full forearm pronation.

UE strength was tested using manual muscle testing (MMT), dynamometer, and pinch meter. MMT was 5/5 in the bilateral UEs, except wrist extensors in the right UE, which were 4/5 with complaints of pain. A dynamometer was used to evaluate grip strength in standard and stressed positions. The standard position is performed with the arm at the side, elbow at 90 degrees of flexion, and forearm in neutral. The stressed position is performed with the elbow fully extended and the forearm pronated. Grip strength was recorded as follows:

STANDARD POSITION		
Average male 45 to 50 years old	Right: 110 lbs	Left: 100 lbs
Grip (David's)	Right: 90 lbs	Left: 120 lbs
STRESSED POSITION		
Grip (David's)	Right: 75 lbs	Left: 135 lbs
Note: The client reports pain with grip on the right more so in the stressed position.		
Pinch (key or lateral)	Right: 28 lbs	Left: 29 lbs
Average	Right: 27 lbs	Left: 25 lbs
Pinch (palmar or three-jaw chuck)	Right: 20 lbs	Left: 26 lbs
Average	Right: 24 lbs	Left: 24 lbs
Note: The client reports pain with right palmar pinch only. lbs = pounds.		

David denies any numbness or tingling in his UEs. There was mild localized edema observed just distal to the right lateral epicondyle and thickness was palpated in this area by the therapist upon evaluation. The client was extremely tender to deep **palpation** over the insertion of the extensor carpi radialis brevis (ECRB) tendon at the right lateral epicondyle at the time of the occupational therapy evaluation.

Goals were established by the occupational therapist in collaboration with David as follows:

Short-Term Goals:

1. Client will be instructed in and comply with a home exercise program within 2 weeks.
2. Client will present with decreased pain from 7/10 to 3/10 at worst during tool use and lifting tasks at work within 4 weeks by using modified lifting techniques, adapting tool handles, using cold modalities, and performing stretches.
3. Client will increase right grip strength by 5 pounds with report of no greater pain within 4 weeks.

4. Client will be able to drive his truck and brush his teeth using his dominant hand with no complaints of pain in the right elbow within 3 weeks.
5. Client will be able to work with a 20-pound lifting restriction on the right UE and fewer complaints of pain in the right elbow within 6 weeks.

Long-Term Goals:

1. Client will demonstrate compliance and independence in a home exercise program at discharge.
2. Client will be independent in self-care and occupational roles using the right UE with no complaints of pain and utilization of ergonomic considerations within 12 weeks.
3. Client will demonstrate MMT and grip pinch strength within normal limits in the right UE within 12 weeks.
4. Client will demonstrate the ability to fish without pain in his right UE at discharge.

The outcome of David's occupational therapy intervention along with treatment techniques and goals achieved can be found in Appendix C.

Body Functions of the Elbow Complex

Joint motions and strength characteristics of the elbow and radioulnar joint as they relate to function will be described in the following section. Also, four common problems seen in the elbow complex and treated in occupational therapy will be defined and discussed. References will be made to David's occupational profile throughout this chapter.

The elbow complex consists of the body structures that provide motion at the elbow and forearm. There are also body structures in the forearm that provide motion at the wrist and the hand; however, these will be discussed in Chapter 9. According to Floyd and Thompson (2001), the elbow consists of two interrelated joints, the humeroulnar and humeroradial joints. The forearm consists of the proximal radioulnar joint. The primary role of the elbow complex is positioning and stabilizing the hand for functional activities, much like the shoulder complex. The elbow complex is made to be strong and stable. Unfortunately, this stability does not allow much room for compensatory adjustments. This makes the elbow complex prone to repetitive stress injuries (Dutton, 2004). A definition of repetitive stress injuries is provided in Box 8-1. The occupational profile demonstrates one of the many overuse injuries seen in the elbow. Fortunately for David and many clients like him, he can return to his prior level of function with the assistance of occupational therapy interventions.

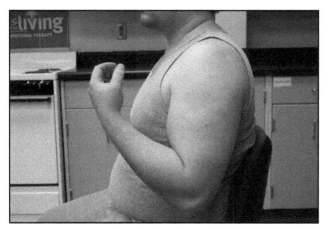

Figure 8-1. Movement of the elbow joint: flexion.

Motions of the Elbow Complex

Movements of the elbow complex include motion at the elbow and forearm of the UE. According to Weiss and Falkenstein (2005), the arc of motion needed to perform most activities of daily living (ADLs) is lower than typical available motion. Elbow ROM required to perform the majority of ADL tasks is between 30 and 130 degrees of flexion and extension. Forearm supination and pronation use is also 50 degrees each for a total arc of motion of 100 degrees. The ROM chart shown later in this chapter provides ROM norms for each of these movements. The movement of elbow flexion and extension involves the humeral articulations. The motion of forearm pronation and supination involves the proximal radioulnar joint.

Motions of the elbow are described as elbow flexion and elbow extension. Elbow flexion occurs when David bends his elbow bringing the hand to the mouth while brushing his teeth. Elbow extension occurs when David straightens his elbow, as in casting a fishing rod.

The motions of the forearm, or proximal radioulnar joint, are called *forearm supination* and *forearm pronation.* Forearm supination happens when David moves his hand from the palm-down position to the palm-up position. Carrying a full bowl of soup in the palm of the hand is an example of forearm supination. Forearm pronation is the opposite motion as when David moves his hand from palm-up to palm-down, as in reaching out to pick up his cellphone

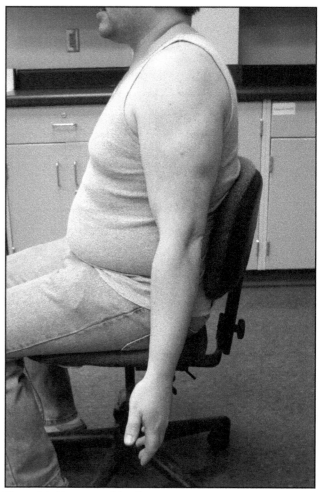

Figure 8-2. Movement of the elbow joint: extension.

from the table. When the movement of forearm rotation occurs, the radius moves around the ulna. The ulna does not rotate, as it is fixed by its bony shape at the proximal end at the olecranon process. Figure 8-1 illustrates elbow flexion, while Figure 8-2 illustrates elbow extension. Figure 8-3 illustrates forearm supination, while Figure 8-4 illustrates forearm pronation.

The **carrying angle** of the elbow provides for improved functional ROM with elbow joint motion. The carrying angle of the elbow is described as the angle formed by the long axis of the humerus and forearm. This angle is evident when the arm is in the anatomical position and the forearm

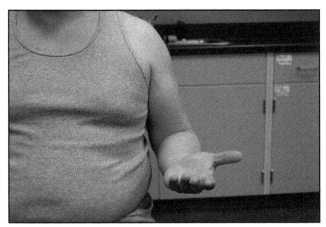

Figure 8-3. Movement of the radioulnar joint: supination.

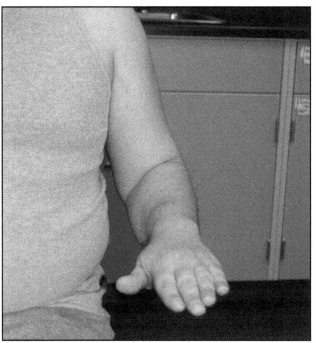

Figure 8-4. Movement of the radioulnar joint: pronation.

and humerus do not display a continuous straight line. The resting angle of the elbow prevents the arms from touching the sides of the trunk as you walk. When the elbow is fully extended, the carrying angle is typically greater in women than men due to the anatomical differences of wider hips and more narrow shoulders in many women. The carrying angle in women is about 10 to 15 degrees, while the carrying angle for men is about 5 degrees (Baskar & Kumar, 2013). When the elbow is flexed, the carrying angle serves to create improved function as the carrying angle assists in bringing the hand to the mouth (Dutton, 2004). Figures 8-5 and 8-6 provide examples of the carrying angle.

Strength Characteristics of the Elbow Complex

The structure of the elbow, as compared to the shoulder, shows increased stability and decreased mobility. The elbow is a strong and stable joint. The tightly fitting bony articulations of the elbow joint and proximal radioulnar joint restrict extreme motion in elbow extension. It is essential for the elbow joint to be strong to withstand forces one to three times the weight of the body (Oatis, 2004). UE weight-bearing activities, such as crutch walking or wheelchair propulsion, can increase forces to the elbow up to one time the body's weight. Forceful, repetitive UE activity, as seen in overhead throwing, has shown to be up to three times the body's weight in force to the elbow joint (Hertling & Kessler, 2006). Additionally, forces may be increased if the individual has weakness in the scapula stabilizers or the rotator cuff muscles of the shoulder complex.

The muscles of the elbow complex provide some joint stability, but their main role is ROM (Oatis, 2004). The four elbow flexors are the biceps, brachialis, brachioradialis, and, to a lesser degree, the pronator teres. The elbow flexors are synergists, as they work together to bend the elbow. The elbow flexor muscles are strongest at the midrange of elbow flexion, or at about 90 degrees. Additionally, the biceps muscle is a stronger flexor muscle when combined with forearm supination. The biceps supinates the forearm along with the supinator muscle. The brachialis muscle is a true elbow flexor, having no effect on forearm rotation. The brachioradialis muscle helps flex the elbow; however, it only aids resisted forearm pronation and supination as the forearm moves to neutral. The pronator teres contributes to elbow flexion only against resistance. The pronator teres assists the pronator quadratus during forearm pronation as well (Dutton, 2004).

The elbow flexors are stronger than their antagonists, the elbow extensors. The muscles that extend the elbow include the triceps and the anconeus muscle. These muscles act as synergists and are the only muscles that work together to straighten the elbow. They have no effect on forearm rotation due to their attachment on the ulna, which does not rotate during forearm pronation or supination. Like the elbow flexors, the elbow extensors are the most powerful at midrange (Hunter et al., 2002). You may notice that most activities that require upper body strength are performed with the elbow at least slightly flexed or flexed at 90 degrees. Functionally, pushing a door open, rising from a chair, or walking with crutches recruit the extensor muscles of the elbow. Opposing muscles, such as the triceps and biceps, can work together to provide elbow joint stability. A good example of this is when the arm is fully extended during weight-bearing activities, such as getting up from the floor or when a gymnast performs a handstand.

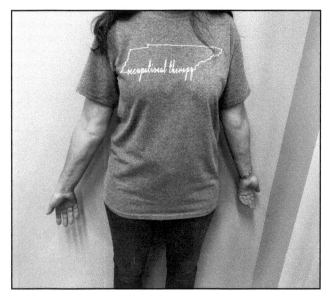

Figure 8-5. Elbow carrying angle: anatomic position.

David's occupational profile will be used to help determine the movement and strength required to complete certain daily activities using the elbow complex. As previously suggested, David is unable to participate in his favorite leisure activity of fishing, which includes casting and reeling the fishing rod, movements that cause pain in his right dominant elbow. As a result, he has stopped performing an occupational role in which he enjoys participating. Refer to Table 8-1 to identify how the joints, muscles, and nerves enable David to participate in fishing.

As you can see, one of David's instrumental activity of daily living (IADL) occupations is casting and reeling the fishing rod. This requires elbow flexion, extension, and forearm pronation. The muscles listed in Table 8-1 work with other muscles in the UE and trunk to enable participation in the fishing activity. According to Dutton (2004), the main function of the elbow complex is to help the shoulder position the hand for ADLs and IADLs. In order for David to return to independent and pain-free use of his right arm, improved coordination of the muscles and joint motion at the elbow complex is required.

Four Problems of the Elbow Complex

Discussed in this section are only four of many injuries or disease of the elbow complex treated by occupational therapists. Therapists work with clients who have a variety of functional impairments. The elbow complex is especially susceptible to overuse injuries, dislocations, fractures, and tendon and ligament tears. Consider David's occupational profile while reading about the following four elbow injuries and diseases seen in occupational therapy. Think about

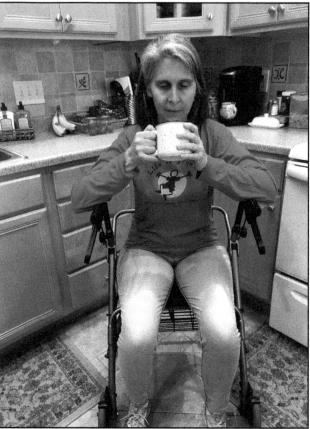

Figure 8-6. Elbow carrying angle: hand-to-mouth functional position.

David's signs and symptoms and functional limitations and see if you can identify his injury. As in the previous chapter, you can find David's epilogue in Appendix C. The epilogue will provide additional information about David's outcomes during and after occupational therapy intervention.

Ulnar Nerve Entrapment (Cubital Tunnel Syndrome)

There are a variety of nerve injuries that occur in and around the elbow. Ulnar nerve entrapment is the most common nerve injury after carpal tunnel syndrome in the UE. The ulnar nerve is the most superficial nerve in the UE as it passes through the cubital tunnel on the medial side of the elbow joint (Dutton, 2004).

Causes of cubital tunnel syndrome include pressure at the medial side of the elbow over the nerve, frequent positioning of the elbow in extreme flexion, and repetitive motion. These activities may cause inflammation and swelling, which in turn limit normal ulnar nerve gliding. The elbow in full flexion can cause pressure on the ulnar nerve at the medial epicondyle and the cubital tunnel retinaculum where the flexor carpi ulnaris inserts (Hertling & Kessler, 2006).

TABLE 8-1
Using a Fishing Rod: Movements, Muscles, and Innervations

MOVEMENT AND MUSCLES	NERVE/INNERVATION	NERVE ROOT
Elbow Flexion		
Biceps brachii	Musculocutaneous	C5, C6
Brachialis	Musculocutaneous	C5, C6
Brachioradialis	Radial	C5, C6
Elbow Extension		
Triceps	Radial	C6, C7, C8
Anconeus	Radial	C6, C7, C8
Forearm Pronation		
Pronator teres	Median	C7, C8
Pronator quadratus	Anterior interosseous, median	C7, C8, T1

Signs and symptoms of cubital tunnel syndrome may include activity-related tingling and numbness in the ring and small fingers of the hand, which may worsen at night. These signs and symptoms are often accompanied by pain in the medial elbow and can progress to include decreased sensation in the ulnar nerve distribution of the hand. Loss of grip, coordination, and muscle atrophy in the involved hand are seen frequently as well (Hunter et al., 2002).

Conservative treatment is very successful if initiated before symptoms progress to include sensory loss in the ulnar nerve distribution and intrinsic weakness of the hand. Occupational therapy treatment may include education about the diagnosis, ergonomic considerations, and restrictions. Clients are instructed to rest the affected extremity, avoid repetitive elbow movement, avoid postures that place the elbow in full flexion, and to protect the medial elbow from pressure or being bumped (Cannon, 2003).

The occupational therapy assistant will instruct the client in a home exercise program that may include nerve gliding exercises and a padded sleeve for protection for use during the day. Towel splinting at night is very effective during early conservative occupational therapy treatment. In this treatment technique, the client uses a towel wrapped around the elbow to prevent full elbow flexion during sleep. When the elbow is not allowed to bend past 90 degrees of flexion during rest, there is less pressure on the ulnar nerve, allowing it to heal. This treatment technique is very effective in decreasing numbness and tingling in the client's small and ring fingers (Cannon, 2003).

If conservative treatment fails, the client may require surgical intervention. The surgery is called *ulnar nerve transposition*. The surgeon releases the ulnar nerve in the cubital tunnel and moves the nerve to the medial side of the medial epicondyle, securing it with a flap of fascia or muscle. The client would then be seen postsurgically in occupational therapy for rehabilitation (Weiss & Falkenstein, 2005).

Distal Biceps Tendon Rupture

In a **distal biceps tendon rupture** the distal portion of the biceps tendon, which attaches at the radial tuberosity, completely tears or ruptures. This sudden injury is most often seen in muscular male clients between the ages of 35 and 60 years. The client usually reports that they were moving a heavy object when their elbow forcibly straightened against the heavy load. This caused increased stress on the biceps muscle and tearing of the tendon from the bone. In most cases, the tear is complete. A distal biceps tear is rarely associated with other medical conditions; however, smokers are more likely to experience the injury due to decreased tendon nutrition caused from the nicotine in the cigarettes (American Academy of Orthopaedic Surgeons, 2022).

The signs and symptoms of a distal biceps tendon rupture or tear may include the following:

- A pop may be heard at the elbow at the time of the injury when the tendon ruptures.
- Pain in the elbow that subsides about 1 to 2 weeks after injury.
- Visible swelling and bruising at the elbow and forearm may occur.
- Weakness with elbow flexion and forearm supination.
- A bulging in the upper arm where the biceps muscle has recoiled.

BOX 8-2

Ergonomics: The study of the interaction between human capabilities and the demands of their occupational roles. Occupational therapy and ergonomics are both concerned with an individual's adaptation to their physical environment.

(Hertfelder & Gwin, 1989)

It is recommended that a distal biceps tendon tear is surgically repaired, especially in a younger, more active individual. Without repair, there is a 30% loss of elbow flexion and a 40% loss of supination strength. After surgical repair, the injured extremity is protected for 6 to 8 weeks. During this protective phase, the client is seen in occupational therapy. The client is referred to therapy approximately 2 weeks postoperatively after the cast is removed. The occupational therapy practitioner will fit the client with a hinged elbow brace locked between 70 and 90 degrees of flexion. The client is then instructed in AROM to the shoulder, wrist, and hand as part of a home exercise program. The client is also instructed in scar and edema management techniques to promote healing and to improve ROM. Only passive range of motion is allowed for elbow flexion and forearm supination. The client is also limited to 40 degrees of elbow extension to protect the repair. At 6 weeks after surgery, the client is allowed to perform AROM out of the brace, but the hinged brace continues to be worn unlocked for protection until 8 weeks postoperatively. The occupational therapy assistant will begin instructing the client in light resistive exercises and light functional tasks at 8 weeks after repair.

The individual with a distal biceps tendon repair has to restrict functional activities somewhat until the tendon is fully healed, which takes 3 to 6 months. Most individuals can return to full ROM and heavy activities, including jobs requiring manual labor, at the end of 6 months (Hertling & Kessler, 2006).

Lateral Epicondylitis (Tennis Elbow)

Lateral epicondylitis, or tennis elbow, commonly presents with inflammation and pain in the elbow caused from overuse. As the term *tennis elbow* suggests, playing racquet sports can cause this condition, as well as other recreational and work-related activities that require repetitive use of the forearm muscles. Carpenters, cooks, painters, and butchers develop tennis elbow more often than other occupations. Individuals between the ages of 30 and 50 years also get tennis elbow more frequently. Men develop the condition more often than women and more frequently in their dominant elbow (American Academy of Orthopaedic Surgeons, 2022).

The symptoms include pinpoint pain at the lateral epicondyle of the elbow that slowly worsens over weeks and months. There is usually no specific injury related to the beginning of symptoms. Individuals will also complain of a weak grip and report more pain with activities that require sustained gripping, such as holding a tool or shaking hands. More pain is also reported in lifting an object with the forearm in pronation (DeSmet & Fabry, 1997).

Inflammation and pain are caused by microscopic tears in the ECRB tendon where it attaches at the lateral epicondyle. Because the ECRB muscle stabilizes the wrist in extension when the elbow is extended, the risk of weakening from overuse increases, causing small tears. When treated conservatively, tennis elbow resolves in approximately 90% of clients (Hertling & Kessler, 2006). Occupational therapy conservative treatment may consist of the following:

- Client education
- Rest
- Ergonomic considerations
- Bracing
- Use of cold and heat
- Stretching
- Scar mobilization
- Strengthening

The occupational therapy goals of conservative treatment in tennis elbow are to decrease pain and inflammation, prevent recurrence of signs and symptoms, and increase functional use of the injured arm. Client education of the diagnosis and the rehabilitation process can increase compliance. The client is taught to rest the injured UE as much as possible and to use cold to decrease inflammation and pain. The client is shown how to adapt tools by making the handles larger and pacing themselves throughout the workday with rest breaks. Clients are educated on how to lift with the weight closer to their center of gravity and with their palms up to lessen the strain on the forearm extensor muscles (Dutton, 2004). These adaptations are a few examples of ergonomic considerations. A definition of **ergonomics** is provided in Box 8-2.

Bracing the wrist in neutral for a time can decrease the tension and avoid additional micro-tearing on the ECRB tendon when extending the wrist and fingers. This is because the ECRB muscle originates on the lateral epicondyle of the humerus and inserts in the hand and fingers. Observe or palpate approximately 1 inch distal to your lateral epicondyle and wiggle your fingers. You can feel or see the movement where the extensor tendon originates at the lateral epicondyle. As a review, palpation is defined as medically examining by touch. As therapists, we use palpation frequently to

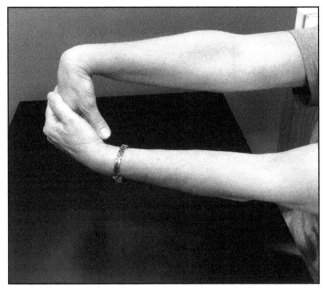

Figure 8-7. Tennis elbow stretch.

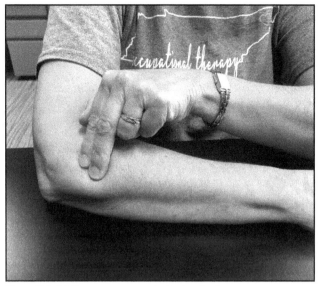

Figure 8-8. Friction massage exercise for tennis elbow.

identify muscles, bony landmarks, and signs and symptoms of injury and disease, such as swelling, scar tissue, and inflammation. You will have an opportunity to practice your palpation skills in the applications section of this chapter.

The occupational therapy assistant would teach the client to perform a home exercise program of passive stretching by bending the wrist into flexion with the elbow extended. This stretch elongates the tendons at the lateral epicondyle to avoid additional micro-tearing and promotes blood flow and healing. A friction massage over the origin of the tendon at the lateral elbow will decrease scar tissue and increase blood flow as well. To perform a friction massage, the client would use two to three fingers and massage perpendicular to the muscle fibers on dry skin with moderate pressure for about 1 minute three times per day or as tolerated. Figures 8-7 and 8-8 illustrate examples of passive stretching and friction massage.

When the client's pain and inflammation have decreased, the treatment would include gradual forearm strengthening. Progression would continue in a home exercise program if signs and symptoms are lessened. Clients tend to do well with conservative treatment due to the fact they now understand what has caused their pain and dysfunction. The epilogue on the occupational profile of David will follow his treatment and progress during occupational therapy and provide the reader with additional information on tennis elbow.

Ulnar Collateral Ligament Tear (Tommy John Injury)

UCL reconstruction, or Tommy John surgery, was first performed by Dr. Frank Jobe in 1974 on Tommy John, a pitcher for the Los Angeles Dodgers. The UCL along with the lateral collateral ligament (LCL) are two of the most important ligaments in the elbow. The UCL is also known as the *medial collateral ligament* because its anterior and posterior bands originate from the medial epicondyle of the humerus and pass over the inner side of the elbow joint. Rupture or tearing of the UCL on the medial side of the elbow can be a result of a fracture, but is more frequently seen among collegiate and professional athletes in several sports, most notably baseball. Factors causing a UCL tear in throwers are most likely overuse, but contributing factors include mechanical faults, shoulder weakness, and laxity.

Symptoms associated with a UCL injury include pain on the medial side of the elbow, a feeling of instability in the elbow, irritation of the ulnar nerve with tingling in the ring and small fingers, and a decreased ability to throw a baseball or other object. UCL reconstruction is recommended if the tear is complete or is incomplete but large. Diagnosis is usually made after magnetic resonance imaging. The surgical procedure requires a tendon graft harvested from the palmaris longus or patellar tendon. Sometimes a cadaveric tendon is used. The graft is woven in a figure-eight pattern between holes drilled in the ulna and humerus bones of the elbow and anchored in place.

Clients recovering from UCL reconstruction will be seen by an occupational or physical therapist specializing in UE orthopedic injuries as well as an athletic trainer. The rehabilitation for throwers is usually a total of 12 to 18 months. Athletes progress from early ROM, focusing on elbow extension, scar management, and reduction of edema and pain. At 8 weeks the thrower can begin strengthening, including dynamic stability and shoulder, scapula, core, and trunk strengthening. Athletes can begin throwing at about 16 weeks. Eighty percent of pitchers return to the same playing level after Tommy John surgery (Healthline, 2018).

TABLE 8-2
Muscle Function and Occupational Roles

MUSCLES	FUNCTION	EXAMPLES OF OCCUPATIONAL ROLES
• Biceps brachii • Brachialis • Brachioradialis	Elbow flexion	Phone to ear, brush teeth, put objects to mouth, shave, button shirt
• Triceps brachii • Anconeus	Elbow extension	Reach for object on table, rise from chair, put arm in sleeve, don/doff socks, tie shoes
• Pronator teres • Pronator quadratus	Forearm pronation	Use keyboard or mouse, write, cut food, pour from cup, wipe table
• Biceps brachii • Supinator	Forearm supination	Carry a bowl in palm, turn page of a book, wash face, peri care, clasp a chain at back of neck

Adapted from Latella, D., & Meriano, C. (2003). *Occupational therapy manual for the evaluation of range of motion and muscle strength.* Delmar Carnage Learning and Weiss, S., & Falkenstein, N. (2005). *Hand rehabilitation: A quick reference guide and review.* Elsevier-Mosby.

Body Structures of the Elbow Complex

Muscles, tendons, ligaments, nerves, and spinal cord levels of the elbow complex as they relate to function will be identified and discussed in this section. The ability to place the hand in space in order to perform personal care and daily activities is important to our independence and self-esteem. The motions of feeding and toileting, for example, are performed by the elbow and radioulnar joints and their supporting neuromuscular system (Hunter et al., 2002). Of course, these activities are made possible by all of the UE structures working together; however, the elbow complex is of vital importance to the performance of these functional activities.

Muscle Actions of the Elbow Complex

The muscles of the elbow complex are divided by function into flexors, extensors, pronators, and supinators. Certain muscles perform more than one action just as other muscles can work differently in combination with each other. An overview of the elbow complex muscles and their functional roles can be found in Table 8-2.

The flexors of the elbow complex are the biceps brachii, brachialis, and the brachioradialis muscles. The biceps brachii is considered a multiarticular muscle. It serves as a weak shoulder flexor, but flexes the elbow and supinates the forearm (Floyd & Thompson, 2001). The biceps muscle is a stronger elbow flexor with the radioulnar joint supinated. When the forearm is in pronation, the effectiveness of the biceps muscle lessens as an elbow flexor. To show this, perform a chin-up holding the bar with the forearms in supination.

Now, try the same chin-up grasping the bar with the forearms in pronation. Your arms do not have as much strength to pull up your body weight in the second position.

The brachialis muscle is the primary elbow flexor and is strong regardless of whether the forearm is in supination or pronation. This is due to its insertion on the ulna, which is stationary during forearm rotation (Lippert, 2000). The brachialis muscle lies deeper in relation to the biceps muscle and contracts whenever the elbow flexes, gaining the nickname the workhorse of elbow flexion (Oatis, 2004).

The brachioradialis muscle is the third elbow flexor. It is strongest when flexing the elbow with the forearm in neutral due to its more lateral and distal attachment at the styloid process of the radius. The brachioradialis also provides stabilization of the elbow joint during rapid elbow flexion, such as pounding a nail into a block of wood with a hammer.

The extensor muscles of the elbow complex are the triceps brachii and the anconeus. The triceps muscle makes up all the muscle mass on the posterior side of the arm and receives its name from its three heads. Because it inserts on the olecranon process of the ulna, it is very effective at extending the elbow. It has no role in forearm rotation because it has no attachment to the rotating radius. The triceps muscle is assisted by a very small muscle called the *anconeus*. The main role of the anconeus is to pull on the annular ligament when it contracts, which keeps the ligament from being pinched in the olecranon fossa with elbow extension. The functional action of the elbow extensors can be seen when using the hand to push open a door, bearing weight on the arm while moving in bed, or rising from a sofa or chair.

The muscles that cause pronation at the radioulnar joint or place the palm facing down are the pronator teres and the pronator quadratus. The pronator teres is primarily a pronator but assists with elbow flexion due to its origin at the medial epicondyle of the humerus, especially when a heavy object is held in the hand. The pronator teres is recruited only with resisted pronation. Elbow position does not affect the action of the pronator teres. The pronator quadratus muscle is the only muscle working when pronation is unresisted. It is a deep, small, flat muscle that cannot be palpated, but it connects the distal portion of the ulna to the radius with a horizontal pull (Lippert, 2000). The pronator muscles hold the forearm in a palm-down position during functional tasks, such as typing or cleaning tabletops.

Supination, or the palm facing up, is accomplished by the biceps brachii and the supinator muscles. The biceps brachii muscle was discussed with the elbow flexors; however, it is important to mention it here as it is the primary supinator of the radioulnar joint. In forearm supination, the biceps is active even if there is no weight in the hand. The supinator muscle is a secondary forearm supinator. It acts alone with unresisted supination, but the biceps is activated with resistance (Hunter et al., 2002). The two muscles combine to rotate the radius around a stable ulna, bringing the hand from a palm-down position to a palm-up position. This action is a good example of a **force couple**, as the biceps and supinator muscles combine to produce rotary movement.

The muscle actions of the elbow complex cannot be separated, even though we try to do so for learning purposes. As in the entire body, rarely is there one muscle that works alone to stabilize or move a joint. To summarize the muscle actions of the elbow and forearm, let's return to David in the occupational profile. Because leisure activities are so important to maintain a balance in our lives, we can look at the meaning of fishing to David. He had stated in the occupational profile that he had been unable to fish due to pain and weakness in his right dominant elbow. Performing an activity analysis of casting and reeling the rod during fishing, think about what movements and muscle actions would be required at the elbow and forearm. You will find that you will use every movement and muscle in the elbow complex along with the joints and muscles of the entire UE to participate in this leisure activity.

Muscles, Nerves, and Spinal Cord Levels

Nerve roots C5, C6, C7, C8, and T1 supply the joints and muscles of the elbow complex. The muscles that flex the elbow and supinate the forearm are innervated by the C5 and C6 nerve roots and the musculocutaneous and radial nerves, respectively. The muscles that extend the elbow receive their innervation from nerve roots C6, C7, and C8 and only from the radial nerve branch. The forearm pronators are supplied by nerve roots C7, C8, and T1. The pronator teres muscle is innervated by the median nerve branch, and the pronator quadratus muscle is innervated by the anterior interosseous branch of the radial nerve (Weiss & Falkenstein, 2005). All of the muscles of the elbow complex are innervated by the terminal nerves of the brachial plexus. Table 8-3 displays the muscles, movements, and innervations of the elbow complex.

The muscles needed for each movement and the innervations required for these movements will be discussed again in relationship to David's favorite leisure activity of fishing. Table 8-1 names the movements, muscles, and nerve innervations necessary to cast and reel a fishing rod. Think about the following questions:

- Which muscles required for casting and reeling a fishing rod are innervated by the radial nerve?
- If David's radial nerve was damaged, where would he have weakness and which elbow movements would be limited?
- If he had a neck injury that affected the nerve roots C5, C6, and C7, which muscles of the elbow complex would be affected?

Elbow flexion and extension are prevalent movements in the activity of fishing. Strengthening the biceps and triceps muscles after decreasing David's pain and inflammation may prevent a recurrence of his tennis elbow. For David to continue his occupational roles in the future and prevent injury as he ages, a structured muscle-strengthening program will be required. He can also preserve his well-being with participation in his chosen leisure activity, fishing.

The elbow complex also serves as protection for the nerve branches that innervate structures more distally. Function of the distal forearm, wrist, and hand can be affected negatively if a peripheral nerve is damaged at the elbow. The radial nerve innervates distal muscles as well as the elbow extensors. If the radial nerve is damaged in the humeral area of the UE, not only will the triceps muscle be weakened, but the wrist, finger, and thumb extensors will also be affected. Referring to one of the common problems of the elbow complex discussed earlier in this chapter, cubital tunnel syndrome is seen when the ulnar nerve becomes compressed or irritated at the medial elbow. Even though the ulnar nerve does not innervate the muscles of the elbow complex, the ulnar nerve's impairment at the elbow can negatively affect the distal muscles.

TABLE 8-3

Motions of the Elbow Complex

MUSCLE	NERVE	NERVE ROOT C5	C6	C7	C8	T1	ELBOW FLEXION 0 to 140 degrees	ELBOW EXTENSION 140 to 0 degrees	FOREARM PRONATION 0 to 80 degrees	FOREARM SUPINATION 0 to 80 degrees
Biceps brachii	Musculocutaneous	X	X				X			X
Brachialis	Musculocutaneous	X	X				X			
Brachioradialis	Radial	X	X				X			
Triceps	Radial		X	X	X			X		
Anconeus	Radial		X	X	X			X		
Pronator teres	Median			X	X				X	
Pronator quadratus	Anterior interosseous (median)			X	X	X			X	
Supinator	Posterior interosseous (radial)		X							X

Adapted from Dutton, M. (2004). *Orthopaedic exam, evaluation and intervention.* McGraw-Hill; Floyd, R. T., & Thompson, C. W. (2001). *Manual of structural kinesiology* (14th ed.). McGraw-Hill; Latella, D., & Meriano, C. (2003). *Occupational therapy manual for the evaluation of range of motion and muscle strength.* Delmar Carnage Learning; and Oatis, C. A. (2004). *Kinesiology: The mechanics and pathomechanics of human movement.* Lippincott Williams & Wilkins.

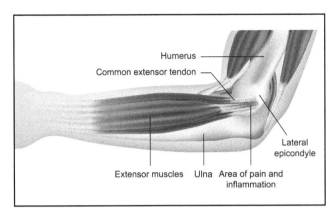

Humerus

Common extensor tendon

Lateral epicondyle

Extensor muscles Ulna Area of pain and inflammation

Figure 8-9. Tennis elbow injury. (medicalstocks/shutterstock.com)

Tendons and Ligaments

The tendons of a muscle are strong and have the ability to elongate during muscle stretch and contraction. The tendons, however, have a decreased blood supply compared to the muscle, which increases risk of injury and slows healing after injury or surgical repair. When a muscle or tendon tears, it is usually where the tendon inserts or originates at the bone or where the tendon and muscle join (the musculotendinous junction). One of the problems of the elbow complex discussed earlier in this chapter, for example, is the distal biceps tendon rupture. The distal tendon of the biceps muscle tears in most cases at the insertion, which is the radial tuberosity. In the case of David's diagnosis, tennis elbow, microscopic tears occurred at the musculotendinous junction where the ECRB attaches at the lateral epicondyle of the humerus. Figure 8-9 provides a view of the musculotendinous junction where pain and inflammation occur at the lateral epicondyle.

In comparison to the shoulder complex, the elbow complex relies on its collateral ligaments for stabilization of mediolateral movement. The ligaments of the elbow also contribute to the limits of elbow extension and prevent subluxation in this more rigid joint (Oatis, 2004). Remember, the shoulder depends on its muscles to stabilize the joints for the most part. Because the ligaments of the elbow complex are so vital for its stability, they will be named and discussed in this section. Table 8-4 identifies the elbow complex ligaments and their functions.

The LCL complex attaches proximally at the lateral epicondyle and distally on the annular ligament and the ulna (Lippert, 2000). This ligament provides stability against excessive varus deviation anywhere in the full range of elbow flexion and extension. Varus is defined as being angled inward or when a distal segment of a joint is adducted. The LCL stabilizes the ulnohumeral and radiohumeral joints when using the elbow resistively, especially when the forearm is supinated (Oatis, 2004).

The medial collateral ligament, also called the UCL, complex is larger than the LCL and attaches proximally at the medial epicondyle of the humerus and distally to the medial sides of the olecranon and coronoid processes of the ulna (Lippert, 2000). The elbow's normal alignment is valgus, as seen in the anatomic position, where the forearm (the joint distal segment) is abducted or angled outward (Oatis, 2004). This predisposes the elbow joint to valgus stress. The UCL complex, which includes the anterior and posterior bands of the UCL, protects the stability of the elbow joint against excessive valgus stress especially with the elbow flexed between 60 and 90 degrees, as in baseball pitchers (Hunter et al., 2002).

The annular ligament is a strong, broad band that surrounds the radial head, like a sling binding it to the ulna (Hunter et al., 2002). The annular ligament is effective in preventing subluxation of the head of the radius and provides protection against dislocation of the proximal radioulnar joint. An injury that is seen involving the annular ligament is known as pulled elbow or **nursemaid's elbow**. It is seen mainly in children younger than 6 years and is caused from a traction force pulling the forearm distally from the elbow. This may occur by swinging or lifting a young child by the hands (Oatis, 2004). It is believed that the weight of the child's body applies traction, pulling the radial head through the underdeveloped, looser annular ligament, causing dislocation. The lateral aspect of the radial head is narrower in a child and can slip through the annular ligament more easily when the elbow is extended and the forearm pronated (Weiss & Falkenstein, 2005). Figure 8-10 shows the mechanics of nursemaid's elbow.

The interosseous membrane is located between the ulna and the radius and helps to keep the two bones from separating through the length of the forearm (Lippert, 2000). It also plays a role in distributing loads applied during weight bearing on the hand. When an individual falls on an outstretched hand, the radius takes the load initially. The orientation of the fibers of the interosseous membrane allows the ulna to receive a portion of the load, lessening the chance of distal radius fractures (Oatis, 2004). As in all the joint movements of the body, the elbow complex relies on the coordination of muscles, the nerves that innervate them, and the supporting soft tissue structures of tendon and ligament for functional movement. All these structures work in harmony to allow clients, such as David, to participate in their preferred occupational roles that may include carpenter, father, or fisherman.

TABLE 8-4
Elbow Complex Ligaments and Their Functions

JOINT	LIGAMENT	FUNCTION
Elbow	LCL	Maintain the ulnohumeral and radiohumeral joints when the elbow is loaded in supination.
	Annular	Prevents subluxation of the radial head. Restrains the radial head and maintains the relationship with the ulna and humerus.
Radioulnar	UCL	Most important to provide stability against valgus stress, especially in the range of 20 to 130 degrees of extension and flexion.
	Annular	Same as ulnar collateral.
	Interosseous membrane	Supports radius and ulna keeping them from separating.

Adapted from Dutton, M. (2004). *Orthopaedic exam, evaluation and intervention*. McGraw-Hill and Lippert, L. S. (2000). *Clinical kinesiology for physical therapist assistants* (3rd ed.). F. A. Davis Company.

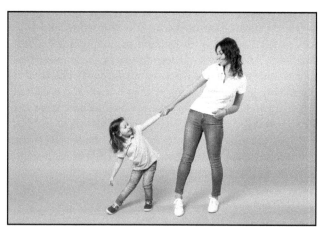

Figure 8-10. Child pulling away from mother, which demonstrates mechanics of nursemaid's elbow. (ViDI Studio/shutterstock.com)

Summary

Utilizing the occupational profile of David, this chapter has explored the movement and function of the elbow complex. The elbow complex provides motion at the elbow and forearm. The elbow allows strength and stability in the UE. These qualities withstand up to three times the body weight during UE weight-bearing activities. Due to this fact, the elbow is prone to injury, including repetitive stress injuries. In this chapter, various diseases and injuries of the elbow complex were discussed. The reader also learned that athletes, especially baseball pitchers, are more prone to elbow injury. The occupational therapy student has been introduced to body structures of the elbow complex as they relate to function. This knowledge will assist in learning how to guide the client to increase their function and independence after an elbow injury or disease process.

References

American Academy of Orthopaedic Surgeons. (2022). Biceps tendon tear at the elbow. http://orthoinfo.aaos.org/en/diseases-conditions/bicep-tendon-tear-at-the-elbow/

Baskar S., & Kumar S. (2013) Variations in carrying angle between two sexes on complete extension. *Journal of Pharmaceutical Sciences and Research, 5*(12), 269.

Cannon, N. M. (2003). *Diagnosis and treatment manual for physicians and therapists: Upper extremity rehabilitation* (4th ed.). The Hand Rehabilitation Center of Indiana.

DeSmet, L., & Fabry, G. (1997). Grip force reduction in patients with tennis elbow: Influence of elbow position. *Journal of Hand Therapy, 10*(3), 229-231.

Dutton, M. (2004). *Orthopaedic exam, evaluation and intervention.* McGraw-Hill.

Floyd, R. T., & Thompson, C. W. (2001). *Manual of structural kinesiology* (14th ed.). McGraw-Hill.

Healthline. (2018). Tommy John Surgery (UCL reconstruction) and recovery. https://www.healthline.com/health/tommy-john-surgery

Hertfelder, S., & Gwin, C. (1989). *Work in progress: Occupational therapy in work programs.* American Occupational Therapy Association.

Hertling, D., & Kessler, R. (2006). *Management of common musculoskeletal disorders: Physical therapy principles and methods.* Lippincott Williams & Wilkins.

Hislop, H. J., & Montgomery, J. (2002). *Daniel's and Worthingham's muscle testing: Techniques of manual examinations* (7th ed.). Saunders.

Hunter, J. M., Maklin, E. J., Callahan, H. D., Skirven, T. M., Schneider, L. H., & Osterman, A. E. (2002). *Rehabilitation of the hand and upper extremity* (5th ed.). Mosby.

Latella, D., & Meriano, C. (2003). *Occupational therapy manual for the evaluation of range of motion and muscle strength.* Delmar Carnage Learning.

Lippert, L. S. (2000). *Clinical kinesiology for physical therapist assistants* (3rd ed.). F. A. Davis Company.

Oatis, C. A. (2004). *Kinesiology: The mechanics and pathomechanics of human movement.* Lippincott Williams & Wilkins.

Rondinelli, R. D., Genoverse, E., Katz, R. T., Mayer, T. G., Mueller, K., & Ranavaya, M. (2008). *Guides to the evaluation of permanent impairment* (6th ed.). American Medical Association..

Weiss, S., & Falkenstein, N. (2005). *Hand rehabilitation: A quick reference guide and review.* Elsevier-Mosby.

Applications

The following activities will help you apply knowledge of the elbow and radioulnar joints in real-life applications. Activities can be completed individually or in a small group to enhance learning.

1. **The Elbow and Radioulnar Joints**: The elbow joint is the articulation of the humerus with the radius, and the ulna and is called a *uniaxial joint* because it allows for only extension and flexion. The radioulnar joint involves the proximal articulation between the ulna and the radius. This is a pivot joint because the radius moves around the ulna, but it is still considered a uniaxial joint because it only allows supination and pronation of the forearm. Complete the following activities to increase your familiarity with the aspects and movements of the elbow and radioulnar joints. Because the elbow is relatively superficial, palpation performed with knowledge of elbow anatomy can lead to significant information. The major bony landmarks are easily palpated just beneath the skin. The medial and lateral epicondyles and the olecranon process are easier to palpate with the elbow flexed to 90 degrees.

   a. Locate and palpate the following landmarks of the humerus, radius, and ulna on a partner or human skeleton model:
      i. Lateral and medial epicondyles
      ii. Radial tuberosity
      iii. Radial head
      iv. Olecranon process
      v. Coronoid process
      vi. Capitulum
      vii. Trochlea
      viii. Olecranon fossa

   b. Identify all motions of the elbow and forearm during the following functional activities:
      i. Blow-drying the hair on the back of your head:
      ii. Bringing your arm back to throw a ball:
      iii. Turning the key in the ignition of your car:
      iv. Doing a chin-up with your palms facing you:
      v. Reaching up to unscrew a light bulb:

2. **ROM of the Elbow and Radioulnar Joints**: Motions of the elbow and radioulnar joints and ROM norms are identified in Table 8-5. ROM norms can vary depending on the reference source. One norm is provided for each motion within this text to increase ease of applications. Additionally, while multiple muscles may influence a particular motion, only the main muscles responsible for a joint motion are included. References for the following information can be found in Box 8-3. With your partner, practice using a goniometer to measure each motion available at the elbow and radioulnar joints. Use Table 8-5 to record ROM for the joints of the elbow complex for both you and your partner.

TABLE 8-5
Elbow Complex Ligaments and Their Functions

JOINT	MOTIONS	AVAILABLE ROM	YOUR ROM	PARTNER'S ROM
Elbow and radioulnar joints	Flexion	0 to 140 degrees		
	Extension	140 to 0 degrees		
	Forearm supination	0 to 80 degrees		
	Forearm pronation	0 to 80 degrees		

BOX 8-3

REFERENCED WORKS FOR RANGE OF MOTION

Sections Referenced (a to e)	Reference
Goniometric landmark, end feel, and start and end positions	Latella & Meriano, 2003
Muscles responsible	Hislop & Montgomery, 2002
Available ROM	Rondinelli, 2008

a. Elbow joint flexion ROM testing
   i. Goniometric landmark: Lateral epicondyle of the humerus
     Moving arm: Midline of the radius
     Stable arm: Midline of the humerus
   ii. Available ROM: 0 to 140 degrees
   iii. End feel: Soft
   iv. Muscles responsible: Biceps brachii, brachialis, brachioradialis
   v. Start and end position: Figure 8-11 displays the start position. The arm is positioned at the side of the body with the arm fully extended and in the anatomical position. Bend the arm at the elbow into maximum flexion with the palm up. Figure 8-12 displays the end position of ROM testing.

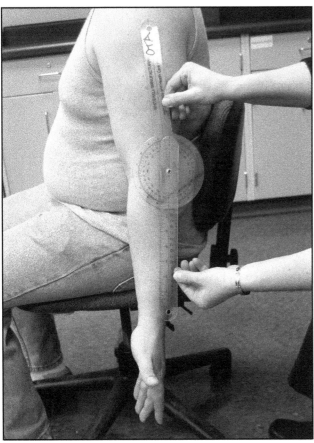

Figure 8-11. Start position for elbow flexion ROM testing.

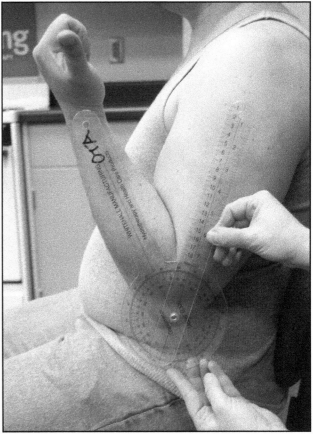

Figure 8-12. End position for elbow flexion ROM testing.

b. Elbow joint extension ROM testing

  i. Goniometric landmark: Lateral epicondyle of the humerus

     Moving arm: Midline of the radius

     Stable arm: Midline of the humerus

  ii. Available ROM: 140 to 0 degrees

  iii. End feel: Hard

  iv. Muscles responsible: Triceps and anconeus

  v. Start and end position: Figure 8-13 displays the start position for goniometric testing of elbow joint extension. During elbow extension, the arm returns to the side of the body after elbow flexion to return to the anatomical position. Figure 8-14 displays the end position.

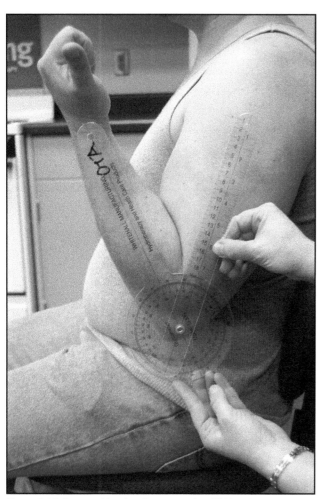

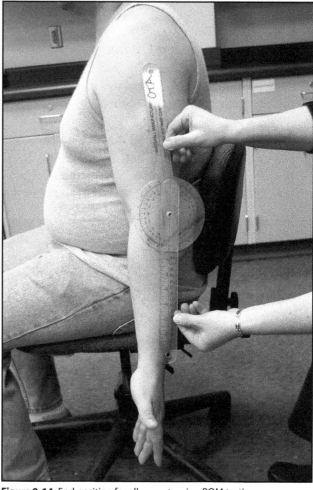

Figure 8-13. Start position for elbow extension ROM testing.

Figure 8-14. End position for elbow extension ROM testing.

c. Forearm supination ROM testing

  i. Goniometric landmark: Anterior surface of the distal forearm, 1 cm proximal to the pisiform

     Moving arm: Across the volar aspect of the distal forearm

     Stable arm: Perpendicular to the floor

  ii. Available ROM: 0 to 80 degrees

  iii. End feel: Firm

  iv. Muscles responsible: Biceps brachii, brachioradialis, supinator

  v. Start and end position: Figure 8-15 displays the start position for goniometric testing of forearm supination. The arm is at the side of the body with the humerus adducted, the elbow flexed to 90 degrees, and the forearm in neutral. The client moves their forearm into full supination or palm up, without moving the shoulder. The end position is pictured in Figure 8-16.

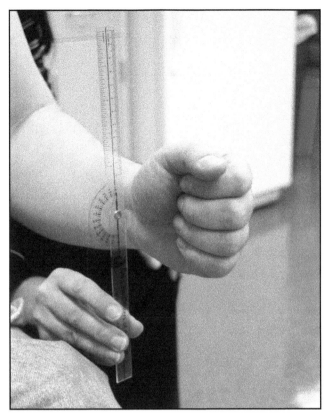

Figure 8-15. Start position for forearm supination ROM testing.

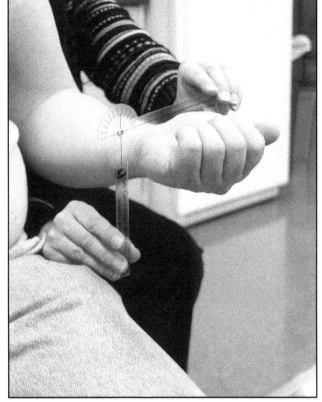

Figure 8-16. End position for forearm supination ROM testing.

d. Forearm supination ROM testing (alternate method). Note: This method requires holding a pen or pencil in the fingers and may be difficult for clients with a limitation in finger flexion.

i. Goniometric landmark: Head of third metacarpal

Moving arm: Parallel to the pen or pencil

Stable arm: Perpendicular to the floor

ii. Available ROM: 0 to 80 degrees

iii. End feel: Firm

iv. Muscles responsible: Biceps brachii, brachioradialis, and supinator

v. Start and end position: Figure 8-17 displays the start position. The client holds a pen or pencil in the fist of the arm being tested. The arm is at the side of the body with the humerus adducted, the elbow flexed to 90 degrees, and the forearm in neutral. The client moves their forearm into full supination, or palm up, without moving the shoulder. Figure 8-18 displays the end position.

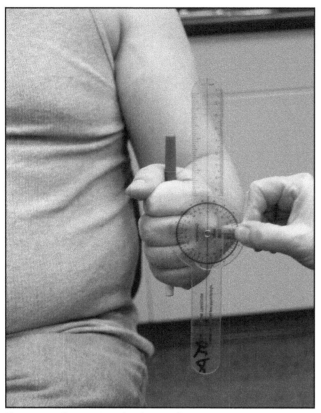

Figure 8-17. Start position for alternate forearm supination ROM testing.

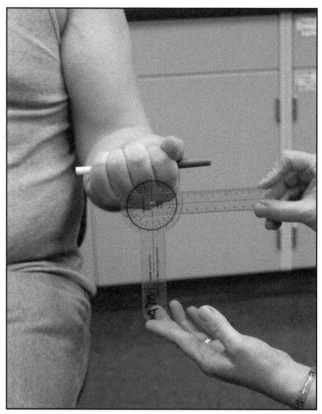

Figure 8-18. End position for alternate forearm supination ROM testing.

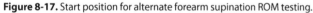

e. Forearm pronation ROM testing
   i. Goniometric landmark: Ulnar styloid process
      Moving arm: Dorsal surface of the distal forearm
      Stable arm: Perpendicular to the floor
   ii. Available ROM: 0 to 80 degrees
   iii. End feel: Firm
   iv. Muscles responsible: Pronator teres, pronator quadratus, brachioradialis
   v. Start and end position: Figure 8-19 displays the start position. The arm is at the side of the body with the humerus adducted, the elbow flexed to 90 degrees, and the forearm in neutral. The client moves their forearm into full pronation, or palm down, without moving the shoulder. Figure 8-20 displays the end position.

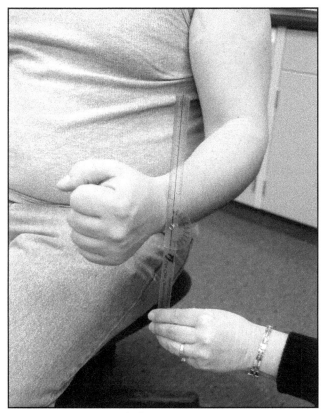

Figure 8-19. Start position for forearm pronation ROM testing.

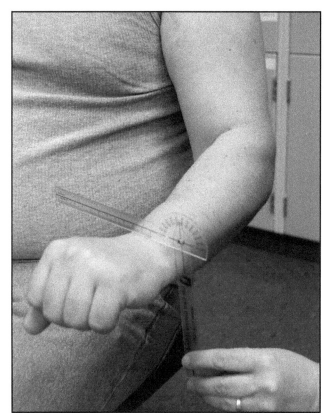

Figure 8-20. End position for forearm pronation ROM testing.

f. Forearm pronation ROM testing (alternate method). Note: This method requires holding a pen or pencil in the fingers and may be difficult for clients with a limitation in finger flexion.

    i. Goniometric landmark: Head of third metacarpal

      Moving arm: Parallel to the pen or pencil

      Stable arm: Perpendicular to the floor

    ii. Available ROM: 0 to 80 degrees

    iii. End feel: Firm

    iv. Muscles responsible: Pronator teres, pronator quadratus, brachioradialis

    v. Start and end position: Figure 8-21 displays the start position. The arm is at the side of the body with the humerus adducted, the elbow flexed to 90 degrees, and the forearm in neutral. The client moves their forearm into full pronation, or palm down, without moving the shoulder. Figure 8-22 displays the end position.

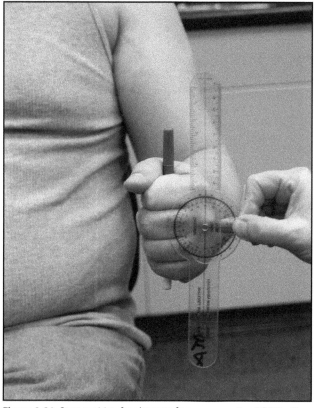

Figure 8-21. Start position for alternate forearm pronation ROM testing.

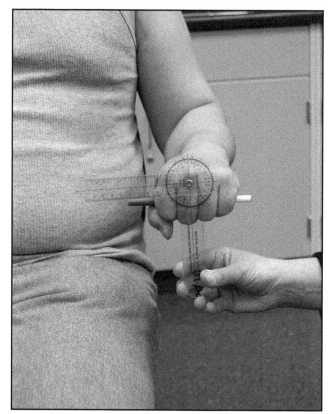

Figure 8-22. End position for alternate forearm pronation ROM testing.

3. **MMT of the Elbow Complex**: Complete gross MMT for motions of the elbow and radioulnar joints using Table 8-6. With your partner, practice the standardized procedure for identifying gross MMT for each elbow and radioulnar joint motion.

TABLE 8-6

Manual Muscle Testing Application Table

JOINT	MOTIONS	PALPATE MUSCLE GROUP/ MUSCLES	GROSS MANUAL MUSCLE TESTING SCORE
Elbow and radioulnar joints	Elbow flexion		
	Elbow extension		
	Forearm supination		
	Forearm pronation		

  a. Elbow joint flexion and extension: Testing procedure: Figure 8-23 displays the start position for elbow joint flexion. The client moves their arm halfway into elbow flexion or to about 90 degrees. The therapist stabilizes the humerus over the biceps muscle to avoid compensation. Resistance is applied to the distal/anterior forearm in the direction of elbow extension. The client is asked to move their arm in the direction of elbow flexion. Figure 8-24 displays the testing position.

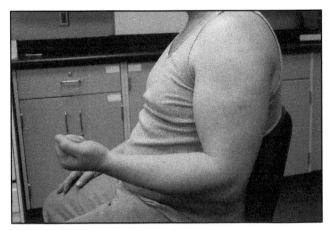

Figure 8-23. Start position for elbow flexion MMT.

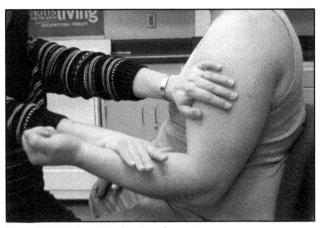

Figure 8-24. Test position for elbow flexion MMT.

Figure 8-25 displays the start position for testing elbow joint extension. The client moves their shoulder to about 120 degrees of flexion with the elbow at 90 degrees of flexion. The therapist stabilizes the humerus over the triceps muscle to avoid compensation. Resistance is applied on the ulnar portion of the distal forearm in the direction of elbow flexion. The client is asked to move their arm in the direction of elbow extension. Figure 8-26 displays the testing position.

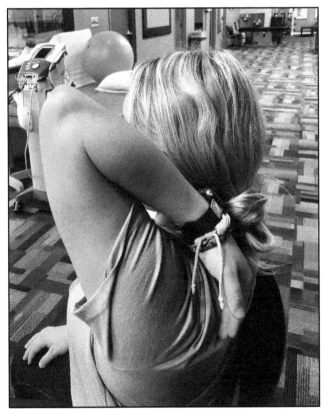

Figure 8-25. Start position for elbow extension MMT.

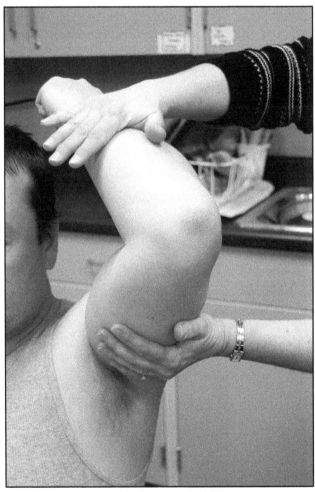

Figure 8-26. Test position for elbow extension MMT.

b. Radioulnar joint supination and pronation: Testing procedure: Figure 8-27 displays the start position for radioulnar joint supination and pronation. The arm is at the side of the body with the humerus adducted, the elbow flexed to 90 degrees, and the forearm in neutral. The therapist stabilizes the arm at the elbow to avoid compensation. To test radioulnar joint or forearm supination, resistance is applied at the distal forearm in the direction of pronation. The client is asked to move their forearm in the direction of supination. Figure 8-28 displays the testing position.

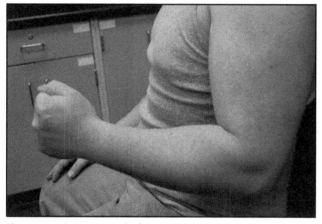

Figure 8-27. Start position for forearm supination and pronation MMT.

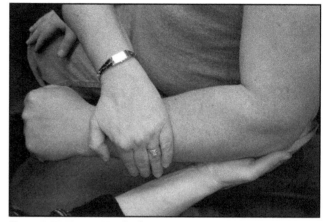

Figure 8-28. Test position for forearm supination MMT.

To test radioulnar joint or forearm pronation, resistance is applied at the distal forearm in the direction of supination. The client is asked to move their forearm in the direction of pronation. Figure 8-29 displays the testing position.

Figure 8-29. Test position for forearm pronation MMT.

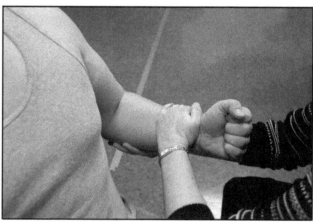

CHAPTER 9

Function and Movement of the Wrist and Extrinsic Hand

Carolyn L. Roller, OTR/L

Key Terms

anatomical snuff box

arthroscopy

attrition rupture

avascular necrosis

biaxial joint

carpometacarpal joint

circumduction

Colles fracture

complex regional pain syndrome

condyloid joint

crepitus

de Quervain's disease

distal radioulnar joint

dorsiflexion

edema

ergonomics

extrinsic muscles of the hand

fall on an outstretched hand

Finkelstein's test

fracture disease

intrinsic muscles of the hand

juncturae tendinae

malunion

open reduction with internal fixation

pointing muscle

radiocarpal joint

reflex sympathetic dystrophy

scaphoid fracture

tendon rupture

thumb spica splint

triangular fibrocartilage complex

Chapter Outline

Introduction

Occupational Profile

Body Functions of the Wrist and Extrinsic Hand

Motions of the Wrist

Motions of the Extrinsic Hand

Strength Characteristics of the Wrist and Extrinsic Hand

Four Problems of the Wrist and Extrinsic Hand

Body Structures of the Wrist and Extrinsic Hand

Muscle Actions of the Wrist

Muscle Actions of the Extrinsic Hand

Muscles, Nerves, and Spinal Cord Levels of the Wrist and Extrinsic Hand

Tendons and Ligaments of the Wrist and Extrinsic Hand

Summary

References

Applications

Sain, S. J., & Roller, C. L. *Kinesiology for the Occupational Therapy Assistant: Essential Components of Function and Movement, Third Edition* (pp. 203-228).
© 2024 Taylor & Francis Group.

Chapter Objectives

After completion of this chapter, students should be able to:

1. Define key terminology.
2. Name motions of the wrist and extrinsic hand and how they affect functional movements.
3. Discuss four problems of the wrist and extrinsic hand seen in occupational therapy.
4. Demonstrate the difference between extrinsic and intrinsic musculature of the hand.
5. Identify joints and supporting soft tissue of the wrist.
6. List the actions and innervations of the muscles in the wrist.

Introduction

This chapter describes the movement and function of the wrist and extrinsic muscles of the hand. The extrinsic muscles have their origin in the forearm but insert in the hand. Motions of the wrist include flexion, extension, and radial and ulnar deviation. Extrinsic muscles of the forearm allow digit flexion and extension. Functional activities performed by the hand and wrist when gripping can generate a high load of force, especially with certain occupations such as hammering a nail, using crutches or swinging a golf club. Throughout this chapter, references will be made to the client in the occupational profile and their functional problems, goals, and treatment. Two of the four problems are mentioned here. Distal radius fracture most often occurs when an individual falls on an outstretched hand and is the most common fracture of the upper extremity (UE). Distal radius fractures are more common in postmenopausal women who have primary osteoporosis. Early intervention to manage **edema** and active range of motion (AROM) of the fingers, elbow, and shoulder can prevent **fracture disease** caused by prolonged immobilization in a cast after wrist fracture. **de Quervain's disease** is inflammation of the tendon sheaths that form the **anatomical snuff box**, which is a small indention just distal to the radial styloid. Clients with de Quervain's disease report pain over the radial wrist and thumb with tasks such as wringing out a washcloth. Lastly, the reader will learn all the structures of the wrist and extrinsic hand and their influence on occupational performance.

Occupational Profile

The following occupational profile is provided to demonstrate occupational therapy intervention as related to the body functions and structures of the wrist and extrinsic hand. This occupational profile of Laura will show how a wrist injury can negatively affect function. References to Laura will be made throughout this chapter.

Laura is a 53-year-old teacher receiving occupational therapy with a physician's referral to increase range of motion (ROM) and decrease edema in her left dominant wrist.

During the occupational therapy evaluation, the following data were gathered.

Subjective: Laura states that 6 weeks ago, she attended a roller skating field trip with her fourth-grade class. While skating, she fell, landing on her left outstretched hand. Laura reports that she noticed immediate pain and swelling in her left wrist and hand. She went to the hospital where x-rays were taken and a cast was applied to her left arm. Laura states she was last seen by her doctor 3 days ago at which time her cast was removed. She was given a wrist brace and was referred to occupational therapy.

Today, Laura complains of stiffness and swelling in her left wrist and hand and pain when she tries to use her arm. She states she cannot drive, write, brush her teeth, feed herself, dry her hair, push a cart in the grocery store, or type on the computer using her left UE. Laura reports, "I need to be able to drive, write, and type to return to my teaching position. The cast is off, and the doctor says the bone is healed, but my wrist is stiff, and my hand is so swollen that I can't make a fist. It hurts when I try to hold the steering wheel while using the turn signal. I don't feel safe driving."

Laura reports a past medical history of high cholesterol and high blood pressure; however, both are controlled with medication. She denies any other health problems and states she lost her husband to cancer 4 years ago. She currently lives alone but has two grown children and four grandchildren who live in the area and have been helpful since her injury. She reports that she has been very active, participating in yoga and walking frequently prior to her injury. Laura states that she loves to knit but has not been able to perform that leisure activity since her injury.

Objective: Laura rates the pain in her left wrist and hand as 0/10 when she is at rest and 5/10 when the pain is at its worst. She states the worst pain is at end ROM with forearm supination, finger flexion, and wrist flexion and extension. She also reports pain as a 5/10 with inadvertent use of her injured wrist and hand.

AROM is within normal limits in both UEs, with the exception of her left forearm, wrist, and hand. Formal AROM measurements are taken with a goniometer where limitations were noted. The joints of the right forearm, wrist, and hand are measured for comparison purposes. AROM is recorded as follows:

FINGERS	MCP JOINTS		PIP JOINTS		DIP JOINTS	
	Right	*Left*	*Right*	*Left*	*Right*	*Left*
Index	0 to 81 degrees	0 to 44 degrees	0 to 98 degrees	0 to 80 degrees	0 to 70 degrees	0 to 45 degrees
Long	0 to 79 degrees	0 to 43 degrees	0 to 108 degrees	0 to 81 degrees	0 to 72 degrees	0 to 35 degrees
Ring	0 to 78 degrees	0 to 49 degrees	0 to 109 degrees	0 to 78 degrees	0 to 68 degrees	0 to 33 degrees
Small	0 to 75 degrees	0 to 35 degrees	0 to 102 degrees	0 to 79 degrees	0 to 74 degrees	0 to 39 degrees
FOREARM			**RIGHT**		**LEFT**	
Supination			0 to 90 degrees		0 to 35 degrees	
Pronation			0 to 90 degrees		0 to 60 degrees	
WRIST			**RIGHT**		**LEFT**	
Extension			0 to 78 degrees		0 to 15 degrees	
Flexion			0 to 93 degrees		0 to 30 degrees	
Radial deviation			0 to 24 degrees		0 to 11 degrees	
Ulnar deviation			0 to 36 degrees		0 to 16 degrees	
THUMB			**RIGHT**		**LEFT**	
MCP flexion			0 to 52 degrees		0 to 20 degrees	
IP flexion			0 to 90 degrees		0 to 15 degrees	

DIP = distal interphalangeal; MCP = metacarpophalangeal; PIP = proximal interphalangeal.
Measurements are recorded as extension/flexion.
Note: The fingers are often referred to as digits one through five beginning with the thumb and ending with the small finger. In this chapter, the digits will be referred to as thumb, index, long or middle, ring, and small fingers.

Laura is unable to make a full fist due to a lack of finger flexion. The linear edge of the goniometer is used to measure the gap from each finger pad to the distal palmar crease and is recorded as follows:

Index finger: 3.5 cm   Ring finger: 3.0 cm

Long finger: 3.0 cm   Small finger: 2.5 cm

Edema is observed to be moderate in the left hand and fingers, with pitting edema noted over the dorsum of the hand. Mild edema is noted in the wrist and distal forearm. Whole hand edema was evaluated using the volumeter with measurements as follows:

Right: 445 mL   Left: 520 mL

Laura complains of unresolved tingling and numbness in her left thumb and index and long fingers, which began when her cast was applied after her injury. Visual examination reveals discoloration of the entire left hand as compared to her uninvolved hand, especially in the thumb and fingers. Manual examination reveals that the fingertips of the left hand feel cold as compared to the fingertips of the right hand. Palpation reveals tenderness over the medial and lateral sides of the PIP and DIP joints of all fingers and over the radial wrist.

Sensory screening is performed, revealing intact two-point discrimination in the left fingertips. Light touch sensation is evaluated using Semmes-Weinstein monofilaments. Findings include normal light sensation (2.83 g) present on the palmar surface of the fingertips of the right hand and the small finger and ulnar portion of the ring finger of the left hand. The left thumb, index finger, long finger, and radial aspect of the ring finger reveal diminished protective light touch sensation (4.31 g). Grip and pinch strength are not tested at this time due to pain and limitations in finger ROM.

Goals were established by the occupational therapist in collaboration with Laura and are presented as follows.

Short-Term Goals:

1. Client will be instructed in and comply with a home exercise program within 2 weeks.

2. Client will tolerate a formal evaluation of left grip and pinch strength when able and appropriate, or within 4 weeks.

3. Client will demonstrate the ability to grade students' papers using the left dominant hand and adaptive writing implements within 3 weeks.

4. Client will demonstrate self-feeding with the left hand and adaptive utensils within 2 weeks.

5. Client will demonstrate decreased edema by 30 mL using edema control techniques of elevation, AROM, and wearing of an Isotoner glove within 3 weeks.

6. Client will demonstrate an increase in AROM in all limited joints by 5 degrees in each joint in 4 weeks.

Long-Term Goals:

1. Client will demonstrate compliance and independence in a home exercise program at discharge.

2. Client will be independent in self-care and occupational roles using the left dominant hand and adaptive equipment within 3 months.

3. Client will demonstrate AROM to within functional limits in left forearm, wrist, and thumb and demonstrate a straight fist in left hand within 3 months.

4. Client will demonstrate a decrease in edema by 50 mL in the left hand volumetrically in 3 months.

5. Client will demonstrate functional ROM in the left dominant hand by resuming her leisure activity of knitting in 3 months.

The outcome of Laura's occupational therapy intervention along with treatment techniques and goals achieved can be found in Appendix C.

Body Functions of the Wrist and Extrinsic Hand

The difference between **extrinsic** and **intrinsic muscles in the hand** is that extrinsic muscles have their origin in the forearm and insert in the hand whereas intrinsic muscles both originate and insert in the hand. Intrinsic muscles and their body functions will be discussed in Chapter 10. In this part of the chapter, joint motions and strength characteristics of the wrist and extrinsic hand as they relate to function will be described. Remember, all the body functions of the UE are interconnected, especially wrist and hand function, both extrinsic and intrinsic. It is difficult to divide the UE into chapters; however, it is necessary for reading and comprehension. Please keep this in mind as you continue. Four problems of the wrist and extrinsic hand commonly treated in occupational therapy will be identified and discussed. Throughout this chapter, references will be made regarding Laura and her functional problems, goals, and treatment.

Motions of the Wrist

The wrist joint is also known as the **radiocarpal joint** and is classified as a **biaxial**, or **condyloid**, **joint** (Lippert, 2000). The wrist joint allows flexion, extension, radial deviation, and ulnar deviation. Because it is a biaxial joint, the wrist also combines these four movements to produce **circumduction**, which is a circular movement of the hand on the forearm (Oatis, 2004).

The amount of wrist motion can vary significantly among clients and even in the same client when comparing the right to the left wrist (Rybski, 2019). Wrist ROM can vary due to ligament tightness or laxity, muscle mass, and articulating surface lubrication (Weiss & Falkenstein, 2005). Normal and functional wrist motions vary significantly according to different references. A table listing wrist ROM for this text and the references cited can be found later in this chapter. Normal wrist ROM can best be determined by comparison of the involved wrist to the uninvolved wrist of the client.

Studies show that individuals can perform independent functional activities with less than normal or full wrist ROM (Oatis, 2004). According to Weiss and Falkenstein (2005), functional wrist ROM for performing most activities of daily living is 40 degrees of combined wrist flexion and extension and 40 degrees of composite radial and ulnar deviation. For example, using a fork or holding a newspaper only requires 35 degrees of wrist extension, whereas weight bearing while using a cane may require 40 degrees of wrist extension (Oatis, 2004). These functional examples demonstrate less-than-normal wrist extension.

Flexion occurs when the client bends their wrist down as if trying to touch the fingers to the anterior aspect of the distal forearm. A daily self-care task that uses wrist flexion is toileting. Wrist extension (occasionally called **dorsiflexion**) occurs when the client bends their wrist back, such as holding a cellphone to the ear. Weight-bearing activities, such as pushing up from a chair or using a walker, are additional examples of functional activities that require wrist extension.

The side-to-side wrist motions are called *radial* and *ulnar deviation*. Wrist radial deviation is seen when the client moves their wrist toward the thumb side of the hand. Wrist ulnar deviation is the opposite of radial deviation and occurs when the client moves their wrist toward the small finger side of the hand. These movements most likely occur when the client casts a fishing rod or uses a hammer. The combination of all four wrist motions together is called *circumduction* and occurs when a client washes their hands or beats an egg with a fork. Figures 9-1 through 9-4 demonstrate wrist flexion, extension, radial deviation, and ulnar deviation.

Motions of the Extrinsic Hand

The wrist and hand motions involve extrinsic musculature only, while fine hand motions involve extrinsic and intrinsic muscles working together. There may, therefore, be some overlap when describing motions of the extrinsic hand in this chapter with motions of the intrinsic hand in Chapter 10.

The thumb is the first digit of the hand and has three joints: the **carpometacarpal** (CMC), MCP, and IP joints (Lippert, 2000). The CMC joint of the thumb is a saddle joint, providing mobility in all directions (Hertling & Kessler, 2006). The thumb CMC joint is formed by the trapezium bone proximally and the first metacarpal bone distally. The trapezium is rotated anteriorly out of the plane of the hand, which facilitates opposition of the thumb (Oatis, 2004). Figure 9-5 illustrates a hand in a relaxed position and the way the thumb is positioned out of the plane of the hand. Motions of the thumb include flexion, radial abduction (also called *extension*), palmar abduction, adduction, and opposition. When the forearm is supinated and the palm is facing up, thumb flexion and radial abduction (extension) is the side-to-side movement across the palm and out. A functional example of thumb radial abduction (extension) and flexion would be turning the page of a book using the left hand. Figure 9-6 demonstrates thumb radial abduction (extension) while Figure 9-7 demonstrates thumb flexion. The MCP joint of the thumb is a hinged uniaxial joint, allowing only flexion and extension. Thumb MCP movement combines with the CMC joint and IP joint of the thumb to provide full opposition and reposition. Reposition is the movement of the thumb as it returns from opposition. Functional movements of the thumb will be covered in more detail in Chapter 10.

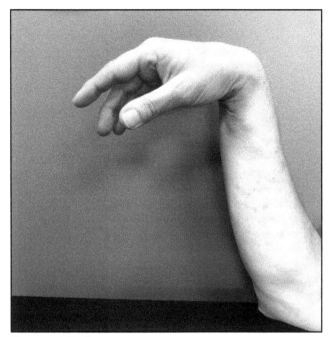

Figure 9-1. Wrist flexion.

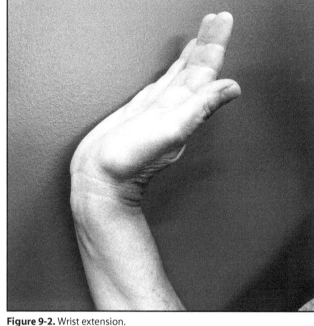

Figure 9-2. Wrist extension.

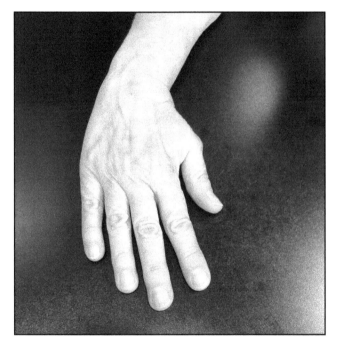

Figure 9-3. Wrist radial deviation.

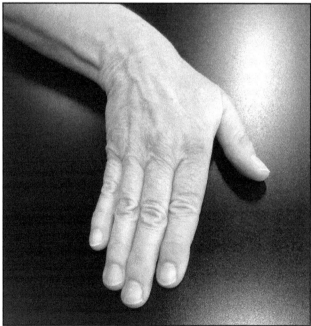

Figure 9-4. Wrist ulnar deviation.

The MCP joints of the fingers are biaxial condyloid joints and are commonly called the *knuckles* when a fist is made (Lippert, 2000). The extrinsic movements that occur at the MCP joints are flexion, extension, and hyperextension. Abduction and adduction also occur at the MCP joint; however, these motions are due to intrinsic musculature and, therefore, will be discussed in Chapter 10. The IP joint of the thumb and the PIP/DIP joints of the fingers are uniaxial

hinge joints that allow only flexion and extension (Hertling & Kessler, 2006). The finger PIP joints are created by the articulations between the proximal and middle phalanges, and the DIP joints are created by the articulations between the middle and distal phalanges. The joints of the fingers and thumb open and close the hand for functional gripping. Figures 9-8 and 9-9 illustrate full finger flexion and extension.

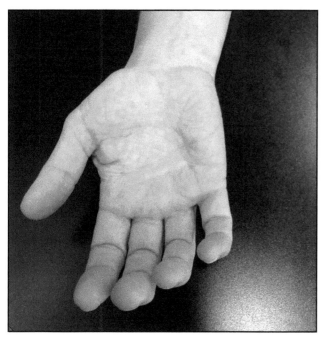

Figure 9-5. Thumb positioned out of the plane of the hand.

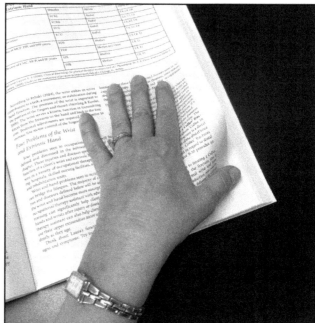

Figure 9-6. Functional thumb radial abduction while turning a page in a book.

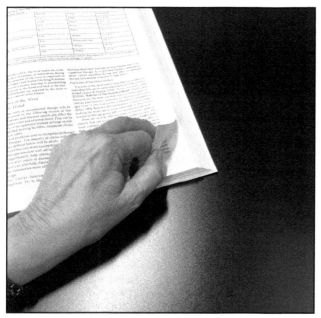

Figure 9-7. Functional thumb flexion while turning a page in a book.

Strength Characteristics of the Wrist and Extrinsic Hand

Functional activities performed by the wrist and hand generate forces. This includes a variety of daily activities, such as digging a hole with a trowel to plant flowers or twisting and tightening a water bottle lid. Sustained gripping or pinching, such as holding the steering wheel or writing, requires strength and stability in the wrist and hand. Another activity that involves higher loads on the wrist and hand is

UE weight bearing. As noted in the chapters on the shoulder and elbow, all the joints and muscles of the UE are used when an individual ambulates with crutches, a walker, or a cane. The UEs must be used in propulsion of a wheelchair when the lower extremities (LEs) are nonfunctional. In forceful, spontaneous hand activities, such as hitting a golf ball, hammering a nail, or using a jackhammer, the wrist is subject to very large loads. During moderate grasping activities involving only a 2-pound weight, the forces to the wrist are found to be up to 35 pounds (Oatis, 2004).

Laura, in the occupational profile, is unable to perform numerous occupational roles, including gripping the steering wheel when driving. In addition to addressing her problems of stiffness, edema, and pain, wrist stability and strength will need to improve before she can drive to work. Table 9-1 identifies the functional roles of the joints, muscles, and nerves of the wrist and extrinsic hand while gripping a steering wheel.

Of course, the activity of driving requires strength and coordination of all the joints of the UEs. Safe driving also requires acute visual and hearing skills and the coordination of the LEs. Clients who may have driving deficits can be evaluated and taught compensatory techniques or can be instructed in the use of adaptive equipment by a trained occupational therapy practitioner.

According to Rybski (2019), the wrist makes an active contribution to a task, a movement, or stabilization during hand function. The position of the wrist is important to the position of the fingers and thumb (Hertling & Kessler, 2006). The wrist serves a kinetic function in transmitting forces from the forearm to the hand and back to the forearm. Positional adjustments are required by the wrist to increase fine motor control of the fingers.

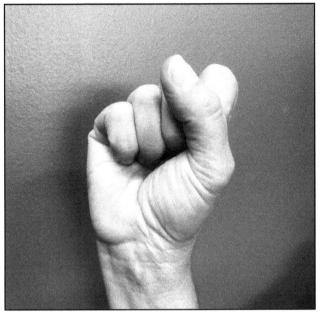

Figure 9-8. Finger flexion.

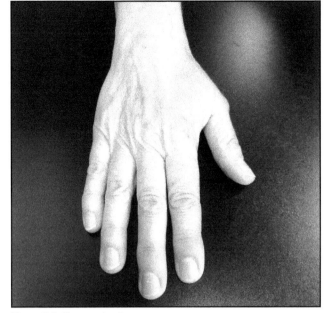

Figure 9-9. Finger extension.

TABLE 9-1
Gripping a Steering Wheel: Movements, Muscles, and Innervations

MOVEMENT	MUSCLES	NERVES	NERVE ROOTS
Wrist extension	Extensor carpi radialis longus	Radial	C6, C7, C8
	Extensor carpi radialis brevis	Radial	C6, C7, C8
	Extensor carpi ulnaris	Radial	C6, C7, C8
Wrist ulnar deviation	Extensor carpi ulnaris	Radial	C6, C7, C8
Finger flexion of MCP, PIP, and DIP joints	Flexor digitorum superficialis	Median	C7, C8, T1
	Flexor digitorum profundus	Median and ulnar	C8, T1
Thumb flexion of CMC, MCP, and IP joints	Flexor pollicis longus	Median	C8, T1
	Flexor pollicis brevis	Median	C8, T1

Adapted from Lippert, L. S. (2000). *Clinical kinesiology for physical therapist assistants* (3rd ed.). F. A. Davis Company and Rondinelli, R. D., Genoverse, E., Katz, R. T., Mayer, T. G., Mueller, K., & Ranavaya, M. (2008). *Guides to the evaluation of permanent impairment* (6th ed.). American Medical Association..

Four Problems of the Wrist and Extrinsic Hand

Four problems seen in occupational therapy will be defined and discussed in the following section of this chapter. These injuries and diseases specifically affect the function of a client's wrist and extrinsic hand. They can be seen in a variety of occupational therapy settings, including hospitals, skilled nursing facilities, outpatient clinics, and rehabilitation units.

Wrist and hand problems seen in occupational therapy can bridge the lifespan. The majority of clients with injuries and diseases defined in the following sections will be adults.

As we age, the wrist and hand become more susceptible to injury. An occupational therapy assistant with advanced competency training can significantly help clients rehabilitate their hands and wrists after injury or disease. The occupational therapy assistant can also help clients learn techniques to use their UEs more efficiently and independently as they age.

Think about Laura's functional limitations and her signs and symptoms. Try to identify her diagnosis while learning about these four injuries and diseases seen in occupational therapy. As in previous chapters, information about Laura's outcomes during and after occupational therapy intervention is located in Appendix C.

Figure 9-10. Colles fracture. (SKYKIDKID/shutterstock.com)

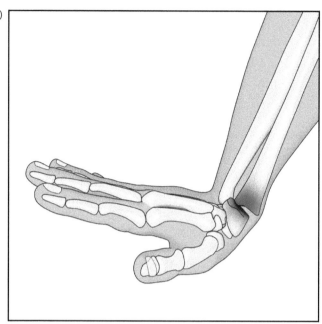

BOX 9-1

Fracture disease: A collection of symptoms caused by prolonged immobilization in a cast. It can lead to unresolved edema, pain, and stiffness even in the unaffected joints of the UE. Muscle atrophy and osteoporosis can occur. Fracture disease can be avoided with early intervention of edema management and AROM of the fingers, elbow, and shoulder while the client is casted.

Fractures of the Distal Radius

Fractures of the distal radius most often occur when an individual falls on an outstretched hand with the wrist extended (Aaron & Stegink, 2000). This is commonly called **fall on an outstretched hand** (FOOSH). Distal radius fractures are the most common fracture of the UE and are more common in postmenopausal women ages 51 to 75 who may present with primary osteoporosis (Riley, 1998). Bone loss after menopause is more prevalent, making the distal radius more vulnerable to fracture if a someone in this group falls on an outstretched hand.

There are several different types of fracture patterns present that can occur with a distal radius fracture. The most common fracture pattern is called a **Colles fracture**, which was first identified by Abraham Colles in 1814 (Aaron & Stegink, 2000). A Colles fracture is a distal radius fracture with dorsal displacement of the distal bone fragment (Weiss & Falkenstein, 2005). Colles fractures will be the only fracture type discussed in regard to distal radius fractures in this chapter. Figure 9-10 provides an illustration of a Colles fracture.

There are a variety of approaches to treating a Colles fracture. It is most important that the fracture site is aligned anatomically to allow normal wrist and forearm movement to return. Closed reduction may require manipulation to align the fracture followed by casting (Cannon, 2003). If the fracture is unstable, fixation may be necessary for the best outcome. Numerous techniques can be used by the surgeon, including percutaneous pin fixation, external fixation, and **open reduction with internal fixation** (ORIF). With ORIF, a plate and screws are utilized by the surgeon to stabilize the radius after fracture. The technique used is contingent upon numerous variables, which may include the surgeon's preference and expertise, the client's age and medical condition, and the type of fracture displacement (Burke et al., 2006). There is a recent trend to perform ORIF more often when appropriate after a Colles fracture so as to begin gentle, controlled ROM earlier and avoid limiting conditions such as fracture disease. Box 9-1 provides a definition of fracture disease.

Occupational therapy treatment techniques will vary according to the fixation techniques used by the physician. Occupational therapy treatment goals for any distal radius fracture should be maximum pain-free forearm and wrist ROM and full ROM of the fingers, thumb, elbow, and shoulder with a return of UE function (Hunter et al., 2002). It is beneficial to initiate occupational therapy while the wrist is still immobilized. The therapist can regain and maintain full shoulder, elbow, finger, and thumb ROM by the time the wrist is ready to be mobilized with early intervention. According to Hurou (1997), occupational therapy intervention assisted clients with distal radius fractures to resume functional activities by significantly increasing wrist and forearm AROM and grip and pinch strength. There is often edema in the thumb and fingers that is more difficult to resolve as it becomes chronic. Edema decreases mobility, reduces circulation, and leads to fibrosis if not resolved early (Hunter et al., 2002). Unfortunately, many clients are not instructed in edema control techniques immediately after casting or surgery. Clients should be individually instructed and provided handouts during occupational therapy. Figure 9-11 illustrates moderate edema in the left hand.

The best way to control edema is through the use of elevation. For elevation to be effective, the elbow should be positioned above the heart and the hand positioned above the elbow. Other edema control techniques include finger ROM exercises, distal to proximal retrograde massage, lymphatic massage, compression garments, such as gloves, and cardiovascular exercise. This is not an all-encompassing list as there are many other approaches used to control edema. Box 9-2 provides an edema control technique handout used in an occupational therapy facility.

A client will be referred to occupational therapy after a Colles fracture has healed and the doctor feels the client can begin treatment. The cast may be removed if surgery was not required, which usually occurs approximately 6 weeks postinjury. If an ORIF was required for proper alignment, the client may be referred to occupational therapy from 2 to 6 weeks after surgery, depending on the referring physician.

Complications can occur after a distal radius fracture. The most common complications are carpal tunnel syndrome (CTS), **malunion**, **complex regional pain syndrome** (CRPS), and **tendon rupture**.

In CTS, the median nerve, which supplies sensation to the thumb and index and middle fingers, becomes compressed or irritated. CTS is sometimes seen after Colles fracture due to edema and misalignment of the bone fragments. This can cause compression of the median nerve in the narrowed carpal tunnel.

Malunion can occur when the proper alignment of fracture slips, causing a deformity. This can occur more often with closed reduction and casting. As the swelling decreases, the cast sometimes loosens, allowing the aligned bone fragments to move. A client's function can be affected negatively due to pain or limited ROM if a malunion occurs. Surgery may be required to align the fracture (Weiss & Falkenstein, 2005).

CRPS, also known as **reflex sympathetic dystrophy**, is a posttraumatic neuropathic syndrome characterized by pain and vasomotor and pseudomotor changes in the involved extremity (Stoykov, 2001). Signs and symptoms may include pain that is disproportionate to the initial injury, excessive edema, discoloration, hypersensitivity, and increased stiffness (Burke et al., 2006). CRPS can be treated successfully if identified early.

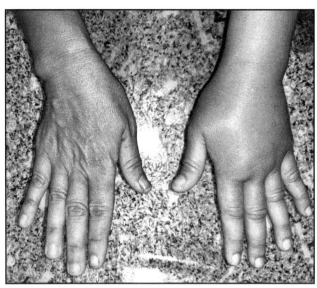

Figure 9-11. Moderate edema in the left hand. (Zay Nyi Nyi/shutterstock.com)

Finally, a tendon rupture may occur as a result of a distal radius fracture. The tendon that ruptures most often after a distal radius fracture is the extensor pollicis longus (EPL). This is due to the position of the tendon located over the distal radius. The healing fracture site is sometimes rough. This can fray the EPL over time and eventually cause a rupture. Box 9-3 identifies this type of tendon rupture (Weiss & Falkenstein, 2005).

Occupational therapy practitioners should be familiar with the signs and symptoms of the most commonly seen complications after a Colles fracture. Occupational therapy assistants can then notify the registered occupational therapist, who will approve notification of the physician in order to aid in early intervention, which can speed recovery and improve function.

de Quervain's Disease

de Quervain's disease is tenosynovitis, or inflammation of the tendon sheaths. de Quervain's disease was first named washer woman's sprain in 1893 and affects the abductor pollicis longus (APL), EPL, and extensor pollicis brevis (EPB) tendons. de Quervain's disease is more prevalent in women than men by a 4:1 ratio, and more common in women 35 to 55 years old. It is typically caused by the combined repetitive movements of the thumb and wrist, combined with forearm rotation during resistive pinching activities (Hunter et al., 2002). Examples of functional tasks in which clients report pain are opening jars, wringing out a wet cloth, cutting with scissors, needlepoint, or playing the piano. The client complains of pain along with localized tenderness and swelling over the anatomical snuff box, which is a depression formed by the APL, EPL, and EPB, found just distal to the radial styloid. Box 9-4 defines the origin of the anatomical snuff box.

BOX 9-2

EDEMA CONTROL TECHNIQUES

The prevention of edema (swelling) is important in the rehabilitation of your hand/arm. These are techniques that can be used to decrease the edema in your hand/arm. Only perform the techniques that are circled and explained to you by your therapist.

1. **Elevation**: For elevation to be effective, the hand must be above the heart. Pillows may be used to elevate the arm and hand at night. During the day, keep your hand elevated as much as possible and not swinging at your side. This is especially important during the first 2 to 3 weeks after surgery or injury.

2. **Cold packs**: Use a gel wrap or frozen vegetables. Apply to affected area to decrease swelling and pain. Avoid placing directly on fingertips.

    Apply _____ times a day for _____ minutes.

3. **Movement**: Perform ROM exercises as prescribed by your therapist. Movement, especially of the fingers and hand, will decrease swelling.

4. **Lymphatic massage**: Light massage proximal to the swollen region encourages the lymphatic system to "unclog," reducing edema. Perform very gently three times daily for 1 minute to the area of your arm your therapist recommends.

5. **Use of an Isotoner glove**: Please wear as directed by your therapist. If it becomes too tight, please remove at once.

(Roller, 2010)

BOX 9-3

Attrition rupture: Can occur when a tendon moves across a roughened bone. This commonly involves the EPL tendon after a distal radius fracture.

(Weiss & Falkenstein, 2005)

BOX 9-4

Anatomical snuff box: A small depression that is formed when the APL, EPL, and EPB tendons contract. The name snuff box originates from tobacco users placing and then sniffing their snuff, or powdered tobacco, in this depression during the 1800s.

(Floyd & Thompson, 2001)

One of the provocative tests used to diagnose de Quervain's disease is called **Finkelstein's test**. The health care provider asks the client to hold their flexed thumb in the palm, extend their arm and ulnarly deviate the wrist. If the test is positive, a sharp pain will be reproduced due to the involved tendons being stretched and compressed over the radial styloid. Figure 9-12 illustrates the position of Finkelstein's test.

Conservative treatment will include activity modification, including ergonomic changes, and the use of adaptive equipment, such as spring-loaded scissors or an electric jar opener, to rest the inflamed wrist and thumb. **Ergonomics** is defined as adapting the environment and tools to the individual. Splinting may be recommended as well to rest the inflamed joints. A wrist and thumb splint, called a **thumb spica splint**, is fabricated with the wrist in neutral to 15 degrees of extension and the thumb in radial abduction, with the thumb MCP and IP joints in extension. The physician may recommend a steroid injection to decrease the inflammation as well. If decreased signs and symptoms are seen in occupational therapy during conservative treatment, the client can progress to AROM exercises, a more flexible brace during the day, and, eventually, hand and wrist strengthening exercises.

If conservative treatment fails, the hand surgeon may recommend release of the compressed tendons. A very small incision is made at the area of the radial head and a portion of the extensor retinaculum is excised in the first dorsal compartment. Figure 9-13 illustrates the first dorsal compartment of the wrist. Postoperative treatment would include

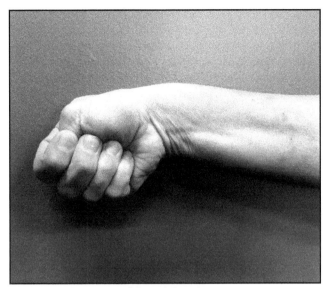

Figure 9-12. The position of the Finkelstein's test.

2 to 4 weeks of splinting, edema and scar management, gentle AROM, and tendon gliding exercises. At approximately 4 weeks, grip and pinch strengthening activities are added, and by 6 to 8 weeks the client should be able to gradually return to normal activities (Hunter et al., 2002).

Triangular Fibrocartilage Complex Tear

The radial and ulnar collateral ligaments provide lateral and medial support, respectively, to the wrist joint. The ulnocarpal complex is more likely to be referred to as the **triangular fibrocartilage complex** (TFCC) and includes the articular disk of the wrist. Figure 9-14 illustrates the TFCC. The TFCC is the major stabilizer of the **distal radioulnar joint** (DRUJ) and can tear after direct compressive force, such as a FOOSH. It is often seen in conjunction with a distal radius fracture. A TFCC tear is most often caused by trauma, but degenerative changes due to aging and/or wear and tear can be a precursor as well. The client will complain of ulnar wrist pain with forearm rotation, ulnar deviation, and gripping. They also may report swelling, loss of grip strength and **crepitus** (a clicking or grating sensation; Weiss & Falkenstein, 2005). The articular disk is found at the distal end of the ulna where it articulates with the triquetrum and lunate. It functions as a shock absorber and spacer, filling the gap created between the ulna and the carpal bones. The gap occurs because the ulna does not extend as far distally as the radius (Lippert, 2000).

There are several ways to help diagnose a TFCC tear. Tenderness to deep palpation over the TFCC may indicate a tear or lesion. Palpate between the extensor carpi ulnaris (ECU) and the flexor carpi ulnaris (FCU) distal to the ulnar styloid and proximal to the pisiform. The piano key sign is a protruding ulnar head that is caused from dorsal DRUJ instability. When you press on the ulnar head and release the pressure, it will spring back like a piano key. An arthrography

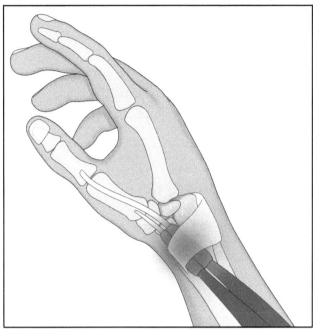

Figure 9-13. Illustrates the first dorsal compartment of the wrist where de Quervain's disease is seen. (SKYKIDKID/shutterstock.com)

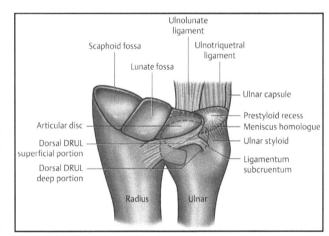

Figure 9-14. The TFCC. (DRUL = distal radioulnar ligament.)

of the wrist, where dye is injected into the joint, can show a TFCC tear because dye will leak from one joint compartment to another. Finally, a wrist **arthroscopy** is performed as a diagnostic tool. In this surgical procedure, portal incisions are made, and the surgeon looks at the joint structures with a small camera. During the wrist scope, the surgeon can debride or repair a TFCC tear if one is discovered (Healthline, 2017).

Conservative treatment may consist of splinting to prevent ulnar deviation and forearm rotation so the tear can heal. The client should be educated on activity modification and the use of ergonomic equipment, such as a special keyboard, to help prevent ulnar deviation. The occupational therapy assistant would also instruct the client in gentle AROM to prevent stiffness. Postoperatively after wrist arthroscopy, treatment may include scar and edema management and

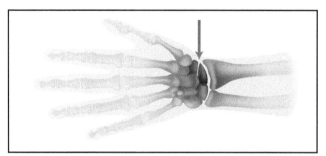

Figure 9-15. Scaphoid wrist fracture. (Alila Medical Media/shutterstock.com)

AROM exercises progressing to grip strengthening as able. Rehabilitation for TFCC debridement will be from 4 to 6 weeks. After TFCC repair, the client's wrist is immobilized for 4 to 6 weeks. Rehabilitation can range from 12 to 16 weeks (Hunter et al., 2002).

Fractures of the Scaphoid

The most common carpal fracture is a **scaphoid fracture**, which is seen in 60% of all carpal fractures. It is more common in male clients ages 15 to 30 years old and happens when there is extreme hyperextension of the wrist combined with radial deviation. A scaphoid fracture is seen frequently in an athlete after a sports-related FOOSH. The client will complain of pain, swelling, and sometimes tenderness with palpation over the anatomical snuff box.

Fractures are categorized by location within the scaphoid bone, which by its shape has a waist, distal pole, and proximal pole. Figure 9-15 illustrates a scaphoid fracture. Waist fractures are the most common at 70%, distal pole fractures comprise 10%, and proximal pole fractures 20%. Overall, the carpal bones do not have a good blood supply because they are covered by articular cartilage. There is a greater risk for **avascular necrosis** (AVN), meaning the death of bone tissue due to lack of blood supply. AVN can lead to a nonunion after scaphoid fracture. In the scaphoid, 90% of its blood vessels are at or distal to the waist so the potential for AVN, especially in the proximal waist and proximal pole, is quite high. A scaphoid fracture can generally be seen in a well-taken x-ray, especially after the initial swelling has decreased; however, a bone scan or magnetic resonance imaging is often required for a proper diagnosis (Richardson & Iglarsh, 1994).

Postinjury treatment depends on the type and location of the fracture. For a nondisplaced distal pole or waist scaphoid fracture, a long arm cast is applied for 4 weeks and then the client wears a short arm cast for an additional 4 weeks. For a nondisplaced proximal pole fracture, casting is from 12 to 24 weeks depending on healing. When the fracture is displaced and in the proximal waist or pole, surgery is performed. The surgeon uses a compression screw to hold the fracture and a long arm cast is applied for 2 to 4 weeks. After the cast is removed, the client will be referred to hand therapy, where a removable splint is fabricated to immobilize the wrist and thumb. The splint is to be worn at all times, with the exception of hygiene and for gentle, controlled AROM exercises several times a day. The AROM can be helpful in increasing blood flow to the fracture, which in turn increases healing. The client is educated to avoid resistive and sport activities. Once the physician ensures a bony union, passive range of motion and strengthening exercises are gradually initiated (Hunter et al., 2002).

Body Structures of the Wrist and Extrinsic Hand

The first part of this chapter introduced the amazing motions and functional input of the wrist and extrinsic hand. This section will explore how all the body structures work together to produce the strong yet intricate functions we possess through the use of our bodies, wrists, and hands. Muscles, nerves, tendons, and ligaments provide the body structures of our hands and arms and will be discussed as they relate to function.

Muscle Actions of the Wrist

The muscles that move the wrist but do not cross the hand to move the fingers and thumb will be presented first. The extrinsic muscles, or the muscles that cross the wrist but have a more significant function at the thumb and fingers will be described in the next section. The six muscles that cause wrist motion are the FCU, flexor carpi radialis (FCR), palmaris longus (PL), extensor carpi radialis longus (ECRL), extensor carpi radialis brevis (ECRB), and the ECU. An overview of the wrist muscles can be found in Table 9-2.

The FCU is a prime mover in wrist flexion and ulnar deviation. Because of its origin at the medial epicondyle of the humerus, it is also a weak flexor of the elbow. Its distal attachment is the fifth metacarpal and the pisiform, making it the only wrist muscle with an attachment to a carpal bone (Lippert, 2000). The FCU is considered the strongest wrist flexor and is active in movements requiring a sustained power grip, such as using an ax or hammer (Rybski, 2019).

The FCR moves the wrist in flexion and radial deviation. It is not as strong as the FCU; however, together with the FCU and PL, the FCR is powerful in stabilizing the wrist against resistance, especially with the forearm in supination (Floyd & Thompson, 2001).

TABLE 9-2

Muscles of the Wrist

ACTION	MUSCLES
Wrist flexion	• Flexor carpi ulnaris • Flexor carpi radialis
Wrist extension	• Extensor carpi radialis longus • Extensor carpi radialis brevis • Extensor carpi ulnaris
Wrist radial deviation	• Flexor carpi radialis • Extensor carpi radialis longus
Wrist ulnar deviation	• Flexor carpi ulnaris • Extensor carpi ulnaris

Adapted from Lippert, L. S. (2000). *Clinical kinesiology for physical therapist assistants* (3rd ed.). F. A. Davis Company.

The PL is the third wrist flexor and the weakest due to its small size and the fact that its distal attachment is the palmar fascia. The insertion on the palmar fascia does allow contribution by the PL to the production of a cupping motion of the hand (Rybski, 2019). This muscle is not present in approximately 15% to 20% of the population either unilaterally or bilaterally, according to Lippert (2000).

Muscles providing extension primarily at the wrist are the ECRL, ECRB, and ECU. These muscles are the most powerful extensors. They also stabilize the wrist against resistance, particularly if the forearm is pronated. Performing the backhand in racquet sports, such as tennis, uses all of these muscles together (Floyd & Thompson, 2001).

The ECRL is a prime mover in wrist extension and radial deviation. It is a more effective wrist extensor when the elbow is also extended. The ECRB is a strong wrist extensor and works with the ECRL to extend the wrist. The ECRB also assists with wrist radial deviation. This is due to its distal attachment at the base of the third metacarpal. The attachment is close to the axis of motion for radial and ulnar deviation (Lippert, 2000).

The ECU moves the wrist in extension and ulnar deviation. According to Oatis (2004), the ECU is more effective in extending the wrist with the forearm in supination. The ECU is also a very weak elbow extensor due to the muscle's origin at the lateral epicondyle of the humerus (Floyd & Thompson, 2001).

It is important to note that of the six muscles primarily responsible for wrist movement, no single muscle moves the wrist in one plane. To produce pure wrist motions of flexion or extension and radial or ulnar deviation, pairs of muscles must contract together. For example, the FCR and the FCU are required to contract for pure wrist flexion (Oatis, 2004). Notice during a functional activity, such as using a hammer, that the wrist commonly moves in a diagonal pattern. This diagonal pattern moves from wrist extension with radial deviation to wrist flexion with ulnar deviation. These muscles are specialized to support and move the wrist and hand in this functional, diagonal pattern.

Muscle Actions of the Extrinsic Hand

Muscles that originate in the forearm and cross the wrist to attach in the hand are called *extrinsic muscles*. These muscles have an assistive role in wrist function, but their primary role is the function of the fingers and thumb. The nine extrinsic muscles are the flexor digitorum superficialis (FDS), flexor digitorum profundus (FDP), flexor pollicis longus (FPL), APL, EPL, EPB, extensor digitorum communis (EDC), extensor digiti minimi (EDM), and extensor indicis proprius (EIP). An overview of these muscles and their motions can be found in Table 9-3.

The FDS muscle divides into four tendons on the palmar aspect of the wrist and hand to insert on each of the four fingers on the sides of the middle phalanx. The FDS is one of only two muscles that produce flexion of all four fingers. The FDS is vital in any type of gripping activity. It is the only muscle that can flex the PIP joints of the fingers without flexing the DIP joints. The FDS also assists in wrist flexion during finger flexion (Oatis, 2004).

The FDP is up to 50% stronger than the FDS but works with the FDS to flex all four fingers. The FDP is the only muscle that produces flexion of the DIP joints of all four fingers.

TABLE 9-3
Extrinsic Muscles of the Hand and Their Movements

MUSCLES	ACTION
Flexor digitorum superficialis	• Finger flexion of the MCP and PIP joints • Wrist flexion
Flexor digitorum profundus	• Finger flexion of the MCP, PIP, and DIP joints • Wrist flexion
Flexor pollicis longus	• Thumb flexion of the CMC, MCP, and IP joints • Wrist flexion
Extensor digitorum communis	• Finger extension of the MCP joints • Wrist extension
Extensor digiti minimi	• Small finger extension of the MCP joints
Extensor indicis proprius	• Index finger extension of the MCP joints
Abductor pollicis longus	• Thumb abduction at the CMC joint
Extensor pollicis longus	• Thumb extension of the CMC, MCP, and IP joints • Thumb CMC adduction • Wrist extension
Extensor pollicis brevis	• Thumb extension of the MCP joint • Wrist extension

Adapted from Floyd, R. T., & Thompson, C. W. (2001). *Manual of structural kinesiology* (14th ed.). McGraw-Hill.

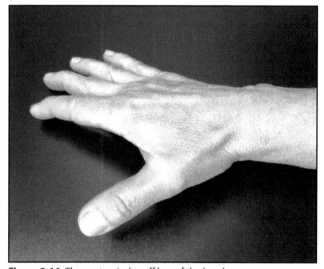

Figure 9-16. The anatomical snuff box of the hand.

It also flexes the PIP and MCP joints of the fingers and assists with wrist flexion. The FDP is the primary flexor of the fingers. The FDS is recruited to work with the FDP when additional strength is required, such as in forceful pinch and grasp (Rybski, 2019).

The FPL muscle is the prime mover of thumb flexion in all three joints: the CMC, MCP, and IP. Because of its palmar relationship to the wrist, it assists in wrist flexion. This muscle plays a vital role in pinching and gripping activities.

The APL muscle effectively abducts the thumb at the CMC joint. It forms the lateral border of the anatomical snuff box with the EPB. The EPL forms the medial border of this landmark. Figure 9-16 illustrates the anatomical snuff box of the hand.

The EPL muscle extends the IP joint of the thumb. The EPL aids in extension of the thumb at the MCP and CMC joints. It also assists with wrist extension and radial deviation. The EPL winds around the dorsal tubercle of the distal radius, which allows it to act as a thumb adductor at the MCP and CMC joints of the thumb.

The EPB extends the thumb at the MCP joint, but because it shares a common tendon sheath with the APL it has nearly the same actions. The EPB assists with CMC extension and wrist radial deviation. Movement of the thumb may alter its effect on wrist flexion and extension. It is one of the three snuff box muscles, forming the lateral border with the APL (Oatis, 2004).

The EDC muscle extends all the joints of the four fingers. It is the only common extensor muscle of the fingers. It originates at the lateral epicondyle of the humerus, passes under the extensor retinaculum at the wrist, and attaches on the distal phalanx of the fingers (Lippert, 2000). The EDC also assists with wrist extension. The extensor tendons of all four fingers are interconnected by fibrous bands at the level of the MCP joints, called **juncturae tendinae**. These bands can impede individual finger extension; however, they provide stabilizing forces to the MCP joints while the fingers are flexed during forceful gripping (Oatis, 2004).

The EDM allows extension of the MCP joint of the small finger. The EDM is located on the ulnar side of the EDC and acts to extend and abduct the PIP and DIP joints of the small finger due to its attachment in the extensor hood (Rybski, 2019). The extensor hood will be discussed in Chapter 10 with the intrinsic hand.

The EIP allows independent extension of the MCP joint of the index finger and, due to a connection to the extensor hood, extends the PIP and DIP joints as well. The EIP is commonly called the **pointing muscle** because it is responsible for extending the index finger, especially when the other fingers are flexed (Floyd & Thompson, 2001). Figure 9-17 illustrates the ability to extend just the index finger while pointing.

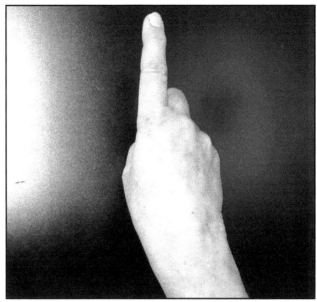

Figure 9-17. Example of the ability to extend the index finger during pointing.

Muscles, Nerves, and Spinal Cord Levels of the Wrist and Extrinsic Hand

When discussing the innervations of the wrist and extrinsic hand, there may be overlap with the innervations of the intrinsic hand, which will be covered in Chapter 10.

Nerve roots C6, C7, C8, and T1 supply the joints and muscles of the wrist and hand. They form the peripheral nerves that innervate the wrist and hand, which are the radial, median, and ulnar nerves. Innervations of the wrist and hand are fairly direct with a few exceptions. Muscles on the posterior surface are mostly innervated by the radial nerve. Muscles on the thumb side are primarily supplied by the median nerve. Muscles on the ulnar side of the hand are supplied by the ulnar nerve. The FDP receives its innervation from both the ulnar and median nerves (Lippert, 2000). Table 9-4 summarizes the motions and innervations of the wrist. The motions and innervations of the hand and thumb, both extrinsic and intrinsic, will be summarized in Chapter 10.

Sensation is extremely important to hand function. If an individual does not have intact sensation in their hand, they must compensate using vision, just as a person who is blind must use the sense of touch. Without intact sensory input, it would be impossible to tell what you are holding in your hand and how much force to use so as not to drop the item if you could not see. Sensory input can also help protect your hands from injury. Examples would be while using tools such as a knife or working on or near a hot stove. Hand sensation is supplied by the median, radial, and ulnar nerves. Figure 9-18 illustrates the pattern of cutaneous nerves of the hand.

Tendons and Ligaments of the Wrist and Extrinsic Hand

The extrinsic tendons of the hand are more susceptible to inflammation due to their length extending from the musculotendinous junction to distal insertion and to the space limitations at the wrist. For example, the FDS, FDP, FCR, and FPL tendons all pass through the carpal tunnel. The tendons of the FDS and FDP share a common synovial sheath as well (Hertling & Kessler, 2006). The flexor tendons of the fingers and thumb, as well as the palm of the hand, are protected their entire length by these sheaths that are lined with synovial fluid. This is to provide protection from impact and repetitive movement during the functional use of daily gripping and pinching.

TABLE 9-4

Motions and Innervations of the Wrist

MUSCLE	NERVE	NERVE ROOT				WRIST FLEXION 0 to 60 degrees	WRIST EXTENSION 0 to 60 degrees	RADIAL DEVIATION 0 to 20 degrees	ULNAR DEVIATION 0 to 30 degrees
		C6	C7	C8	T1				
Extensor carpi radialis longus	Radial	X	X				X	X	
Extensor carpi radialis brevis	Radial	X	X				X		
Extensor carpi ulnaris	Ulnar		X	X			X		X
Flexor carpi radialis	Median	X	X			X		X	
Palmaris longus	Median	X	X			X			
Flexor carpi ulnaris	Ulnar			X	X	X			X

Adapted from Lippert, L. S. (2000). Clinical kinesiology for physical therapist assistants (3rd ed.). F. A. Davis Company and Rondinelli, R. D., Genoverse, E., Katz, R. T., Mayer, T. G., Mueller, K., & Ranavaya, M. (2008). Guides to the evaluation of permanent impairment (6th ed.). American Medical Association.

The flexor tendons are secured at the fingers by annular, oblique, and cruciate fibers called *pulleys*. These pulleys prevent bowstringing of the tendons during composite finger flexion and gripping. The flexor tendons are cordlike in shape, which adds to their strength. In comparison, the extensor tendons are flatter and weaker and do not have synovial sheaths. The extensor tendons of the fingers and thumb do not have to work against resistance, so they require less strength. Both the extensor and flexor tendons of the hands are prone to laceration because the tendons are superficial and exposed to many dangers as the hands perform their duties. If an individual completely lacerates a tendon in their thumb or fingers, it will have to be surgically repaired to regain function. There will be a time of immobilization to allow healing, then rehabilitation to regain ROM and strength for return to functional use. To learn more about tendon repairs of the hand and occupational therapy treatment, see the e-Hand website listed in Appendix A.

The ligaments of the wrist can be divided into two large categories: extrinsic and intrinsic. Please refer to Table 9-5, which illustrates the ligaments of the wrist and their functions.

The extrinsic ligaments consist of the palmar radiocarpal ligament, dorsal radiocarpal ligament, ulnar collateral ligament, radial collateral ligament, and ulnocarpal complex. The palmar radiocarpal ligament is a tough, thick ligament that limits wrist extension. It attaches from the radius to the scaphoid, lunate, and triquetrum. Because most activities require wrist extension, this ligament is more likely to be sprained or stretched (Lippert, 2000). The dorsal radiocarpal ligament attaches to the same structures as the palmar radiocarpal ligament but on the posterior surface. It limits the amount of flexion at the wrist. This ligament is not as strong as its counterpart.

The intrinsic ligaments of the wrist include the palmar and dorsal midcarpal ligaments and the interosseous ligaments. The palmar and dorsal midcarpal ligaments form and stabilize the proximal and distal rows of the carpal bones. The interosseous ligaments stabilize the individual carpal bones to each other within their proximal or distal row. Like the extrinsic ligaments, the palmar midcarpal ligaments are stronger than the dorsal. The interosseous ligaments are considered the strongest in the wrist but are less rigid, which may allow larger loads of force to be sustained when falling on an outstretched hand. Despite the protective mechanical properties of the ligaments of the wrist, numerous sprains are reported (Oatis, 2004).

The transverse carpal ligament, or flexor retinaculum, supports the carpal arch, creating the carpal tunnel. It attaches medially on the pisiform and the hook of the hamate and laterally on the tubercles of the trapezium and scaphoid (Oatis, 2004).

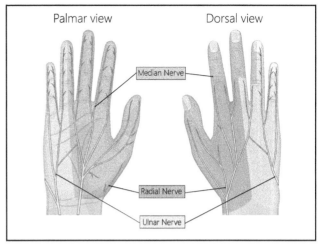

Figure 9-18. Pattern of cutaneous nerves in the hand. (Aksanaku/shutterstock.com)

The ligaments of the hand will be limited to discussion of the CMC and MCP joints of the thumb. A brief general description of the ligaments of the IP joints of the thumb and fingers and their main functions will follow. Ligaments affecting the intrinsic hand as well as the fascia and arches of the hand will be described in Chapter 10.

Providing support at the CMC joint of the thumb are the radial, dorsal, and volar oblique ligaments. These ligaments stabilize the CMC joint but also play a role in guiding the movement of the CMC joint. The pull of the oblique ligaments rotates the metacarpal during flexion/abduction and extension/adduction of the thumb (Oatis, 2004). The ligaments of the MCP joints of the thumb and fingers consist of collateral ligaments, which are thick bands running obliquely from the metacarpal to the proximal phalanges and the volar plate. The volar plate consists of fibrous connective tissue and fibrocartilage and limits hyperextension. The collateral ligaments protect the joints against radial and ulnar movement (Oatis, 2004). The ulnar collateral ligament of the thumb MCP joint is prone to strain or rupture when an individual falls on the hand, forcing the thumb into abduction. This injury will be discussed in detail under the four problems of the hand and thumb in Chapter 10 and is commonly called *skier's thumb* (Weiss & Falkenstein, 2005).

The ligaments of the IP joint of the thumb and the PIP and DIP joints of the fingers are quite similar. They consist of collateral ligaments and a volar plate. They also have a fan-shaped accessory ligament that attaches to the proximal portion of the volar plate. The collateral ligaments provide stabilization of the joints from the radioulnar direction throughout flexion and extension excursion. The accessory ligaments provide additional support to the joints, especially when the distal joints of the thumb and fingers are extended. The IP joints also receive stability from the surrounding tendons and their related connective tissue structures (Oatis, 2004).

TABLE 9-5
Ligaments of the Wrist and Their Function

EXTRINSIC LIGAMENTS	FUNCTION
Palmar radiocarpal	Volarly stabilizes radius to carpal bones; limits excessive wrist extension.
Dorsal radiocarpal	Dorsally stabilizes radius to carpal bones; limits excessive wrist flexion.
Ulnar collateral	Provides lateral stability of ulnar side of wrist between ulna and carpals.
Radial collateral	Provides lateral stability of radial side of wrist between radius and carpals.
Ulnocarpal complex and articular disk (or TFCC)	Stabilizes and helps glide the ulnar side of wrist; stabilizes DRUJ.
INTRINSIC LIGAMENTS	**FUNCTION**
Palmar midcarpal	Forms and stabilizes the proximal and distal rows of carpal bones.
Dorsal midcarpal	Forms and stabilizes the proximal and distal rows of carpal bones.
Interosseous	Intervenes between each carpal bone contained within its proximal or distal row.
ACCESSORY LIGAMENT	**FUNCTION**
Transverse carpal	Stabilizes carpal arch and contents of the carpal tunnel.

Adapted from Hertling, D., & Kessler, R. (2006). *Management of common musculoskeletal disorders: Physical therapy principles and methods.* Lippincott Williams & Wilkins; Oatis, C. A. (2004). *Kinesiology: The mechanics and pathomechanics of human movement.* Lippincott Williams & Wilkins; and Weiss, S., & Falkenstein, N. (2005). *Hand rehabilitation: A quick reference guide and review.* Mosby-Elsevier.

Summary

The two preceding chapters discussed the structure and function of the shoulder and elbow. The resulting functional relevance for both joint complexes, along with the wrist, is to position the hand. The mobility of the shoulder creates an immense space through which the hand can be moved. The elbow, while less mobile, stabilizes the hand along with the forearm and wrist for a variety of functional tasks. The hand carries out the performance of the UE, including reaching nearly all parts of the body. Hand and wrist function shows variety and diversity, gentleness and strength, precision and emotion. This diversity requires structural complexity with a comparative ease of performance. If there is no pathology, there is complete synergy among the structures of the UE, which allows efficient completion of functional activities.

Through Laura, this chapter has explored how the wrist and extrinsic hand move, grasp, and pinch. Knowledge of the normal wrist and extrinsic hand and their supporting structures is necessary to understand the injuries and diseases that can affect them. Restoration of function is the objective of occupational therapy treatment. Effective wrist and hand function is a direct and critical link to independence.

References

Aaron, D. H., & Stegink, C. W. (2000). Hand rehabilitation: Matching patient priorities and performance with pathology and tissue healing. *Occupational Therapy Practice, 5*(8), 11-15.

Burke, S. L., Higgins, J. P., McClinton, M. A., Saunders, R., & Valdata, L. (2006). *Hand and upper extremity rehabilitation: A practical guide* (3rd ed.). Elsevier-Mosby.

Cannon, N. M. (2003). *Diagnosis and treatment manual for physicians and therapists: Upper extremity rehabilitation* (4th ed.). The Hand Rehabilitation Center of Indiana.

Floyd, R. T., & Thompson, C. W. (2001). *Manual of structural kinesiology* (14th ed.). McGraw-Hill.

Healthline. (2017). Understanding TFCC tears. https://www.healthline.com/tfcc-tear#causes-and-risk-factors

Hertling, D., & Kessler, R. (2006). *Management of common musculoskeletal disorders: Physical therapy principles and methods.* Lippincott Williams & Wilkins.

Hunter, J. M., Maklin, E. J., Callahan, H. D., Skirven, T. M., Schneider, L. H., & Osterman, A. E. (2002). *Rehabilitation of the hand and upper extremity* (5th ed.). Mosby.

Hurou, J. R. (1997). Fractures of the distal radius: What are the expectations of therapy? A two year retrospective study. *Journal of Hand Therapy, 10*(4), 269-276.

Latella, D., & Meriano, C. (2003). *Occupational therapy manual for the evaluation of range of motion and muscle strength.* Delmar Carnage Learning.

Lippert, L. S. (2000). *Clinical kinesiology for physical therapist assistants* (3rd ed.). F. A. Davis Company.

Oatis, C. A. (2004). *Kinesiology: The mechanics and pathomechanics of human movement.* Lippincott Williams & Wilkins.

Pendleton, H. M., & Schultz-Krohn, W. (2006). *Pedretti's occupational therapy practice skills for physical dysfunction* (6th ed.). Mosby-Elsevier.

Richardson, J., & Iglarsh, Z. (1994). *Clinical orthopaedic physical therapy.* W. B. Saunders Company.

Riley, M. A. (1998). The effects of medical conditions and aging on hand function. *Occupational Therapy Practice, 3*(6), 24-27.

Rondinelli, R. D., Genoverse, E., Katz, R. T., Mayer, T. G., Mueller, K., & Ranavaya, M. (2008) *Guides to the evaluation of permanent impairment* (6th ed.). American Medical Association.

Rybski, M. (2019). *Kinesiology for occupational therapy* (3rd ed.). SLACK Incorporated.

Stoykov, M. E. (2001). OT treatment for complex regional pain syndrome. *Occupational Therapy Practice, 6*(15), 10-14.

Roller, C. (2010). *Edema (swelling) control techniques* (Brochure). Author.

Weiss, S., & Falkenstein, N. (2005). *Hand rehabilitation: A quick reference guide and review.* Elsevier-Mosby.

Applications

The following activities will help you apply knowledge of the wrist and extrinsic hand in real-life applications. Activities can be completed individually or in a small group to enhance learning.

1. **Joints and Motions of the Wrist and Hand**: Complete the following activities to increase your familiarity with the functional aspects and movements of the wrist and hand.
   a. Using your anatomy skills, locate and palpate the following landmarks on yourself or a partner:
      i. Radial styloid process
      ii. Ulnar styloid process
      iii. Hook of hamate
      iv. Thenar eminence
      v. Hypothenar eminence
      vi. Anatomical snuff box
   b. Identify all motions of the wrist and hand during the following functional activities:
      i. Button a shirt:
      ii. Text using a cellphone:
      iii. Remove a textbook from a backpack:
      iv. Remove a glass from an overhead cupboard:
      v. Cut a piece of food using a knife and fork:
      vi. Brush your teeth with a manual toothbrush:
   c. The PL is a small muscle that assists with wrist flexion. It is absent in approximately 15% to 20% of the population. The PL tendon is superficial and can be found in the volar distal forearm. Find and palpate the PL tendon in yourself and your partner. Is it present in you and your partner? What motions of the wrist and hand make the tendon more prominent?

2. **Strength of the Wrist and Hand**: Complete the following activities to familiarize yourself with functional stability, grip, and prehension of the wrist and hand.
   a. Perform push-ups using several different styles. Which style feels easier or more difficult? See how many you or your partner can perform of each style:
      i. Palms flat on floor, forearms pronated
      ii. Weight bearing on fingertips
      iii. Hands in a fist, weight bearing on knuckles
      iv. Palms flat, forearms in mid-position
   b. Many clients you treat as an occupational therapy assistant will have LE deficits that will require them to use an assistive device to ambulate. Demonstrate the use of the wrists and hands during the following:
      i. Ambulate using a standard or quad cane
      ii. Ambulate using a standard walker with left LE weight bearing only
      iii. Ambulate using crutches with no weight bearing through the LE bilaterally
      iv. Propel yourself using a manual wheelchair

3. **Goniometric Measurements of the Wrist**: ROM norms can vary depending on the reference source. One norm is provided for each motion within this text to increase ease of applications. Additionally, while multiple muscles may influence a particular motion, only the main muscles responsible for a joint motion are included. References for the following information can be found in Box 9-5. With your partner, practice using a goniometer to measure each motion available at the joints of the wrist. You may record the available ROM in Table 9-6. For ease of practice, all goniometric measurements of the hand will appear in Chapter 10. This will include the extrinsic and intrinsic movements of the hand and thumb.

BOX 9-5

REFERENCED WORKS FOR RANGE OF MOTION

Sections Referenced (a to e)	Reference
Goniometric landmark, end feel, and start and end positions	Latella & Meriano, 2003; Pendleton & Schultz-Krohn, 2006
Muscles responsible	Floyd et al., 2001; Oatis, 2004
Available ROM	Rondinelli et al., 2008

TABLE 9-6

Range of Motion Application Table

JOINT	MOTIONS	AVAILABLE ROM (DEGREES)	ROM OF YOUR PARTNER
Wrist	Flexion	0 to 60	
	Extension	0 to 60	
	Radial deviation	0 to 20	
	Ulnar deviation	0 to 30	

Adapted from Rondinelli, R. D., Genoverse, E., Katz, R. T., Mayer, T. G., Mueller, K., & Ranavaya, M. (2008). *Guides to the evaluation of permanent impairment* (6th ed.). American Medical Association.

a. Wrist flexion ROM
   i. Goniometric landmark: Dorsal aspect of the wrist and forearm at the wrist crease
      Stable arm: Midline of the dorsal forearm
      Moving arm: Midline of third metacarpal
   ii. Available ROM: 0 to 60 degrees
   iii. End feel: Firm
   iv. Muscles responsible: FCR, PL, FCU
   v. Start and end position: Figure 9-19 displays the start position for wrist flexion and extension. The client is seated with the elbow resting on a table. The fingers are relaxed or extended. Bend the wrist down or into maximum flexion. Figure 9-20 displays the end position of ROM.

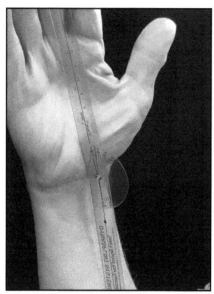

Figure 9-19. Start position for ROM testing of wrist flexion and extension.

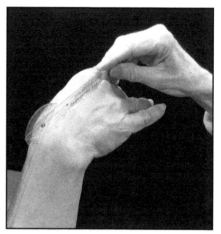

Figure 9-20. End position for ROM testing of wrist flexion.

b. Wrist extension ROM
   i. Goniometric landmark: Volar aspect of the wrist and forearm at the wrist crease
      Stable arm: Midline of the volar forearm
      Moving arm: Midline of third metacarpal
   ii. Available ROM: 0 to 60 degrees
   iii. End feel: Firm
   iv. Muscles responsible: ECRL, ECRB, ECU
   v. Start and end position: Figure 9-19 displays the start position for wrist extension. The client is seated with the elbow resting on a table. Bend the wrist back or into maximum extension. Figure 9-21 displays the end position of ROM testing.

Figure 9-21. End position for ROM testing of wrist extension.

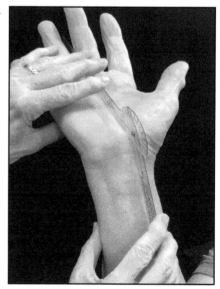

c. Wrist radial deviation ROM

  i. Goniometric landmark: Base of third metacarpal over the capitate

     Stable arm: Midline of forearm

     Moving arm: Midline of third metacarpal

  ii. Available ROM: 0 to 20 degrees

  iii. End feel: Firm

  iv. Muscles responsible: ECRL, FCR

  v. Start and end position: Figure 9-22 displays the start position for radial and ulnar deviation. The client is seated with the arm pronated and resting on a table, wrist neutral, and palm flat. Bend the wrist toward the thumb side or into maximum radial deviation. Figure 9-23 displays the end position of ROM testing.

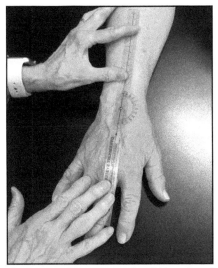

Figure 9-22. Start position for ROM testing of wrist radial and ulnar deviation.

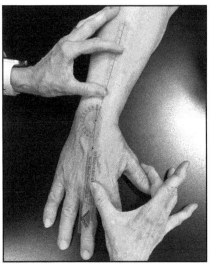

Figure 9-23. End position for ROM testing of wrist radial deviation.

d. Wrist ulnar deviation ROM

  i. Goniometric landmark: Base of third metacarpal over capitate

     Stable arm: Midline of forearm

     Moving arm: Midline of third metacarpal

  ii. Available ROM: 0 to 30 degrees

  iii. End feel: Firm

  iv. Muscles responsible: ECU, FCU

  v. Start and end position: Refer to Figure 9-22 for the start position. Client is seated with arm pronated and resting on a table, wrist in neutral, and palm flat. Bend wrist toward the small finger side or into maximum ulnar deviation. Figure 9-24 displays the end position of ROM testing.

Figure 9-24. End position for ROM testing of wrist ulnar deviation.

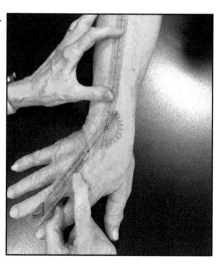

4. **Manual Muscle Testing (MMT) of the Wrist and Hand**: Complete gross MMT of the joints of the wrist and hand using Table 9-7. MMT of the hand and thumb will appear in Chapter 10, including both extrinsic and intrinsic musculature.

TABLE 9-7

Manual Muscle Testing Application Table

JOINT	MOTIONS	PALPATE MUSCLE GROUP/MUSCLE	GROSS MMT SCORE
Wrist	Flexion		
	Extension		
	Radial deviation		
	Ulnar deviation		

Adapted from Rondinelli, R. D., Genoverse, E., Katz, R. T., Mayer, T. G., Mueller, K., & Ranavaya, M. (2008). *Guides to the evaluation of permanent impairment* (6th ed.). American Medical Association.

a. Wrist flexion and extension
   i. Muscle palpation (if applicable)
   ii. Testing procedure: Figure 9-25 displays the start position for wrist joint flexion. The client is seated with arm resting on a table, forearm supinated, and wrist and fingers relaxed. The client moves their wrist into flexion. The therapist stabilizes the distal forearm to avoid compensation, and resistance is applied to the palm of the hand in the direction of wrist extension. Figure 9-26 displays the testing position.

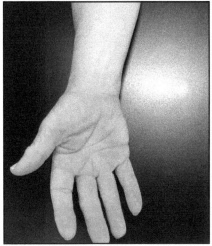

Figure 9-25. Start position for MMT of wrist flexion.

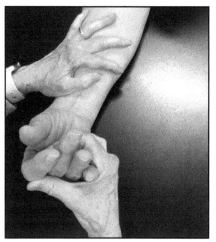

Figure 9-26. Testing position for MMT of wrist flexion.

Figure 9-27 displays the start position for testing wrist joint extension. The client is seated with the arm resting on a table, forearm pronated, and wrist and fingers relaxed. The client moves their wrist into extension. The therapist stabilizes the distal forearm to avoid compensation. Resistance is applied to the dorsum of the hand in the direction of wrist flexion. Figure 9-28 displays the testing position.

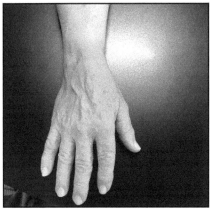

Figure 9-27. Start position for MMT of wrist extension.

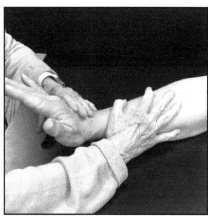

Figure 9-28. Testing position for MMT of wrist extension.

b. Wrist radial and ulnar deviation
   i. Muscle palpation (if applicable)
   ii. Testing procedure: Figure 9-29 displays the start position for wrist radial and ulnar deviation. The client is seated with arm resting on a table, forearm pronated, wrist in neutral, and fingers and thumb relaxed. The therapist stabilizes the distal forearm to avoid compensation. To test radial deviation, the client moves their wrist into radial deviation. Resistance is applied at the second metacarpal in the direction of ulnar deviation. Figure 9-30 displays the testing position. To test ulnar deviation, the client moves their wrist into ulnar deviation. Resistance is applied at the fifth metacarpal in the direction of radial deviation. Figure 9-31 displays the testing position.

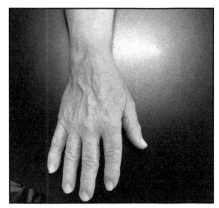

Figure 9-29. Start position for MMT of wrist radial and ulnar deviation.

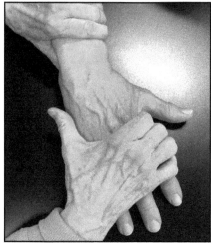

Figure 9-30. Testing position for MMT of wrist radial deviation.

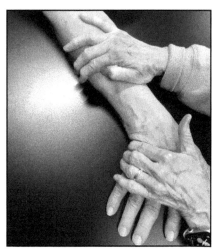

Figure 9-31. Testing position for MMT of wrist ulnar deviation.

CHAPTER 10

Function and Movement of the Intrinsic Hand

Carolyn L. Roller, OTR/L

Sain, S. J., & Roller, C. L. *Kinesiology for the Occupational Therapy Assistant: Essential Components of Function and Movement, Third Edition* (pp. 229-266).
© 2024 Taylor & Francis Group.

Chapter Objectives

After completion of this chapter, students should be able to:

1. Define key terminology.
2. Name motions of the intrinsic hand and how they affect functional movements.
3. Discuss four problems of the hand and thumb seen in occupational therapy.
4. Demonstrate the difference between extrinsic and intrinsic musculature of the hand and thumb.
5. Identify the arches of the hand and their function.
6. Understand the grasp patterns of the hand and thumb and how they relate to occupational roles.
7. List the actions and innervations of the intrinsic hand and thumb.

Introduction

In this chapter, functional movement of the intrinsic hand and thumb will be explored. Intrinsic muscles of the hand are muscles that originate and insert on the hand distal to the carpal bones. The function of the hand and thumb depends on all the joints and muscles of the upper extremity (UE) working together. The shoulder places the hand in space, the elbow extends the hand away from the body, the wrist moves the hand and flexes the fingers in a **functional position** for grip and precision tasks. Four problems seen frequently in occupational therapy are **rheumatoid arthritis** (RA) and **osteoarthritis** (OA) of the hand and thumb, **repetitive stress injuries** (RSIs), **Dupuytren's disease**, and **skier's thumb**. OA of the thumb or carpometacarpal (CMC) OA and Dupuytren's disease will be discussed here. OA is caused from wear and tear of the joints. The CMC joint of the thumb is the most common site for surgical reconstruction of OA in the hand. OA may cause deformity and pain with daily function, especially with pinch, because 50% of hand use is in the thumb. When surgery is indicated, a tendon is used to replace the trapezium carpal bone which cushions the joint between the metacarpal of the thumb and the wrist. The goals are to create a stable, pain-free joint with full thumb function. Dupuytren's disease causes a flexion contracture of the small and/or ring fingers. Clients will report an inability to straighten those fingers to don a glove, for example. The surgical treatment is a palmer **fasciotomy** where the thickened tissue is removed, correcting the deformity. Finally, the reader will learn the structures of the thumb and hand, including muscles, ligaments, tendons, and nerve innervations, and their influence on occupational performance.

Occupational Profile

The following occupational profile is provided to demonstrate occupational therapy intervention as related to the body functions and structures of the intrinsic hand and thumb. This profile will show how a thumb injury can negatively affect function. References to Sara, the client in this profile, will be addressed throughout the chapter.

Sara is a 43-year-old food service worker receiving occupational therapy with a physician's referral to increase functional range of motion (ROM) and grip/pinch strength in her right dominant hand and thumb.

During the occupational therapy evaluation, the following data were gathered.

Subjective: Sara states that approximately 5 months ago, while hiking with her family, she fell with her hiking poles in her hands. When she landed, her weight came down on her right thumb, causing it to bend back, or hyperextend. The next day she went to a walk-in clinic where x-rays revealed no fracture. She was given a wrist and thumb brace and advised to see her doctor. Her doctor referred her to a hand surgeon who ordered magnetic resonance imaging. The results showed a complete tear in the ulnar collateral ligament (UCL) of her right thumb. She received surgical repair and was casted for 10 weeks.

Today, Sara complains of stiffness, swelling, and pain in her injured thumb. She reports functional limits with the use of her dominant hand. She states she is unable to cut with a knife or scissors, write with a pencil, button her pants, or tie her shoes. She reports difficulties with pulling up her pants, brushing her teeth, vacuuming the floors, and driving.

Sara denies any other health problems and does not take any prescription medications. She lives with her husband and three teenage children, ages 19, 16, and 13. She reports that her husband and 19-year-old daughter have been helpful since her injury. She works full time at the nearby high school as a cook and delivery driver. Duties include food preparation, cooking, serving, and clean up, as well as pick up, delivery, and putting up the food orders. Her job requires lifting up to 80 pounds.

BOX 10-1

The Numeric Pain Rating Scale is a diagnostic tool to assist in assessing the severity of pain being experienced by a client. The client is asked to rate the intensity of their pain over the past 24 hours on a scale of 0 (no pain) to 10 (worst pain imaginable).

0	1	2	3	4	5	6	7	8	9	10	
No pain					Moderate pain					Worst pain	possible

At home she runs a busy household, caring for the home and the family pets. In her rare leisure time, she enjoys reading, knitting, and crocheting. "Right now, I can't move my thumb; it is stiff, swollen, and painful when I try to use my hand. I've missed 6 weeks of work and I need to get back!"

Objective: Sara states she has no pain in her right hand or thumb at rest but if she tries to move or use her right thumb, the pain is rated a 5/10. Pain is rated using the 0 to 10 Numeric Pain Rating Scale. Please see Box 10-1 for a definition and key for the Numeric Pain Rating Scale.

Formal active range of motion (AROM) and passive range of motion (PROM) are taken with a goniometer where limitations were noted. The joints of the left thumb were measured for comparison.

AROM and PROM is recorded as follows:

THUMB	RIGHT		LEFT	
	AROM	*PROM*	*AROM*	*PROM*
MCP flexion	0 to 10 degrees	0 to 15 degrees	0 to 55 degrees	0 to 60 degrees
IP flexion	0 to 15 degrees	0 to 20 degrees	0 to 5 degrees	0 to 90 degrees
Palmar abduction	0 to 20 degrees	0 to 25 degrees	0 to 50 degrees	0 to 55 degrees
Radial abduction	0 to 30 degrees	0 to 35 degrees	0 to 45 degrees	0 to 50 degrees
IP = interphalangeal; MCP = metacarpophalangeal.				

Sara is unable to touch her thumb to her small finger. The linear edge of the goniometer is used to measure the gap from her thumb pad to her small finger pad.

- Opposition: Lacks 3 cm from thumb to small finger on the right.
- End stage opposition is measured using the Kapandji scale
  - Score: Right is 3/10. Left is 10/10.

Please see Box 10-2 for a definition and illustration of the Kapandji scoring of end stage opposition.

Sara is unable to bring her thumb completely in to touch the radial side of her index finger. CMC adduction is measured using the linear edge of the goniometer to record the gap from the ulnar side of the IP joint of the thumb to the radial side of the hand at the base of the index finger.

- CMC adduction: Lacks 1 cm on right, left is intact.
- Edema is observed to be mild in the right thumb.
  - Localized edema was measured circumferentially at the IP joints of both thumbs: Right is 7 cm, left is 6 cm.
- Grip and pinch strength were not tested at this time due to pain and ROM limitations.

Goals were established by the occupational therapist in collaboration with Sara and are presented as follows.

Short-Term Goals:

1. Client will be instructed in and comply with a home exercise program within 2 weeks.

2. Client will tolerate a formal evaluation of right grip and pinch strength when able and appropriate or within 3 weeks.

3. Client will be able to brush teeth with right hand using a toothbrush with an adapted handle within 2 weeks.

4. Client will demonstrate self-feeding with the right hand using adaptive utensils within 1 week.

5. Client will demonstrate decreased edema by 0.5 cm in right thumb to help with buttoning within 3 weeks.

6. Client will demonstrate an increase in AROM in right thumb by 5 degrees in MCP and IP flexion and radial and palmar abduction. To be able to fully adduct thumb and to increase end stage opposition on the Kapandji scale from 3/10 to 6/10 to assist with dressing activities within 3 weeks.

Long-Term Goals:

1. Client will demonstrate compliance and independence in a progressive home exercise program at discharge.

2. Client will be independent in self-care tasks and occupational roles using right dominant hand and adaptive tools within 6 weeks.

3. Client will demonstrate an increase in AROM in MCP and IP joint flexion by 30 degrees within 6 weeks to be independent in buttoning pants and tying shoes.

BOX 10-2

The Kapandji scoring tool measures the end stage of opposition and is useful for assessing opposition of the thumb. It is based on where the client can touch their hand with the tip of their thumb. Scoring is as follows:

1. Radial side of the proximal phalanx of the index finger
2. Radial side of the middle phalanx of the index finger
3. Tip of the index finger
4. Tip of the middle finger
5. Tip of the ring finger
6. Tip of the small finger
7. Distal interphalangeal (DIP) joint crease of the small finger
8. Proximal interphalangeal (PIP) joint crease of the small finger
9. MCP joint crease of the small finger
10. Distal palmar crease

(Kapandji, 1986)

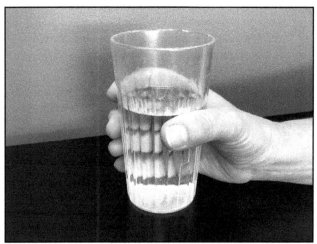

Figure 10-1. Functional thumb palmar abduction while holding a glass.

4. Client will be able to return to work with a 40-pound lifting restriction within 6 weeks.
5. Client will demonstrate the ability to knit and crochet for 30 minutes at a time with no pain within 6 weeks.

The outcome of Sara's occupational intervention along with treatment techniques and goals achieved can be found by reading the Epilogue in Appendix C.

Body Functions of the Intrinsic Hand

In this part of the chapter, joint motions and strength characteristics of the intrinsic hand as they relate to function will be explained. Four problems of the intrinsic hand and thumb treated in occupational therapy will be identified and described. Throughout this chapter references will be made to Sara and her functional problems, goals, and treatment.

Motions of the Intrinsic Hand and Thumb

It is important to reiterate here that the movement of the hand and thumb depends on many factors, including the synchronized motion of the entire UE. The scapula and shoulder place the hand in space and the elbow adds additional movement away from the body when it extends. Both the shoulder and elbow complex help to stabilize the wrist and hand. The wrist moves the hand and fixes the fingers in a functional position for grip and precision tasks. Intrinsic motions of the hand and thumb will be described in this section as they relate to function.

The **thenar** group of the intrinsic muscles provides thumb movement along with the extrinsic thumb motions covered in Chapter 9. Intrinsic motions of the thumb are identified as CMC joint abduction and adduction, CMC joint opposition, and CMC and MCP joint flexion. With the forearm supinated and the palm facing up, the movement of the thumb in palmar or CMC abduction and adduction can be displayed. The thumb moves up toward the ceiling for palmar abduction and returns to touch the second digit, or index finger, for adduction. Functionally, palmar or CMC abduction can be seen when a client prepares to pick up a glass of water, as illustrated in Figure 10-1. Adduction is seen when a client uses a lateral pinch to hold a coin, as illustrated in Figure 10-2. Thumb opposition is a combination of thumb flexion and abduction. This combined movement positions the pad of the thumb to oppose or touch the pad of a finger. The ability to oppose the thumb is what separates humans from other animals. A functional task that requires

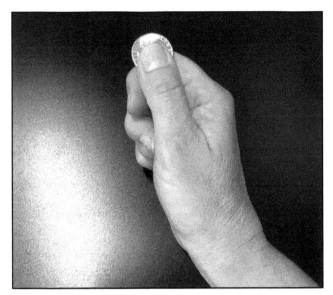

Figure 10-2. Functional thumb adduction while holding a coin.

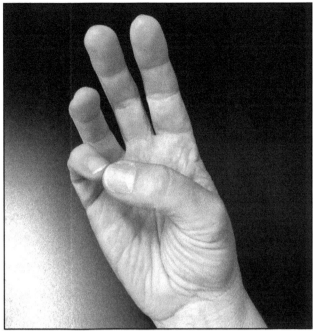

Figure 10-3. Opposition to the fifth digit.

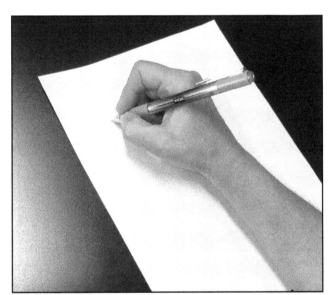

Figure 10-4. Functional opposition while writing.

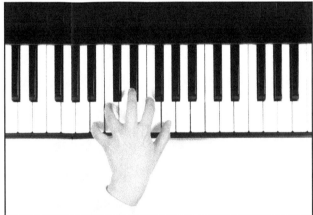

Figure 10-5. Small finger abduction on piano. (Veja/shutterstock.com)

opposition is writing. Figure 10-3 illustrates opposition to the fifth digit while Figure 10-4 illustrates functional opposition during writing. Sara in the occupational profile presents with functional limitations due to her injury. She is unable to flex, abduct, adduct, or oppose her thumb fully and, as such, is not able to hold a pen or pencil to write. Do you think she could hold a coin as illustrated in Figure 10-2?

The **hypothenar** group of intrinsic muscles provides motion to the small finger, or fifth digit. Intrinsic movements of the small finger are opposition, abduction, and flexion of the MCP joint. Functionally, opposition of the fifth digit assists thumb opposition as seen in Figure 10-3. The movement of small finger joint abduction is seen in Figure 10-5, which shows the motion as in reaching for a chord while playing the piano. MCP joint flexion of the small finger is crucial in many functional activities. In-hand manipulation is the ability to linearly move an object from the palm to the fingers or the fingers to the palm. In-hand manipulation skills are divided into three major categories: translation, shift, and rotation. Stabilization of an object is required in each category. A good functional example of in-hand manipulation is moving coins from the palm of the hand to the fingertips to insert into a bank, as pictured in Figure 10-6.

Another functional example of small finger MCP flexion is found while playing a guitar or a violin. The small finger must secure a string of the instrument while the remainder of the hand holds the neck and secures other strings. As seen in Figure 10-4, MCP flexion of the fifth digit is required for writing. The hypothenar muscles hold the small finger in flexion so the ulnar side of the hand can rest on the table, stabilizing the hand while the thumb, index, and middle finger move the pen or pencil to write.

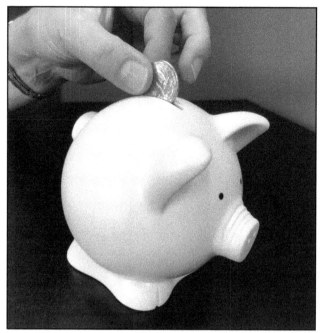

Figure 10-6. Moving coins from palm to fingertips to insert in bank.

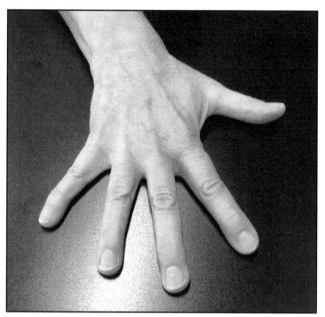

Figure 10-7. Finger abduction.

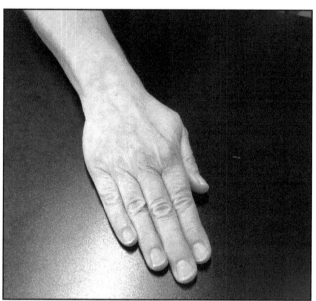

Figure 10-8. Finger adduction.

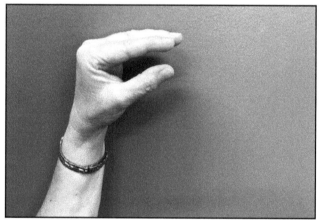

Figure 10-9. The intrinsic plus position of the hand.

The palmar and **dorsal interossei** provide the movements of the MCP joint in abduction and adduction of the fingers. MCP joint abduction occurs when the second, fourth, and fifth digits move away from the middle finger, or third digit, which is used as a reference point for abduction and adduction of the other three digits. Adduction is the return from abduction of the second, fourth, and fifth digits. Only the middle finger abducts in either direction and does not adduct. Figures 10-7 and 10-8 illustrate full finger abduction and adduction.

The ability to abduct the fingers allows us to pick up and hold many different sized objects in our hands. The dorsal interossei also provide MCP joint flexion with PIP/DIP joint extension of the digits along with the **lumbricals**. This motion can be seen in the intrinsic plus position of the hand as seen in Figure 10-9.

Think about these intrinsic movements and their function as you continue this chapter. Grasp patterns and how they develop from infancy will be discussed in the next section of this chapter. Keep in mind the functional motions as you examine the muscle actions in the body structures portion of this chapter. As before, consider Sara in the occupational profile, her occupational roles, and their movements.

Strength Characteristics of the Intrinsic Hand and Thumb

Positional adjustments are required by the wrist to increase fine motor control of the fingers. This, in turn, can allow fine degrees of prehension as well as a powerful grasp. There is an ideal position for the wrist and hand. The functional position is most effective in terms of strength and precision during activities (Lippert, 2000). In the functional position the wrist is slightly extended to approximately 20 degrees, the fingers are slightly flexed at all their joints, with the degree of flexion increasing slightly from the index to the small finger, and the thumb is in opposition with the MCP joint moderately flexed and the IP joint slightly flexed (Hertling & Kessler, 2006). Figure 10-10 illustrates the functional position of the hand and wrist.

Because humans have the ability to oppose the thumb to the fingers, they exhibit a wide variety of prehension grasping patterns. These patterns are classified by the position of the fingers, area of contact between the thumb and fingers, and object grasped. Prehension can be either pinching or grasping. Pinching is primarily used for precision manipulation and involves the thumb and the pads of the index and long fingers. Grasping typically involves all of the hand, including the palm and the fingers (Oatis, 2004).

The grasp is sometimes called the *power grip* and is used when an object needs to be held forcefully while being moved by more proximal joints. The power grip involves an isometric contraction with very little movement occurring between the hand and the object. The most common power grips are the cylindrical, spherical, and hook. In the cylindrical grip, all of the fingers are flexed around the object in one direction, and the thumb is flexed in the opposite direction. Examples of the cylindrical grip include holding a golf club, steering wheel, or hammer. A spherical grip has all the fingers and thumb abducted around the object with the fingers more apart. Activities requiring a spherical grip include holding an orange, turning a doorknob, and opening a jar. The hook grip involves the fingers flexed around an object in a hook-like manner. The thumb is not necessarily involved. Examples of a hook grip are seen when holding onto a handle, such as in carrying a briefcase or bucket (Lippert, 2000). Figures 10-11 through 10-13 illustrate the three power grips of cylindrical, spherical, and hook.

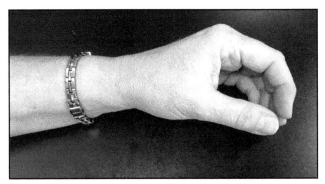

Figure 10-10. Functional position of the hand and wrist.

A precision grip, commonly called a *pinch*, provides finer movements and accuracy. The object is usually small and the palm is not always involved. The intrinsic muscles of the hand are used more with pinching. The precision grip needs to be developed normally when one is a child to work efficiently in adulthood. **Pincher grasp** is a developmental milestone at about 9 to 12 months of age. It enables a young child to pick up small objects using the thumb, index finger, and, often, the middle finger. The pincher grasp allows a more refined, neater way of getting food to the mouth. Over time the child will use variations of the pincher grasp for other important tasks, such as holding a pencil; holding and using eating utensils; fastening zippers and buttons; using scissors; and transferring small items, such as coins, within the palm out to the fingers (Case-Smith, 2005).

There are three commonly recognized pinches used to assess occupational therapy clients. The lateral, or key pinch, holds the object between the thumb and the radial side of the index finger. This is the strongest pinch used and is seen during activities such as turning a key to start a car or unlocking a door. The three-jaw chuck, three-point, or palmar pinch involves the thumb and two fingers, usually the index and middle fingers. This pinch is used the most in functional activities. A good example of a specialized three-point pinch is referred to as a *tripod grasp* and is used for holding a pen during writing (Benbow, 2001). The tip or two-point pinch (pincher grasp) holds the object between the tips of the index finger and thumb. This pinch is used often when a very small object is picked up, such as a sewing needle or small coin. Figures 10-14 through 10-16 illustrate the three most common pinches.

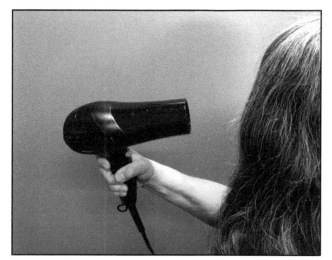

Figure 10-11. Cylindrical grip.

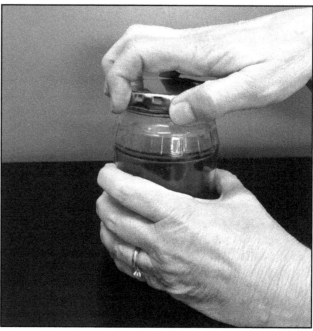

Figure 10-12. Spherical grip.

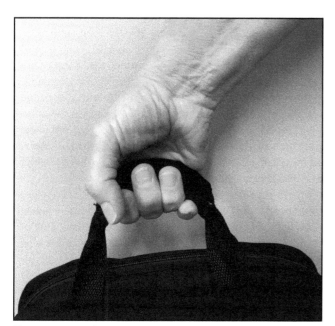

Figure 10-13. Hook grip.

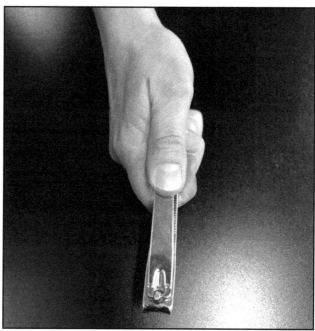

Figure 10-14. Lateral or key pinch.

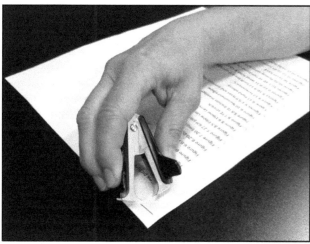

Figure 10-15. Three-jaw chuck or three-point pinch.

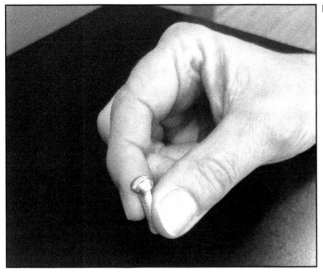

Figure 10-16. Pincher, tip, or two-point pinch.

TABLE 10-1			
Frequency Patterns of Prehension Pinch			
	LATERAL PINCH	**THREE-POINT PINCH**	**TWO-POINT PINCH**
Functional pick-up	33%	50%	17%
Hold during functional use	10%	88%	2%
Adapted from Rybski, M. (2019). *Kinesiology for occupational therapy* (3rd ed.). SLACK Incorporated.			

Table 10-1 shows the frequency of functional patterns of prehension pinch.

Hand strength can be assessed by the occupational therapy practitioner using a dynamometer for grip strength and a pinch gauge for pinch strength. Comparisons to the uninvolved hand along with consideration of dominance and normative data are used during the assessment. Please refer to Appendix D for averages in pounds for varying age groups of men and women. Figures 10-17 and 10-18 show the dynamometer and pinch gauge.

Four Problems of the Intrinsic Hand and Thumb

Four problems seen in occupational therapy will be defined and discussed in the following sections. These injuries and diseases specifically affect the function of a client's intrinsic hand and thumb. They can be seen in a variety of occupational therapy settings, including hospitals, outpatient clinics, rehabilitation facilities, and skilled nursing facilities. Hand and thumb problems seen in occupational therapy can bridge the lifespan but as we age, the UEs become more susceptible to injury and disease. As with all specialties, treatment of the hand and wrist requires advanced competency training by the occupational therapy practitioner. With additional training, the occupational therapy assistant can help clients rehabilitate their hands after injury or disease. The occupational therapy assistant can also teach clients skills to use their hands more independently and efficiently.

Think about Sara's functional limitations and her signs and symptoms, and then try to identify which diagnosis fits her occupational profile. Read her Epilogue in Appendix C to discover her outcomes in occupational therapy.

Rheumatoid Arthritis and Osteoarthritis

RA is a systemic autoimmune disorder. The cause of RA is unknown, and it most commonly affects women between 20 and 50 years of age. RA most commonly affects the joints of the hands, wrists, elbows, shoulders, hips, and ankles. Signs and symptoms include fatigue, joint pain, inflammation, edema, warmth, and redness. The distinctive factors in RA are **synovitis** of the peripheral joints, causing progressive joint destruction, deformity, and disability. Synovitis is a thickening and inflammation of the synovial lining of the joints. Synovitis from RA can cause ligament and tendon destruction as well, leading to ligament laxity and possible tendon rupture. Hand involvement may include ulnar deviation of the MCP joints and swan neck or boutonniere deformities of the fingers and thumb. A **swan neck deformity** describes a

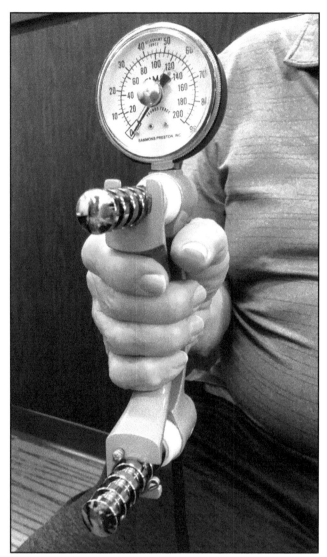

Figure 10-17. Dynamometer.

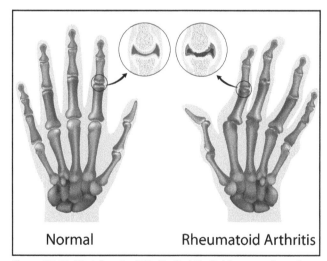

Figure 10-19. RA deformity. (Alila Medical Media/shutterstock.com)

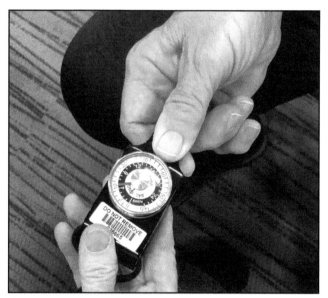

Figure 10-18. Pinch gauge.

finger with a hyperextended PIP joint and a flexed DIP joint. A **boutonniere deformity** describes a finger with a flexed PIP joint and a hyperextended DIP joint. Clients with RA of the hand, wrist, and thumb may be seen in occupational therapy for conservative management and postoperatively following joint replacement (Cannon, 2003).

Occupational therapy goals for conservative treatment of hand and wrist RA may include preventing further deformity and providing instruction in joint protection and energy conservation. Occupational therapy practitioners may provide instruction in the use of assistive devices, instruct the client in pain control techniques, and provide instruction to maintain or increase strength (Hunter et al., 2002).

Clients may require static splinting of the hand and wrist for support, to decrease pain, and to avoid further deformities of the joints through positioning. A common deformity pattern seen in the wrist and hand of RA clients is the zigzag or Z pattern. This pattern is characterized by carpal supination with a secondary radial shift of the metacarpals followed by an ulnar deviation of the digits (Weiss & Falkenstein, 2005). Figure 10-19 illustrates the zigzag deformity of the hand and wrist in RA. Figure 10-20 illustrates static splinting to prevent further deformity of the zigzag pattern.

Clients with RA may benefit from instruction in gentle ROM exercises to help maintain or increase flexibility. Because of the inflammatory nature of RA, gentle resistive exercises should be introduced gradually to maintain or increase grip strength. A soft ball or sponge squeezed in a bowl of warm water is a gentle way to add resistance. Clients also benefit from instruction in basic joint protection, proper lifting, and energy conservation techniques, which are included in basic protection principles. Table 10-2 gives an overview of protection principles.

Occupational therapists may also see clients with RA in hand therapy postoperatively. The most common surgery performed on the hand of clients with RA seen in occupational therapy is MCP joint implant **arthroplasty**. The indications for performing flexible MCP joint implant arthroplasty are severe RA of the MCP joints of the hands that result in deforming disability and pain, limiting function in daily activities (Cannon, 2003). The surgeon uses a flexible silicone spacer to replace the MCP joint. This allows for good alignment of the joint as well as proper tendon repositioning, enabling return of effective finger function (Burke et al., 2006).

Usually, the client will present with implants in four digits postoperatively. Therapy is indicated to maintain MCP joint alignment, reduce pain and edema, and enhance functional performance. Treatment consists of static and dynamic splinting and AROM and PROM exercises. At approximately 3 to 7 days after surgery the therapist will fabricate a dynamic splint for continuous daytime wear for 4 to 6 weeks. The splint will hold the wrist in 15 degrees of extension and the MCP joints between 0 and 10 degrees of flexion with light rubber band traction at a 60-degree angle. The client should perform active finger flexion within the splint every hour. A static resting splint is also fabricated with the wrist at 0 to 15 degrees of extension and the MCP joints at neutral and slight radial deviation. The IP joints are placed in neutral as well. If finger flexion is very limited, PROM to the digits can be initiated. Very light activities of daily living (ADLs) may be completed without the splint, gradually starting about 6 weeks after surgery. The client may be allowed to fold clothes for 15 minutes then return to the splint, for example. At approximately 10 weeks after surgery the client can stop wearing the dynamic splint and begin gentle strengthening exercises. The client should continue to avoid lateral pinching, which stresses the MCP joints in ulnar deviation. The MCP joints are most stable and functional at 60 to 70 degrees of flexion after this surgery (Cannon, 2003).

Unlike RA, OA is caused by wear and tear of the joints. Degenerative changes from overuse or trauma cause destruction of joint surfaces. This results in pain and stiffness in the joints (Burke et al., 2006). OA is more prevalent in women older than 50. It is commonly seen in the PIP and DIP joints of the digits, CMC joint of the thumb, cervical and lumbar spine, shoulders, knees, and hips (Riley, 1998). Figure 10-21 illustrates OA joint deformities of the hand.

Conservative treatment for clients with OA in occupational therapy is quite similar to treatment for clients with RA. Clients with OA who have pain and stiffness in their hands will benefit from protection principles that include assistive devices, gentle ROM, strengthening exercises, splinting, and the use of heat or other modalities. It is important to

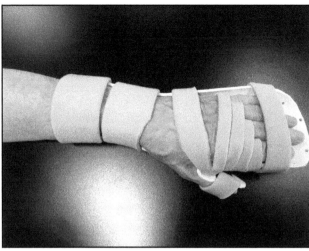

Figure 10-20. Resting splint with ulnar deviation correction to prevent further deformity.

consider the client's needs when developing a home program for clients with RA or OA. A home program should also include treatment techniques that will be easy and cost-effective to increase compliance and carryover at home. Older adults with arthritis can use assistive devices at home to increase their independence in leisure, self-care, and home management activities (Mann et al., 1995). According to Mann and colleagues (1995), clients with RA and OA used reachers, magnifying glasses, grab bars, jar openers, and other assistive devices in their homes and found them to be helpful in performing ADLs and instrumental activities of daily living (IADLs). The clients were instructed in the use of the assistive devices by an occupational therapy practitioner (Mann et al., 1998). Because RA and OA are chronic and progressive diseases, clients seen in any setting will benefit from protection principles prior to discharge. Appendix A provides suggestions for online references that you can share with your clients when you practice occupational therapy in the future.

The CMC joint of the thumb is the most common site for surgical reconstruction of OA in the hand and UE (Hunter et al., 2002). Indications for surgery include pain or deformity that interferes with daily function. Clients who present with severe symptomatic CMC OA usually complain of pain at the base of their thumb and weakness, especially with gripping and pinching. Clients often state they can no longer open their thumbs enough to pick up a bottle or glass for drinking. Clients may also report an inability to open jars or medication bottles or pinch their thumbs to hold a book.

When surgery is indicated, soft tissue reconstruction is performed using a tendon as the soft tissue arthroplasty. Arthroplasty is joint replacement surgery. There are a variety of different styles of soft tissue arthroplasty depending on the surgeon and the anatomy and physiology of the client.

TABLE 10-2

Protection Principles

Respect pain	• Stop activities before the point of discomfort. • Decrease activities that cause pain that lasts more than 2 hours. • Avoid activities that put strain on painful joints.
Balance rest and activity	• Rest before exhaustion and take frequent breaks. • Avoid activities that cannot be stopped. • Avoid staying in one position for a long time. • Alternate heavy and light activities. • Take more breaks when inflammation is active. • Allow extra time for activities; avoid rushing. • Plan your day ahead of time. • Eliminate unnecessary activities.
Reduce the effort	• Avoid excessive loads with carts, get help, and use appliances. • Keep items near where they are used. • Use prepared foods; freeze leftovers for later use. • Avoid low chairs. • Maintain proper body weight. • Try to eliminate trips up and down stairs by completing work on each floor. • Sit to work when possible.
Avoid positions of deformity	• Avoid bent elbows, knees, hips, and back while sleeping. • Practice good posture during the day. • Use workstation evaluation for proper posture.
Use the larger joints	• Slide heavy objects on kitchen counters. • Use palms, rather than fingers, to lift or push. • Carry a backpack instead of a handheld purse. • Keep packages close to the body; use two hands. • Push swinging doors open with side of body instead of the hands.
Use adaptive equipment	• Use jar openers, button hooks, etc. that are specific to each client's needs.
Distribute pressure	• Use both hands, leverage, carts, etc.

Adapted from Hunter, J. M., Maklin, E. J., Callahan, H. D., Skirven, T. M., Schneider, L. H., & Osterman, A. E. (2002). *Rehabilitation of the hand and upper extremity* (5th ed.). Mosby.

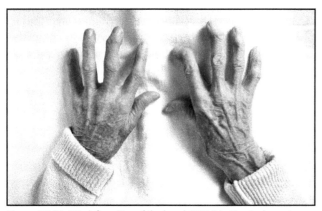

Figure 10-21. OA deformities of the hand. (LIAL/shutterstock.com)

Generally, CMC arthroplasty includes the removal of the diseased trapezium and the use of a tendon or portion of a tendon as the joint. According to Cannon (2003), the two tendons commonly harvested for this type of surgery are the flexor carpi radialis or the abductor pollicis longus. The goals of this highly successful surgery are to create a stable, pain-free joint with full function of the thumb. Box 10-3 shows the basic guidelines for rehabilitation after CMC arthroplasty for OA of the CMC joint.

BOX 10-3

CARPOMETACARPAL ARTHROPLASTY PROTOCOL

1. A cast is applied for the initial 4 weeks to immobilize the wrist and thumb.
2. After cast removal, a thumb spica splint is applied to be worn between exercise sessions and at night for protection.
3. Edema, pain, and scar management techniques are used after cast removal.
4. AROM of the thumb and wrist is initiated at 4 weeks.
5. Gentle PROM is initiated at 6 weeks where joints are limited.
6. Gentle gripping and pinching, as well as use of the hand in light resistive ADLs, is initiated at 6 to 8 weeks.
7. The splint is discontinued at 6 to 8 weeks (and used as needed).
8. Resistive use as tolerated is initiated at 10 to 12 weeks.
9. Clients will continue to notice some discomfort, stiffness, and weakness for 6 to 12 months after this surgery.

(Cannon, 2003; Weiss & Falkenstein, 2005)

Repetitive Stress Injuries

RSIs, also known as **cumulative trauma disorders**, affect the wrist, hand, and thumb more often than any other part of the body. As an analogy of our hands compared to tires on a car, we replace the tires after about 50,000 miles or the car will have a blow-out or flat tire. Unfortunately, we cannot replace our hands when they get tired, injured, or worn out. *Repetitive stress injury* is an umbrella term that encompasses many specific conditions of the UE including lateral epicondylitis (tennis elbow), which was described in Chapter 8. Conditions limited to the hand will be discussed here including **carpal tunnel syndrome** (CTS), **tendinitis**, and **trigger finger**. OA of the CMC joint is considered an RSI as well, but was covered in the previous section under arthritis.

Repetitive motion is required in many work and leisure activities. Jobs that require repetition include assemblers, mechanics, carpenters, computer programmers, and landscapers. Leisure activities such as gardening, quilting, reading, and baking are repetitive. The use of communication devices, such as **handheld electronic devices** (HEDs), is a described IADL in the *Occupational Therapy Practice Framework: Domain and Process, Fourth Edition* (American Occupational Therapy Association [AOTA], 2020). HEDs, including cellphones, BlackBerrys (TCL Corporation), computer notepads, and electronic readers, require repetitive hand movements, according to the *Occupational Therapy Practice Framework: Domain and Process, Fourth Edition* (AOTA, 2020). The era we live in demands a fast-paced exchange of information in all areas of life, including work, leisure, and ADLs. The ability to connect with coworkers, family, and friends around the world through social media is not without its drawbacks. The use of HEDs and the repetitive hand movements required can place individuals at increased risk for developing RSIs (Amini, 2006). Factors that may increase the risk of RSIs include repetitive activities,

poor posture and body mechanics, an inherited predisposition to a health condition, and poor lifestyle choices (Weiss & Falkenstein, 2005). Clients cannot do anything about their inherent risk of arthritis, but they do have more control over their lifestyle choices. Making smart lifestyle changes can decrease the risk of developing or acquiring an RSI. Those changes should include no tobacco use, limiting caffeine and alcohol, and weight control, which include a healthy diet and more aerobic exercise. After briefly describing two RSIs of the hand and thumb frequently seen in occupational therapy, a discussion of preventative treatment will follow.

Tendinitis, as the name infers, is an irritation or inflammation of the tendons. Tendinitis is prevalent in the hand and wrist and can be a precursor to other RSIs. For example, tendinitis of the flexor tendons, which run through the carpal tunnel, can cause swelling in this small space, exerting pressure on the median nerve. This ultimately could lead to CTS. In tendinitis of the hand and wrist, microscopic tears of the tendons can occur, especially at the area where the tendon and muscle join (the **musculotendinous junction**). This junction is a weaker section of the tendon–muscle complex and is more stressed during repetition and overuse of the hands and arms (Amini, 2006). The signs and symptoms of tendinitis are pain and swelling. The most common tendons affected are the flexor and extensor tendons of the wrist and the extensor tendons of the thumb. CTS is a compression of the median nerve at the level of the wrist. It is believed to be caused by chronic tenosynovitis of the flexor tendons that run through the carpal tunnel. Chronic, progressive CTS can lead to sensory loss and motor weakness of the intrinsic muscles of the hand and, consequently, in a loss of hand function (Cannon, 2003). It is thought to be most common in women who perform repetitive tasks. Women generally have a smaller carpal tunnel and more flexibility in their wrists than men, which increases the risk of developing CTS. Numbness and tingling, more so at night, is the complaint that distinguishes CTS from other RSIs. Clients will complain of numbness and tingling in the median nerve distribution. Other signs and symptoms include pain, swelling, weakness in grip and pinch, and dropping objects (Novak & Mackinnon, 1997). The good news regarding CTS is that surgical intervention can relieve the signs and symptoms. The surgeon completely releases the transverse carpal ligament, which forms the ceiling of the carpal tunnel. When this thickened ligament is divided, pressure on the median nerve is relieved, decreasing signs and symptoms of numbness and pain. Clients frequently recover strength and function of their hands after surgery. The client may benefit from several sessions of occupational therapy and a home exercise program. The client may complain of tenderness or pillar pain surrounding the small incision in the palm of the hand after surgery. There may also be weakness during gripping activities after carpal tunnel release surgery. These complaints usually resolve within 3 months after surgery.

Trigger finger is defined as pathological thickening of the sheath of the flexor tendon at or around the A1 pulley. If there is enough swelling in this area, the tendon can become locked in flexion, causing a snap with pain as the swollen tendon and its sheath slide under the pulley. A knot can be palpated at the distal palmar crease of the injured digit. The affected digit can become very stiff in PIP flexion. The thumb is the most affected digit, followed by the ring and long fingers (Weiss & Falkenstein, 2005). Clients with a history of RA or diabetes are more likely to be affected. Treatment of trigger finger varies depending on severity and duration. Conservative treatment in occupational therapy may consist of instruction in rest, use of home cold modalities, splinting, and stretching exercises. The client will need to avoid repetitive gripping and the use of vibrating handheld equipment for at least 3 to 4 weeks. Icing the palm three times per day may improve the pain and inflammation. A splint to hold the finger in extension at night may rest the tendon and keep the fingers from curling into a fist while sleeping, which may decrease pain and triggering. Gentle stretching exercises will help maintain finger mobility. If the symptoms become worse or conservative treatment fails, the doctor may recommend a steroid injection, which is the most common treatment and is effective in 90% of individuals. If trigger finger release surgery is required, a small incision is made at the distal palmar crease in order to clip the A1 pulley and release the swollen tendon. Occupational therapy after surgery may include edema and scar management, stretching, and ROM exercises, progressing to grip and pinch strengthening exercises as tolerated (Hunter et al., 2002).

Conservative treatment of RSI is always preferable to surgery, and this is where occupational therapy practitioners can make a difference through intervention. A comprehensive plan should include improving the symptoms of an existing RSI and preventing future trauma through education. After the occupational therapy evaluation, occupational therapy assistants may use physical agent modalities (PAMs) according to state licensure and the AOTA (2008) guidelines in preparation for purposeful activity (Amini, 2006). PAMs, which may include ultrasound or electrical stimulation, assist tissue healing, enhance movement, and decrease pain. PAMs also include the use of cold to reduce inflammation and pain during conservative treatment of RSIs. Splinting to rest the inflamed joints along with tendon and nerve gliding exercises are also helpful in alleviating the symptoms of RSI and improving functional use of the client's UEs.

Client education is the key for prevention of RSIs in the future. Occupational therapy practitioners possess the knowledge base to teach clients general protection principles as well as specific body mechanics and tool adaptations that can be utilized at home and work and in leisure activities. See Box 10-4 for specific adaptations used in client education to prevent RSIs.

Dupuytren's Disease

Dupuytren's disease is a contracture of the **palmar aponeurosis** named after French surgeon, Baron Guillaume Dupuytren, who first operated on it in 1831. The palmar aponeurosis is the thickened, central portion of the deep palmar fascia. Its main function is mechanical as it protects the flexor tendons of the palm and gives firm attachment to the skin of the palm to help with grip. Dupuytren's disease is seen more frequently in men more than 50 years old who are of Northern European descent. It generally runs in families, as individuals who have it can remember a father or grandfather with the same signs and symptoms. The disease begins with a thickening in the palm just under the skin on either side of the distal palmar crease at the base of the small finger. Dupuytren's disease will often affect both hands, but signs and symptoms are generally worse in one hand. The disease is a benign process, and the individual typically does not seek treatment until the contracture negatively affects function. The most common complaint is an inability to completely straighten the small or ring fingers. This is due to the flexion contracture at the MCP and/or PIP joints (Hertling & Kessler, 2006). Functional deficits can include difficulty reaching into a pocket, donning a glove, and shaking hands or the inability to receive change.

Unfortunately, conservative treatment does not seem to help the signs and symptoms. There are two main treatment options available to people with disabling contracture from

BOX 10-4

PREVENTION OF REPETITIVE STRESS INJURIES

For healthy computer and HED use:

- Maintain neutral wrists.
- Take short, frequent rest breaks.
- Stretch frequently to enhance blood flow.
- Investigate the use of a cordless keyboard and mouse.
- Use hands-free headsets with phone use.
- Use a stylus (an inverted pencil) for tapping on miniature keyboards.
- Be selective when responding to emails and text messages; use abbreviations or use the voice activation key if available.

Additional prevention principles:

- Avoid a sustained grip or pinch in daily activities.
- Avoid repetitive overuse of the wrist and hand in activity.
- Avoid positioning the wrists in a flexed posture (fetal position) while sleeping.
- Use ergonomic tools where possible (i.e., larger, cushioned handles and tool designs that avoid awkward wrist positions).
- Use vibratory diminishing devices or antivibratory gloves when using tools with high-frequency vibration.

(Amini, 2006; Cannon, 2003; Keller et al., 1998; Weiss & Falkenstein, 2005)

Dupuytren's disease. The nonsurgical option is a **XIAFLEX** (collagenase *Clostridium histolyticum*) injection. XIAFLEX is an enzyme drug that is injected into the contracture in the palm. The enzyme quickly dissolves a portion of the thickened fascia, making it possible for the surgeon to manipulate the contracture, straightening the finger the next day in the office.

The surgical treatment for Dupuytren's disease is called a *palmar fasciotomy*. This procedure involves removing the thickened fascia, or connective tissue, which releases the palmar contracture through a single, larger incision. Occupational therapy after either of these procedures is very important to a good outcome. The surgeon wants therapy to maintain the ROM gains made by the injection with manipulation or the surgery. The therapist's intervention includes splinting to maintain digit extension; wound, edema, and scar management; AROM and PROM; and, eventually, strengthening (Cannon, 2003).

Skier's Thumb

Skier's thumb is an acute injury to the UCL of the thumb. The condition is called skier's thumb because an injury to this ligament is often seen among skiers who fall with the ski pole still in hand. Forty-nine percent of injuries to the UCL of the thumb result from a fall on an outstretched hand. You will recall this acronym from a discussion of the distal radius fracture in Chapter 9. During a fall that results in a skier's thumb injury, force to the outstretched thumb may cause hyperextension of the proximal phalanx, tearing the UCL, especially if the fingers are still closed around the handle of a ski or hiking pole. Individuals with this injury will complain of tenderness, bruising, and swelling along the ulnar side of the thumb MCP joint. Signs and symptoms also may include side-to-side instability at the MCP joint, and the inability to tear a piece of paper or tie one's shoes (Hunter et al., 2002).

UCL tears are categorized from grades I to III, and treatment depends on the extent of the tear. A grade I UCL tear is the most common and involves microscopic tears in the ligament fiber but no instability. Rest and immobilization using a splint or taping may be the only treatment. Grade II tears involve a partial ligament disruption, but the overall integrity is still intact. The rehabilitation is virtually the same but with a slower recovery time due to a longer phase of immobilization. When the UCL is completely ruptured, the tear is considered grade III. Magnetic resonance imaging may help the surgeon discover the grade of the tear, especially if they notice instability at the MCP joint upon examination. It is recommended that a grade III UCL tear be surgically repaired. In 80% of grade III UCL tears, a **Stener lesion** is present. A Stener lesion happens when the aponeurosis of the adductor pollicis (AP) muscle is interposed between the bones of the MCP joint and the torn UCL. This prevents adequate healing of the ligament and is why surgical repair is so important in complete UCL tears. The repair involves direct suturing of the ligament to itself or to an adjacent bone (Strittmatter & Preston, 2022). If there is an **avulsion fracture** present, the surgeon will repair it with wires or screws. An avulsion fracture is an injury to the bone at an attachment when the ligament or tendon tear and pull off a piece of the bone. After surgery for a grade III skier's thumb repair the individual is casted 4 to 6 weeks. When the cast is removed, therapy is recommended for 6 to 8 weeks with intervention focused on functional movement, grip, and pinch, as well as edema and scar management. The therapist will fabricate an MCP thumb splint to be worn with activities for up to 3 months. The client may be required to wait 3 to 5 months before returning to heavy lifting or sports activities. Tenderness and thickening at the repair site may persist for up to 1 year.

Please refer to the occupational profile of Sara at the beginning of this chapter and in Appendix C for more information on occupational therapy intervention for skier's thumb.

Body Structures of the Intrinsic Hand

Muscles, tendons, ligaments, nerves, and spinal cord levels of the intrinsic hand will be identified and discussed as they relate to function in this section. These structures are responsible for the precise movements required by our hands to perform fine motor tasks during self-care, work, and leisure activities.

Muscle Actions of the Intrinsic Hand and Thumb

The intrinsic muscles of the hand are named as such because they originate and insert on the hand distal to the carpal bones. These muscles have a function on the thumb and fingers. They are also responsible for precise movements and fine motor control of the hand (Lippert, 2000). Although this text has separated the extrinsic and intrinsic muscle groups of the hand for learning purposes, it is important to understand how their function is interwoven. The hand functions by using a blended combination from the extrinsic and intrinsic groups of muscles (Oatis, 2004).

This section arranges the intrinsic muscles of the hand into four functional groups to help the student understand how the intrinsic muscles interact. The four functional groups include the thenar, hypothenar, interossei, and lumbrical muscles. Table 10-3 presents an overview of the intrinsic muscles of the hand.

The four thenar muscles (the primary movers of the thumb), are the abductor pollicis brevis (APB), flexor pollicis brevis (FPB), opponens pollicis (OP), and AP. These intrinsic muscles form the thenar eminence of the hand.

The APB abducts the CMC joint of the thumb. Active abduction of the thumb is needed to position the thumb for grip or pinch. APB atrophy from median nerve palsy can lead to decreased strength in pinch and grip (Oatis, 2004).

The primary function of the FPB is to flex the MCP joint of the thumb. The FPB assists the flexor pollicis longus (FPL) in CMC flexion only because it crosses the CMC joint. The FPB assists the APB in CMC joint abduction (Lippert, 2000).

The OP produces opposition of the CMC joint. Thumb opposition is the most important function of the hand, which probably explains why thumb movement is known to make up approximately 50% of hand function. The FPB and APB assist in this function because opposition is a combination of flexion, abduction, and rotation of the thumb. The OP is the second largest muscle of the thenar intrinsic group and reinforces the actions of the other thenar muscles. Weakness in the OP muscle affects positioning and stabilization of the CMC joint during pinching activities (Oatis, 2004).

The AP is the largest of the thenar muscles and adducts the CMC joint of the thumb. The AP is a deep muscle, so it does not make up the bulk of the thenar eminence. It also flexes the thumb MCP joint. The AP adducts the thumb only to the palm, then the extensor pollicis longus (EPL) continues adduction through its full excursion (Oatis, 2004). This muscle supplies much of the force in pinch.

The hypothenar muscles are the intrinsic muscles of the hand that act on the small finger. They are the opponens digiti minimi (ODM), abductor digiti minimi (ADM), and flexor digiti minimi brevis (FDMB). All the joints of the small finger are influenced by these three muscles.

The ODM is the largest and strongest of the hypothenar muscles and opposes the small finger at the MCP joint. Opposition of the small finger contributes to the volar arch, which is formed while cupping the hand. The ADM abducts the small finger at the MCP joint and assists with MCP flexion as well. The FDMB flexes the small finger at the MCP joint. It is the smallest and weakest of the hypothenar muscles. Weakness of this muscle group could impair the intricate function of the small finger, especially in abduction. Individuals whose careers depend on finger movements, such as computer programmers or musicians, may be more negatively affected by hypothenar muscle weakness (Oatis, 2004).

The **palmar interossei** adduct the MCP joints of the index, ring, and small fingers to the long finger (Hunter et al., 2002). With the long finger as a central axis of the hand, the dorsal interossei muscles abduct the fingers. There are four palmar interossei muscles and four dorsal interossei muscles. If the client presents with weakness in the interossei muscles, they will not be able to completely spread the fingers or bring them tightly together. The client may also present with weakness in functional grip and pinch.

The lumbrical muscles are the last of the intrinsic muscles discussed. There are four lumbrical muscles located deep within the hand. The lumbrical muscles are unique because they have no bony attachments in the hand. They attach proximally to the tendons of the flexor digitorum profundus (FDP) and distally to the tendons of the extensor digitorum communis (EDC), which are antagonists (Oatis, 2004). The

TABLE 10-3
Intrinsic Muscles of the Hand and Their Movements

THENAR MUSCLE GROUP	MOVEMENT
Abductor pollicis brevis	• CMC abduction of the thumb
Flexor pollicis brevis	• CMC flexion and abduction • MCP flexion of the thumb
Opponens pollicis	• CMC opposition of the thumb
Adductor pollicis	• CMC adduction • MCP flexion of the thumb
HYPOTHENAR MUSCLE GROUP	**MOVEMENT**
Opponens digiti minimi	• MCP opposition of the small finger
Abductor digiti minimi	• MCP abduction of the small finger
Flexor digiti minimi brevis	• MCP flexion of the small finger
Palmar interossei	• MCP adduction of the index, ring, and small fingers
Dorsal interossei	• MCP flexion and abduction • PIP/DIP extension of the index, long, and ring fingers • MCP adduction of the long finger
Lumbricals	• MCP flexion and PIP/DIP extension of the index, long, ring, and small fingers

Adapted from Floyd, R. T., & Thompson, C. W. (2001). *Manual of structural kinesiology* (14th ed.). McGraw-Hill.

lumbricals flex the MCP joints and extend the PIP and DIP joints of all four fingers. This combined motion is called the *intrinsic plus position* (Lippert, 2000). If the intrinsic musculature is weakened due to an ulnar nerve injury, a "claw hand" deformity, or intrinsic minus position, can occur, negatively affecting hand function. The intrinsic plus position is the ultimate hand position for healing after injury because it maintains MCP joint flexion and a good hand posture for recovery of function. A good example of functional intrinsic plus hand posture is seen while an individual is holding a book by the binding. Figures 10-22 and 10-23 illustrate the functional intrinsic plus position and the claw hand deformity.

Muscles, Nerves, and Spinal Cord Levels of the Intrinsic Hand and Thumb

Tables 10-4 and 10-5 summarize both extrinsic and intrinsic motions and innervations of the hand and thumb. The hand is supplied by the median, ulnar, and radial nerves. The motor fibers to the intrinsic muscles of the hand are carried by the median and ulnar nerves and are derived from the C7-T1 segments of the spinal cord. The median nerve enters the hand by passing through the carpal tunnel. A superficial branch enters just distal to the flexor retinaculum and innervates the APB, FPB, OP, and the first and second lumbrical muscles. These thenar muscles give the hand fine precision and pinch function. The median nerve is known as the *nerve of function* to the hand due to its sensory innervations to the palmar surface of the thumb and index and middle fingers, and the radial portion of the ring finger.

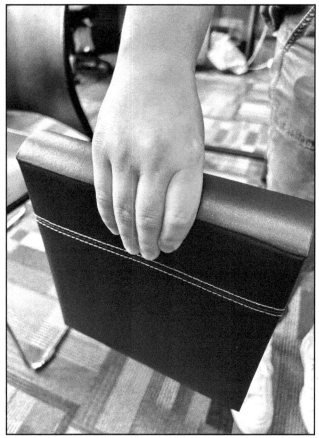

Figure 10-22. Functional intrinsic plus position while holding a book.

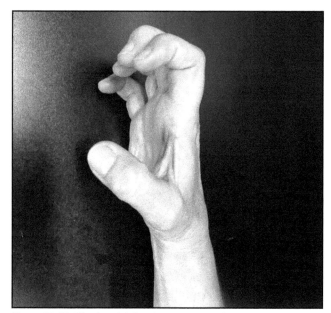

Figure 10-23. Claw hand deformity or intrinsic minus position.

The ulnar nerve enters the hand anterior to the flexor retinaculum and lateral to the pisiform. It descends from spinal roots C8-T1 and divides into superficial and deep branches. The superficial branch supplies the palmaris brevis muscle. The deep branch passes between the ADM and FDMB, which it innervates. It then supplies the ODM and curves around the hook of the hamate and across the palm of the hand. There it innervates all the interossei muscles, the third and fourth lumbrical muscles, and the AP. It gives sensation to the posterior of the small finger, ring finger, the ulnar portion of the middle finger, the anterior portion of the small finger, and the anterior/ulnar portion of the ring finger. Injury to the ulnar nerve can cause severe disabilities to the hand because it supplies the muscles responsible for the finer movements of the fingers and the power grasp of the hand.

The radial nerve supplies dorsal, digital nerves to the thumb, index finger, middle finger, and the radial half of the ring finger. The radial nerve innervates the wrist and digit extensors, which control the position of the hand (Cleveland Clinic, 2021).

Tendons and Ligaments of the Intrinsic Hand and Thumb

The tendons of the intrinsic muscles function by their origins and where they attach. The thenar muscles, OP, APB, and FPB, are located at the base of the thumb and produce the thenar eminence. They are responsible for fine movements of the thumb. The OP and FPB originate from the trapezium, along with the APB, which also originates from the scaphoid. All three tendons also originate from the flexor retinaculum. The OP inserts into the thumb metacarpal. The APB and FPB attach to the proximal phalanx of the thumb. The hypothenar muscles produce the hypothenar eminence on the ulnar side of the palm. The ODM and the FDMB originate at the hook of the hamate and the flexor retinaculum. The ADM originates from the pisiform and the flexor carpi ulnaris tendon. The ODM attaches at the small finger metacarpal and the ADM and FDMB insert at the base of the small finger proximal phalanx. The lumbricals of each finger originate from the tendon of the FDP and insert into the extensor hood. The four dorsal interossei muscles originate from the lateral and medial metacarpals of the corresponding finger. They attach to the extensor hood and proximal phalanx of each finger. The three palmar interossei muscles and their tendons originate from a medial or lateral surface of a metacarpal and attach into the extensor hood and proximal phalanx of the same finger (Hunter et al., 2002).

The ligaments of the CMC joints of the wrist, hand, and thumb were discussed in Chapter 9. In this chapter, the ligaments of the MCP, PIP, and DIP joints of the fingers as well as the MCP and IP joints of the thumb will be covered briefly.

TABLE 10-4   Motions and Innervations of the Thumb

MUSCLE	NERVE	SPINAL NERVE ROOT				THUMB				
		C6	C7	C8	T1	Flexion* CMC (Palmar Abduction) 0 to 50 degrees MCP: 0 to 60 degrees IP: 0 to 80 degrees	Extension* CMC (Radial Abduction) 0 to 20 degrees MCP: 60 to 0 degrees IP: 80 to 0 degrees	Abduction CMC 0 to 50 degrees	Adduction CMC 50 to 0 degrees	Opposition CMC Measured in centimeters lacking
Extensor pollicis longus (E)	Radial	X	X	X			X			
Extensor pollicis brevis (E)	Radial	X	X				X			
Abductor pollicis longus (E)	Radial	X	X					X		
Flexor pollicis longus (E)	Median			X	X	X				
Flexor pollicis brevis (I)	Median	X	X			X				
Abductor pollicis brevis (I)	Median	X	X					X		
Opponens pollicis (I)	Median	X	X							X
Adductor pollicis (I)	Ulnar			X	X				X	

* Some muscles do not have actions at all joints listed in the category. For example, the FPB does not act at the IP joint as it inserts proximal to this joint.

E = extrinsic; I intrinsic.

Adapted from Lippert, L. S. (2000). *Clinical kinesiology for physical therapist assistants* (3rd ed.). F. A. Davis Company and Rondinelli, R. D., Genoverse, E., Katz, R. T., Mayer, T. G., Mueller, K., & Ranavaya, M. (2008). *Guides to the evaluation of permanent impairment* (6th ed.). American Medical Association.

TABLE 10-5

Motions and Innervations of the Fingers

MUSCLE	NERVE	SPINAL NERVE ROOT				FINGERS				
		C6	C7	C8	T1	Flexion MCP 90 degrees PIP: 0 to 100 degrees DIP: 0 to 70 degrees	Extension MCP 90 to +20 degrees PIP: 100 to 0 degrees DIP: 70 to 0 degrees	Abduction MCP 0 to 25 degrees	Adduction MCP 25 to 0 degrees	Opposition Small finger not tested
Extensor digitorum communis (E)	Radial	X	X	X			X			
Extensor indicis (E)	Radial	X	X	X			X			
Extensor digiti minimi (E)	Radial	X	X	X			X			
Flexor digitorum superficialis (E)	Median		X	X	X	X				
Flexor digitorum profundus (E)	Median and ulnar			X	X	X				
Lumbricals 1 and 2 (I)	Median	X	X			X (MCP)	X (DIP, PIP)			
Lumbricals 3 and 4 (I)	Ulnar			X	X	X (MCP)	X (DIP, PIP)			
Flexor digit minimi brevis (I)	Ulnar			X	X	X				
Abductor digiti minimi (I)	Ulnar			X	X			X		
Opponens digit minimi (I)	Ulnar			X	X					X
Dorsal interossei (I)	Ulnar			X	X			X		
Palmar interossei (I)	Ulnar			X	X				X	

E = extrinsic; I = intrinsic.

Adapted from Rondinelli, R. D., Genoverse, E., Katz, R. T., Mayer, T. G., Mueller, K., & Ranavaya, M. (2008) Guides to the evaluation of permanent impairment (6th ed.). American Medical Association.

TABLE 10-6
Intrinsic Ligaments and Their Function

LIGAMENT	FUNCTION
Ulnar collateral	Provides lateral stability during motion on ulnar side of joint
Radial collateral	Provides lateral stability during motion to radial side of joint
Accessory collateral	Fan-shaped part of UCL and RCL, provides more stability when joint is extended
Volar plate	Prevents hyperextension
Retinacular	Retains and positions common extensor mechanism during PIP and DIP joint flexion
Deep transverse metacarpal	Prevents metacarpal heads from excessive abduction
Superficial transverse metacarpal (natatory)	Resists abduction
Sagittal bands	Keeps extensor mechanism tracking in midline during MP joint flexion
Expansion hood	Along with central slip and lateral bands helps extend PIP and DIP joints
Digital cutaneous	Stabilizes skin to fascia and bone. Stabilizes neurovascular bundle during finger flexion and extension

Adapted from Hertling, D., & Kessler, R. (2006). *Management of common musculoskeletal disorders: Physical therapy principles and methods.* Lippincott Williams & Wilkins; Oatis, C. A. (2004). *Kinesiology: The mechanics and pathomechanics of human movement.* Lippincott Williams & Wilkins; and Weiss, S., & Falkenstein, N. (2005). *Hand rehabilitation: A quick reference guide and review.* Elsevier-Mosby.

The lesser-known ligaments of the hand and their functions are not discussed in the body of this chapter but are named in Table 10-6. They are the retinacular, deep transverse metacarpal, natatory or superficial transverse metacarpal, sagittal band, expansion hood, and digital cutaneous ligaments. Please refer to Table 10-6, which illustrates the ligaments of the hand and their functions.

The radial and ulnar collateral ligaments can be found on both sides of each joint in the fingers and thumb. They are thick bands running obliquely from the metacarpal to the proximal, middle, and distal phalanges and to the volar plate. The collateral ligaments also have a fan-shaped accessory ligament that attaches to the proximal portion of the volar plate. There is a volar plate located under each joint of the fingers and thumb and is comprised of fibrous connective tissue and fibrocartilage that limits hyperextension. The collateral ligaments provide stabilization of the joints from the radioulnar direction throughout flexion and extension excursion. The accessory ligaments provide additional support to the joints, especially when the distal joints of the thumb and fingers are extended. The UCL of the thumb MCP joint is prone to strain or rupture when an individual falls on the hand, forcing the thumb into abduction and extension. Please refer to the skier's thumb portion under the four problems of the hand and thumb in this chapter for more detailed information.

The IP joints receive additional stability from the surrounding tendons and their related connective tissue structures (Oatis, 2004). In the hand, the connective tissue or fascia is quite different on the dorsum or the back of the hand than the palm. Dorsally, the fascia is loose, thin, and mobile leaving it prone to avulsion injury and/or an accumulation of edema. The palmar fascia, often called the *palmar aponeuroses*, is deep, thick, and fibrous. The palmar aponeuroses fibers are oriented in many different directions, including vertical, longitudinal, transverse, and oblique (Hunter et al., 2002). This thick and varied fascia stabilizes the skin to underlying structures and provides protection, more so during resistive grasping activities (Oatis, 2004).

When the hand is relaxed, the palm forms a cupped position. This posture is maintained by the skeleton, the ligaments, and the use of the intrinsic muscles in the hand. There are three arches that form this cupped shape. These arches enable the hand to grasp objects of different sizes and shapes. They direct the skilled motion of the fingers and control the power of the grasp. The first arch in the developed adult hand is the proximal transverse arch that is formed by the base of the metacarpals and the carpal bones and is maintained by the flexor retinaculum. The distal transverse arch is formed by the metacarpal heads. The longitudinal arch runs from the wrist to the length of the fingers (Lippert, 2000). Figure 10-24 illustrates the functional arches of the hand.

The development of hand arches in babies is important for skilled movement of the fingers and controlled strength of the hand in adults. Using the hands to crawl is important toward developing the arches on the small finger side of the hand because most weight bearing occurs on that side of the hand. The infant learns that they can hold something with the thumb, index finger, and middle finger and continue to crawl. This is the beginning of hand separation development, which is critical for hand manipulation and writing skills (Case-Smith, 2005).

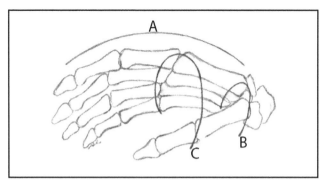

Figure 10-24. Functional arches of the hand and wrist. (A) The top curved horizontal line is the longitudinal arch. (B) The proximal half circle is the proximal transverse arch. (C) The distal half circle is the distal transverse arch. (Reproduced with permission from Angela Hartman.)

Summary

Through Sara, this chapter has explored how the intrinsic hand and thumb move and function. Knowledge of the normal hand and thumb and their supporting structures is necessary to understand the pathology that can affect them. Hands are a complex structure of intricate nerves, tendons, muscles, and bones. There are 27 bones in each hand and wrist alone. Hands enable us to move our fingers in ways machines cannot. However, those very components that enable us to play the cello, use a tool to tighten a screw, paint a masterpiece, or simply brush our teeth and tie our shoes, also make our hands susceptible to numerous injuries. These injuries and diseases can be painful and debilitating, causing us to lose our valued independence. As occupational therapy practitioners, we have the knowledge to help our clients return to a healthy and independent lifestyle and maintain it as long as possible throughout the lifespan.

References

American Occupational Therapy Association. (2008). Occupational therapy practice framework: Domain and process (2nd ed.). *American Journal of Occupational Therapy, 62,* 625-683.

American Occupational Therapy Association. (2020). Occupational therapy practice framework: Domain and process (4th ed.). *American Journal of Occupational Therapy, 74*(Suppl. 2), Article 7412410010. https://doi.org/10.5014/ajot.2020.74S2001

Amini, A. (2006). Repetitive stress injuries and the age of communication. *Occupational Therapy Practice, 11*(9), 10-15.

Benbow, M. (2001). Hand skills and handwriting. In S. A. Cermark & D. Larkin (Eds.), *Developmental coordination disorders.* Singular Thomson Learning.

Burke, S. L., Higgins, J. P., McClinton, M. A., Saunders, R., & Valdata, L. (2006). *Hand and upper extremity rehabilitation: A practical guide* (3rd ed.). Elsevier-Mosby.

Cannon, N. M. (2003). *Diagnosis and treatment manual for physicians and therapists: Upper extremity rehabilitation* (4th ed.). Hand Rehabilitation Center of Indiana.

Case-Smith, J. (2005). *Occupational therapy for children.* Elsevier-Mosby.

Cleveland Clinic. (2021). Radial nerve. https://my.clevelandclinic.org/health/body/21617-radial-nerve

Floyd, R. T., & Thompson, C. W. (2001). *Manual of structural kinesiology* (14th ed.). McGraw-Hill.

Hertling, D., & Kessler, R. (2006). *Management of common musculoskeletal disorders: Physical therapy principles and methods.* Lippincott Williams & Wilkins.

Hunter, J. M., Maklin, E. J., Callahan, H. D., Skirven, T. M., Schneider, L. H., & Osterman, A. E. (2002). *Rehabilitation of the hand and upper extremity* (5th ed.). Mosby.

Kapandji, A. (1986). [Clinical test of apposition and counter-apposition of the thumb]. *Annales de Chirurgie de la Main et du Membre Supérieur, 5*(1), 67-73.

Keller, K., Corbett, J., & Nichols, D. (1998). Repetitive strain injury in computer keyboard users: Pathomechanics and treatment principles in individual and group intervention. *Journal of Hand Therapy, 11*(1), 9-26.

Latella, D., & Meriano, C. (2003). *Occupational therapy manual for the evaluation of range of motion and muscle strength.* Delmar Carnage Learning.

Lippert, L. S. (2000). *Clinical kinesiology for physical therapist assistants* (3rd ed.). F. A. Davis Company.

Mann, W. C., Hurren, D., & Tomita, M. (1995). Assistive devices used by home-based elderly persons with arthritis. *American Journal of Occupational Therapy, 49*(8), 810-820.

McCaffery, M., & Pasero, C. (1999). *Pain: Clinical manual.* Mosby.

Novak, C. B., & Mackinnon, S. E. (1997). Repetitive use and static postures: A source of nerve compression and pain. *Journal of Hand Therapy, 10*(2), 151-159.

Oatis, C. A. (2004). *Kinesiology: The mechanics and pathomechanics of human movement.* Lippincott Williams & Wilkins.

Pendleton, H. M., & Schultz-Krohn, W. (2006). *Pedretti's occupational therapy practice skills for physical dysfunction* (6th ed.). Mosby-Elsevier.

Riley, M. A. (1998). The effects of medical conditions and aging on hand function. *Occupational Therapy Practice, 3*(6), 24-27.

Rondinelli, R. D., Genoverse, E., Katz, R. T., Mayer, T. G., Mueller, K., & Ranavaya, M. (2008) *Guides to the evaluation of permanent impairment* (6th ed.). American Medical Association

Rybski, M. (2019). *Kinesiology for occupational therapy* (3rd ed.). SLACK Incorporated.

Strittmatter, J., & Preston, C. (2022). Skier's thumb. *eMedicineHealth.* https://www.emedicinehealth.com/skiers_thumb/article_em.htm

Weiss, S., & Falkenstein, N. (2005). *Hand rehabilitation: A quick reference guide and review.* Elsevier-Mosby.

Applications

The following activities will help you apply knowledge of the hand and thumb in real-life applications. Activities can be completed individually or in a small group to enhance learning.

1. **Joints and Motions of the Hand and Thumb**: Complete the following activities to increase your familiarity with the functional aspects and movements of the hand and thumb.
    a. Demonstrate how the thumb and fingers work individually. First, produce the American Sign Language sign for "I love you" by performing the following steps:
        i.   Fully extend the index and small fingers
        ii. Flex the long and ring fingers
        iii. Radially abduct the thumb
        iv. Move the wrist from radial to ulnar deviation

    Did one hand seem easier than the other? Do you know why you cannot flex the DIP joints of the long and ring fingers? Second, lace the fingers together, and supinate the forearms. Twiddle the thumbs in isolation from the fingers, rotate thumbs away from your body, and then rotate thumbs toward your body.
    b. Reliable and useful landmarks in the hand are skin creases. They are more prominent on the palmar surface and change during movement. The creases are valuable to the occupational therapy practitioner during observation, evaluation, and especially during splint fabrication. Observe and identify the following creases found in the palm of your hand:
        i.   Thenar
        ii. Distal palmar
        iii. Proximal palmar
        iv. Proximal phalangeal
        v.   Distal phalangeal
    c. The arches of the hand are formed by bones and ligaments in the wrist and hand. Intrinsic muscles and the nerves that innervate them help to hold objects in the hand by means of cupping the palm. With the forearm supinated and the hand cupped, place small objects in your palm (try vitamins, coins, dried beans, or marbles). Now, without closing your fingers around the objects, shake your arm and hand side to side. How many small objects can you and your partner hold in the cup of your hand without dropping them?

2. **Strength and Dexterity of the Hand and Thumb**: Complete the following activities to familiarize yourself with functional stability, grip, and prehension of the hand and thumb.
    a. Note how the ring and small fingers appear inactive while the thumb, index, and middle fingers perform skilled activities during the following:
        i.   Cut with scissors.
        ii. Snap your fingers.
        iii. Seal a sandwich bag.
    b. Demonstrate the precision of the thumb and fingertips during the following:
        i.   Thread a needle.
        ii. Hold a dime between the thumb, index finger, and middle finger, flipping it from heads to tails and back using one hand.
        iii. Continue to hold the dime as in ii., tails up, now rotate it to read the text using one hand.
    c. As occupational therapy practitioners, you will educate clients in protection principles. Complete the following, noting which task was easier on your hands:
        i.   Hold a bag of groceries with your fingers and your elbow extended next to your side; now place the handles over your forearm with your elbow bent to 90 degrees.
        ii. Carry a pillow by pinching it between your thumb and fingers, your elbow extended, arm to your side; now carry the pillow under your arm.
        iii. Carry a filled coffee mug in your hand using the handle; now, carry it with both hands avoiding the handle.

    iv. Write using a ballpoint pen; now write using a gel pen with a built-in rubber grip.

    v. Open a door with a round doorknob; now open a door with a lever-type handle.

d. In-hand manipulation is the ability to move and position objects within one hand without using the other hand. It is probably the most complex fine motor skill. Demonstrate in-hand manipulation with the following activities:

    i. Hold at least 12 coins in your hand, now place the coins one at a time in a bank.

    ii. Hold a pencil in your fingertips, ready for writing, then "walk" the fingers to the eraser end of the pencil, then back to the tip.

    iii. Turn dice within the fingertips to see different sides using one hand.

e. Note the way your hand works in the following tasks:

    i. Write a sentence on a piece of paper that is placed on a table.

    ii. Now write the same sentence with your nondominant hand.

    iii. Now write the sentence again with your dominant hand but keep your ring and small fingers extended.

3. **Goniometric Measurements of the Intrinsic Hand and Thumb**: ROM norms can vary depending on the reference source. One norm is provided for each motion within this text to increase ease of application. Additionally, while multiple muscles may influence a particular motion, only the main muscles responsible for a joint motion are included. References for the information can be found in Box 10-5. With your partner, practice using a goniometer to measure each motion available at the joints of the hand. You may record the available ROM in Table 10-7.

BOX 10-5

REFERENCED WORKS FOR RANGE OF MOTION

Sections Referenced (a to e)	Reference
Goniometric landmark, end feel, and start and end positions	Latella & Meriano, 2003; Pendleton & Schultz-Krohn, 2006
Muscles responsible	Floyd et al., 2001; Oatis, 2004
Available ROM	Rondinelli et al., 2008

TABLE 10-7

Range of Motion Application Table

JOINT	MOTIONS	AVAILABLE ROM (DEGREES)	ROM OF YOUR PARTNER
Finger MCP	Flexion	0 to 90	
	Extension	90 to 0	
	Hyperextension	0 to 20	
	Abduction	0 to 25	
	Adduction	25 to 0	
Finger PIP	Flexion	0 to 100	
	Extension	100 to 0	
Finger DIP	Flexion	0 to 70	
	Extension	70 to 0	
Thumb MCP	Flexion	0 to 60	
	Extension	60 to 0	

(continued)

TABLE 10-7 (CONTINUED)
Range of Motion Application Table

JOINT	MOTIONS	AVAILABLE ROM (DEGREES)	ROM OF YOUR PARTNER
Thumb IP	Flexion	0 to 80	
	Extension	80 to 0	
Thumb CMC	Radial abduction (extension)	0 to 20	
	Palmar abduction	0 to 50	
	Adduction	50 to 0	
	Opposition	Measured in centimeters lacking	

a. Finger MCP flexion ROM
   i. Goniometric landmark: Dorsal surface of the MCP joint of the finger

   Stable arm: Midline of dorsal surface of finger metacarpal

   Moving arm: Midline of dorsal surface of proximal phalanx of finger
   ii. Available ROM: 0 to 90 degrees
   iii. End feel: Firm
   iv. Muscles responsible: Flexor digitorum superficialis, FDP, lumbricals
   v. Start and end position: Figure 10-25 displays the start position for finger MCP flexion. The client is seated with the arm resting on a table on the ulnar border with the wrist in neutral and the MCP joints straight. The client bends the MCP joint into maximum flexion. Figure 10-26 displays the end position of ROM testing.

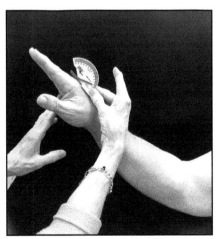

Figure 10-25. Start position for ROM testing of finger MCP flexion/end position for finger MCP extension.

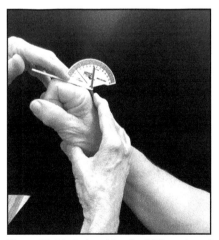

Figure 10-26. End position for ROM testing of finger MCP flexion/start position for finger MCP extension.

Note: Because MCP extension is simply a return from MCP flexion, the start position for MCP flexion will be the same as the end position for MCP extension. Similarly, the start position for MCP extension will be the same as the end position for MCP flexion (see Figures 10-25 and 10-26).

b. Finger MCP extension ROM

   i. Goniometric landmark: Dorsal surface of the MCP joint of the finger

      Stable arm: Midline of dorsal surface of finger metacarpal

      Moving arm: Midline of dorsal surface of proximal phalanx of the finger

   ii. Available ROM: 90 to 0 degrees

   iii. End feel: Firm

   iv. Muscles responsible: EDC, extensor indicis, extensor digiti minimi (EDM), lumbricals

   v. Start and end position: See Figure 10-26 for start position. The client is seated with the arm resting on a table on the ulnar border with the wrist in neutral and the MCP joints flexed. The client straightens or moves the MCPs into maximum extension as in Figure 10-25 or end position.

c. Finger MCP hyperextension ROM

   i. Goniometric landmark: Dorsal surface of the MCP joint of the finger

      Stable arm: Midline of dorsal surface of finger metacarpal

      Moving arm: Midline of dorsal surface of proximal phalanx of the finger

   ii. Available ROM: 0 to 20 degrees

   iii. End feel: Firm

   iv. Muscles responsible: EDC, extensor indicis, EDM, lumbricals

   v. Start and end position: Figure 10-27 displays the start position for finger MCP hyperextension. The client is seated with the arm resting on a table on the ulnar border with the wrist in neutral and MCP joints straight. The client extends or moves the MCP joints into maximum hyperextension. Figure 10-28 displays the end position of ROM testing.

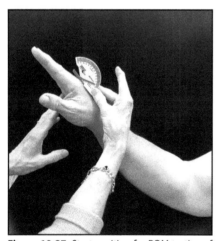

Figure 10-27. Start position for ROM testing of finger MCP hyperextension.

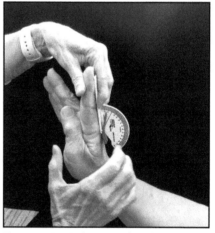

Figure 10-28. End position for ROM testing of finger MCP hyperextension.

d. Finger MCP abduction ROM

   i. Goniometric landmark: Dorsal aspect of the MCP joint of the finger

      Stable arm: Dorsal and parallel to the corresponding metacarpal

      Moving arm: Dorsal and parallel to the proximal phalanx

   ii. Available ROM: 0 to 25 degrees

   iii. End feel: Firm

   iv. Muscles responsible: ADM, dorsal and palmar interossei

   v. Start and end position: Figure 10-29 displays the start position for finger MCP abduction. The client is seated with the arm resting on a table with the forearm pronated, wrist neutral, palm flat, and the MCP joints adducted. The client moves the fingers into maximum MCP abduction. Figure 10-30 displays the end position of ROM testing.

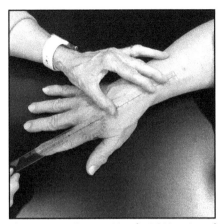

Figure 10-29. Start position for ROM testing of finger MCP abduction.

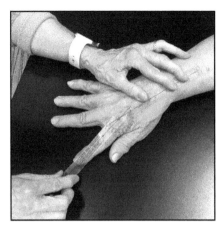

Figure 10-30. End position for ROM testing of finger MCP abduction.

e. Finger PIP joint flexion ROM
   i. Goniometric landmark: Dorsal surface of the PIP joint of the finger tested
      Stable arm: Dorsal and midline of proximal phalanx of the finger
      Moving arm: Dorsal and midline of the middle phalanx of the finger
   ii. Available ROM: 0 to 100 degrees
   iii. End feel: Firm
   iv. Muscles responsible: Flexor digitorum superficialis, FDP, lumbricals
   v. Start and end position: Figure 10-31 displays the start position for PIP flexion. The client is seated with the arm resting on a table on the ulnar border with the forearm and wrist in neutral and the PIP joints straight. The client bends or moves the PIP joints into maximum flexion. Figure 10-32 displays the end position of ROM testing.

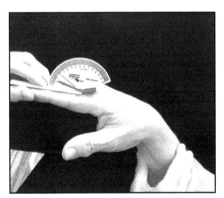

Figure 10-31. Start position for ROM testing of finger PIP flexion/end position for finger PIP extension.

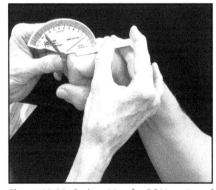

Figure 10-32. End position for ROM testing of finger PIP flexion/start position for finger PIP extension.

Note: Because PIP extension is simply a return from PIP flexion, the start position for PIP flexion will be the same as the end position for PIP extension. Similarly, the start position for PIP extension will be the same as the end position for PIP flexion (see Figures 10-31 and 10-32).

f. Finger PIP joint extension ROM
   i. Goniometric landmark: Dorsal surface of the PIP joint of the finger tested
      Stable arm: Dorsal and midline of proximal phalanx of the finger
      Moving arm: Dorsal and midline of the middle phalanx of the finger
   ii. Available ROM: 100 to 0 degrees
   iii. End feel: Firm
   iv. Muscles responsible: EDC, extensor indicis, EDM, lumbricals

v. Start and end position: See Figure 10-32 for start position. The client is seated with the arm resting on a table on the ulnar border with the forearm and wrist in neutral and the PIP joints flexed. The client straightens or moves the PIP joints into maximum extension as in Figure 10-31 or the end position.

g. Finger DIP joint flexion ROM

i. Goniometric landmark: Dorsal surface of the DIP joint of finger tested

Stable arm: Dorsal and midline of the middle phalanx of finger tested

Moving arm: Dorsal and midline of distal phalanx of finger tested

ii. Available ROM: 0 to 70 degrees

iii. End feel: Firm

iv. Muscles responsible: FDP

v. Start and end position: Figure 10-33 displays the start position for DIP flexion. The client is seated with the arm resting on a table on the ulnar border with the forearm and wrist in neutral and DIP joints straight. The client bends or moves the DIP joints into maximum flexion. Figure 10-34 displays the end position of ROM testing.

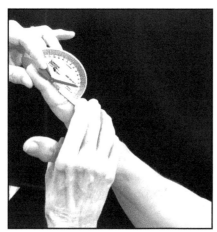

Figure 10-33. Start position for ROM testing of finger DIP flexion/end position for finger DIP extension.

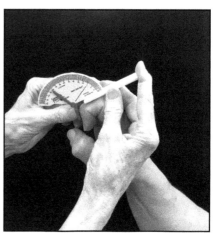

Figure 10-34. End position for ROM testing of finger DIP flexion/start position for finger DIP extension.

Note: Because DIP extension is simply a return from DIP flexion, the start position for DIP flexion will be the same as the end position for DIP extension. Similarly, the start position for DIP extension will be the same as the end position for DIP flexion (see Figures 10-33 and 10-34).

h. Finger DIP joint extension ROM

i. Goniometric landmark: Dorsal surface of the DIP joint of finger tested

Stable arm: Dorsal and midline of the middle phalanx of finger tested

Moving arm: Dorsal and midline of distal phalanx of finger tested

ii. Available ROM: 70 to 0 degrees

iii. End feel: Firm

iv. Muscles responsible: EDC, extensor indicis, EDM

v. Start and end position: See Figure 10-34 for start position. The client is seated with the arm resting on a table on the ulnar border with the forearm and wrist in neutral and the DIP joints flexed. The client straightens or moves the DIP joints into maximum extension or the end position as in Figure 10-33.

i. Thumb MCP joint flexion ROM

i. Goniometric landmark: Dorsal surface of the thumb MCP joint

Stable arm: Midline dorsal surface of the thumb MCP joint

Moving arm: Midline dorsal surface of the proximal phalanx

ii. Available ROM: 0 to 60 degrees

iii. End feel: Firm

iv. Muscles responsible: FPL, FPB

v. Start and end position: Figure 10-35 displays the start position for thumb MCP flexion. The client is seated with the arm resting on a table on the ulnar border with the forearm and wrist in neutral and the thumb MCP joint straight. The client bends or moves the thumb into maximum flexion. Figure 10-36 displays the end position of ROM testing.

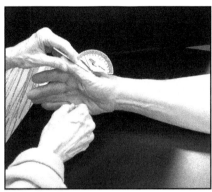

Figure 10-35. Start position for ROM testing of thumb MCP flexion/end position for thumb MCP extension.

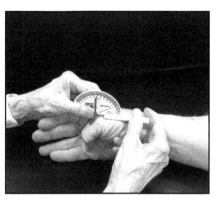

Figure 10-36. End position for ROM testing of thumb MCP flexion/start position for thumb MCP extension.

Note: Because thumb MCP extension is simply a return from MCP flexion, the start position for thumb MCP flexion will be the same as the end position for MCP extension. Similarly, the start position for thumb MCP extension will be the same as the end position for MCP flexion (see Figures 10-35 and 10-36).

j. Thumb MCP joint extension ROM

   i. Goniometric landmark: Dorsal surface of the thumb MCP joint

     Stable arm: Midline dorsal surface of the thumb MCP joint

     Moving arm: Midline dorsal surface of the proximal phalanx

   ii. Available ROM: 60 to 0 degrees

   iii. End feel: Firm

   iv. Muscles responsible: Extensor pollicis longus, extensor pollicis brevis

   v. Start and end position: See Figure 10-36 for start position. The client is seated with the arm resting on a table on the ulnar border with the forearm and wrist in neutral and the thumb MCP joint flexed. The client straightens or moves the thumb into maximum extension as in Figure 10-35 or end position.

k. Thumb IP joint flexion ROM

   i. Goniometric landmark: Dorsal surface of the thumb IP joint

     Stable arm: Midline dorsal surface of the proximal phalanx

     Moving arm: Midline dorsal surface of the distal phalanx

   ii. Available ROM: 0 to 80 degrees

   iii. End feel: Firm

   iv. Muscles responsible: FPL

   v. Start and end position: Figure 10-37 displays the start position for thumb IP joint flexion. The client is seated with the arm resting on a table on the ulnar border with the forearm and wrist in neutral and the thumb IP joint straight. The client bends or moves the thumb into maximum flexion. Figure 10-38 displays end position for ROM testing.

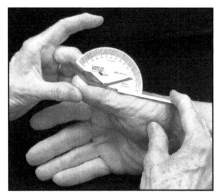

Figure 10-37. Start position for ROM testing of thumb IP flexion/end position for thumb IP extension.

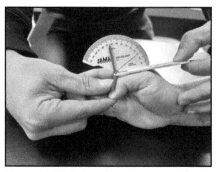

Figure 10-38. End position for ROM testing of thumb IP flexion/start position for thumb IP extension.

Note: Because thumb IP extension is simply a return from IP flexion, the start position for thumb IP flexion will be the same as the end position for IP extension. Similarly, the start position for thumb IP extension will be the same as the end position for IP flexion (see Figures 10-37 and 10-38).

l. Thumb IP joint extension ROM

    i. Goniometric landmark: Dorsal surface of the thumb IP joint

       Stable arm: Midline dorsal surface of the proximal phalanx

       Moving arm: Midline dorsal surface of the distal phalanx

    ii. Available ROM: 80 to 0 degrees

    iii. End feel: Firm

    iv. Muscles responsible: EPL

    v. Start and end position: See Figure 10-38 for start position. The client is seated with the arm resting on a table on the ulnar border with the forearm and wrist in neutral, and the thumb IP joint flexed. The client straightens or moves the IP joint of the thumb into maximum extension as in Figure 10-37 or the end position.

Note: It is common to see hyperextension at the thumb IP joint; however, unless the injury involves the IP joint directly, it is not typically measured. Instructions for ROM testing of the IP joint hyperextension of the thumb are not provided in this chapter.

m. Thumb CMC joint radial abduction (also called *CMC extension*) ROM

    i. Goniometric landmark: Over the CMC joint at the base of the thumb metacarpal

       Stable arm: Parallel to the index finger metacarpal

       Moving arm: Parallel to the thumb metacarpal

    ii. Available ROM: 0 to 20 degrees

    iii. End feel: Firm

    iv. Muscles responsible: EPL, extensor pollicis brevis

    v. Start and end position: See Figure 10-39 for start position. The client is seated with the arm resting on a table with the forearm pronated, palm flat, and fingers and thumb adducted. The client moves the thumb into maximum CMC radial abduction or CMC extension. Figure 10-40 displays the end position of ROM testing.

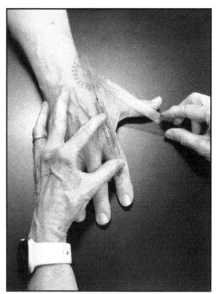

Figure 10-39. Start position for ROM testing of thumb CMC radial abduction (extension).

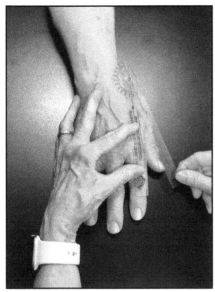

Figure 10-40. End position for ROM testing of thumb CMC radial abduction (extension).

n. Thumb CMC joint palmar abduction ROM

   i. Goniometric landmark: Over the CMC joint at the base of the thumb metacarpal

      Stable arm: Parallel to the second or index finger metacarpal

      Moving arm: Parallel to the first or thumb metacarpal

   ii. Available ROM: 0 to 50 degrees

   iii. End feel: Firm

   iv. Muscles responsible: Abductor pollicis longus, APB

   v. Start and end position: See Figure 10-41 for start position. The client is seated with the arm resting on a table on the ulnar border with the forearm and wrist in neutral, and the fingers straight with the thumb adducted. The client moves the thumb into maximum CMC abduction. Figure 10-42 displays the end position of ROM testing.

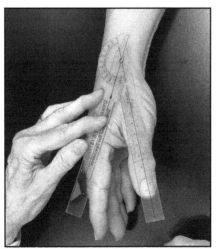

Figure 10-41. Start position for ROM testing of thumb CMC palmar abduction.

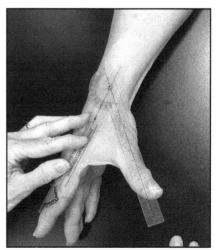

Figure 10-42. End position for ROM testing of thumb CMC palmar abduction.

o. Thumb CMC adduction: Deficits in thumb adduction may be recorded by measuring the distance between the index finger MCP joint and the thumb IP joint with a centimeter ruler, as displayed in Figure 10-43. The muscle responsible is the AP.

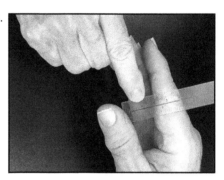

Figure 10-43. Position for measuring lack of thumb CMC adduction.

p. Opposition: Deficits in opposition may be recorded by measuring the distance between the centers of the pads of the thumb and the small finger using a centimeter ruler as displayed in Figure 10-44. The muscles responsible are the OP, ODM, and ADM.

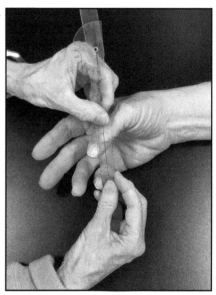

Figure 10-44. Position for measuring lack of opposition.

4. **Manual Muscle Testing (MMT) of the Hand and Thumb**: Complete gross MMT of the joints of the hand and thumb using Table 10-8.

TABLE 10-8
Manual Muscle Testing Application Table

JOINT	MOTIONS	PALPATE MUSCLE GROUP/MUSCLE	GROSS MMT SCORE
Finger MCP	Flexion		
	Abduction		
	Adduction		

(continued)

TABLE 10-8 (CONTINUED)
Manual Muscle Testing Application Table

JOINT	MOTIONS	PALPATE MUSCLE GROUP/MUSCLE	GROSS MMT SCORE
Finger PIP	Flexion		
	Extension		
Finger DIP	Flexion		
	Extension		
Thumb MCP	Flexion		
	Extension		
Thumb IP	Flexion		
	Extension		
Thumb CMC	Radial abduction (extension)		
	Palmar abduction		
	Opposition		

Adapted from Rondinelli, R. D., Genoverse, E., Katz, R. T., Mayer, T. G., Mueller, K., & Ranavaya, M. (2008) *Guides to the evaluation of permanent impairment* (6th ed.). American Medical Association.

a. Finger MCP flexion
   i. Muscle palpation (if applicable)
   ii. Testing procedure: Figure 10-45 displays the start position. The client is seated with the arm resting on a table, forearm supinated, wrist in neutral, and fingers extended. The therapist stabilizes proximal to the MCP joints at the metacarpals to avoid compensation. The client moves their fingers in the direction of MCP flexion. Resistance is applied at the proximal phalanges in the direction of MCP extension. Figure 10-46 displays the testing position.

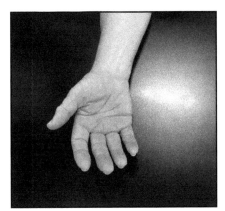

Figure 10-45. Start position for MMT of finger MCP flexion.

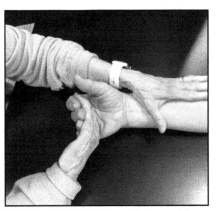

Figure 10-46. Testing position for MMT of finger MCP flexion.

b. Finger PIP/DIP flexion
   i. Muscle palpation (if applicable)
   ii. Testing procedure: Figure 10-47 displays the start position. The client is seated with the arm resting on a table, forearm supinated, wrist in neutral, and fingers extended. The therapist stabilizes at the MCP joints and metacarpals. The client moves their fingers in the direction of PIP/DIP flexion while keeping MCP joints in extension. Resistance is applied at the middle and distal phalanges in the direction of PIP/DIP extension. Figure 10-48 displays the testing procedure.

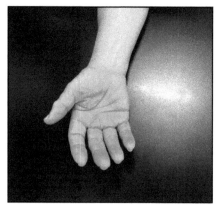

Figure 10-47. Start position for MMT of finger PIP/DIP flexion.

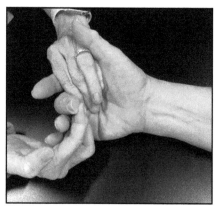

Figure 10-48. Testing position for MMT of finger PIP/DIP flexion.

c. Finger MCP/PIP/DIP extension
    i. Muscle palpation (if applicable)
    ii. Testing procedure: Figure 10-49 displays the start position. The client is seated with the arm resting on a table, forearm pronated, wrist in neutral, and fingers flexed. The therapist stabilizes at the wrist and metacarpals to avoid compensation. The client moves the fingers in the direction of MCP/PIP/DIP extension. Resistance is applied to each finger individually on the dorsum of the proximal, middle, or distal phalanges in the direction of MCP/PIP/ DIP flexion. Figure 10-50 displays the testing position.

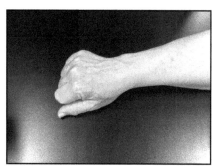

Figure 10-49. Start position for MMT of finger MCP/PIP/DIP extension.

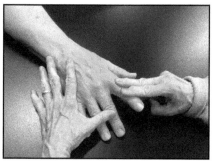

Figure 10-50. Testing position for MMT of finger MCP/PIP/DIP extension.

d. Finger MCP abduction and adduction
    i. Muscle palpation (if applicable)
    ii. Testing procedure: Figure 10-51 displays the start position for finger MCP abduction. The client is seated with arm resting on a table, forearm pronated, wrist in neutral, fingers in extension, and MCP joints adducted. The client then moves the fingers in the direction of MCP abduction. The therapist stabilizes at the metacarpals to avoid compensation. Resistance is applied at the side of each individual finger in the direction of adduction. The long finger should be tested in both directions because it only abducts. Figure 10-52 displays the testing position.

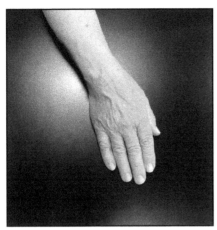

Figure 10-51. Start position for MMT of finger MCP abduction.

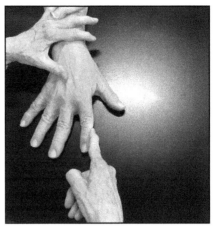

Figure 10-52. Testing position for MMT of finger MCP abduction.

Figure 10-53 displays the start position for testing finger MCP adduction. The client is seated with arm resting on a table, forearm pronated, wrist in neutral, fingers in extension, and MCP joints abducted. The client then moves their fingers into adduction. The therapist stabilizes at the metacarpals to avoid compensation. Resistance is applied at the side of the index, ring, and small fingers into abduction. Figure 10-54 displays the testing position.

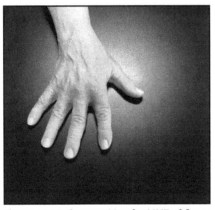

Figure 10-53. Start position for MMT of finger MCP adduction.

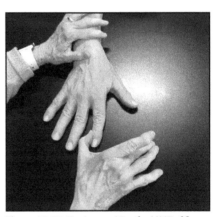

Figure 10-54. Testing position for MMT of finger MCP adduction.

e. Opposition of the thumb to the small finger
   i. Muscle palpation (if applicable)
   ii. Testing procedure: Figure 10-55 displays the start position for opposition. The client is seated with the arm resting on a table, forearm supinated, wrist in neutral, and fingers and thumb extended in a relaxed position. The client's wrist and forearm are stabilized against the table. The client moves in the direction of thumb opposition to the small finger. Resistance is applied at the thumb and small finger in the direction of extension. Figure 10-56 displays the testing procedure.

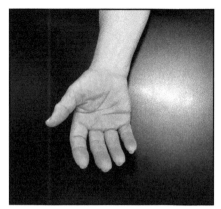

Figure 10-55. Start position for MMT of opposition.

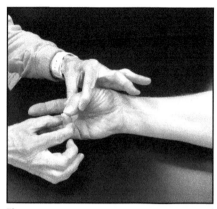

Figure 10-56. Testing position for MMT of opposition.

f. Thumb MCP flexion and extension
   i. Muscle palpation (if applicable)
   ii. Testing procedure: Figure 10-57 displays the start position of thumb MCP flexion. The client is seated with arm resting on a table on the ulnar border, forearm in mid-position, wrist in neutral, and fingers and thumb extended in a relaxed position. The client's wrist and forearm are stabilized against the table. The client moves the thumb MCP in the direction of flexion. The therapist stabilizes the wrist and first metacarpal. Resistance is applied at the proximal phalanx in the direction of extension. Figure 10-58 displays the test position.

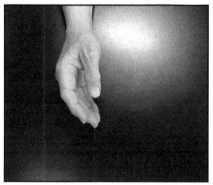

Figure 10-57. Start position for MMT of thumb MCP flexion.

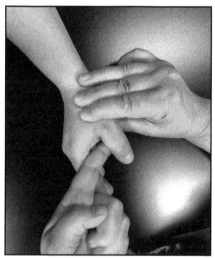

Figure 10-58. Testing position for MMT of thumb MCP flexion.

Figure 10-59 displays the start position for thumb MCP extension. The client is seated with the arm resting on a table on the ulnar border, forearm in mid-position, wrist in neutral, fingers extended, and thumb flexed into the palm at the MCP joint. The client moves the thumb MCP in the direction of extension. The therapist stabilizes the wrist and first metacarpal. Resistance is applied at the proximal phalanx in the direction of flexion. Figure 10-60 displays the test position.

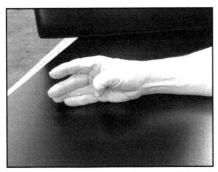

Figure 10-59. Start position for MMT of thumb MCP extension.

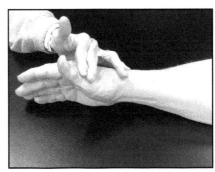

Figure 10-60. Testing position for MMT of thumb MCP extension.

g. Thumb IP flexion and extension
   i. Muscle palpation (if applicable)
   ii. Testing procedure: Figure 10-61 displays the start position of thumb IP flexion. The client is seated with the arm resting on a table on the ulnar border, forearm in mid-position, wrist in neutral, fingers and thumb in a relaxed position. The client moves the thumb IP in the direction of flexion. The therapist stabilizes the thumb at the proximal phalanx, and resistance is applied at the distal phalanx in the direction of extension. Figure 10-62 displays the testing position.

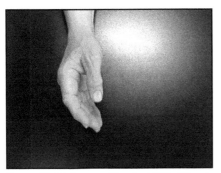

Figure 10-61. Start position for MMT of thumb IP flexion.

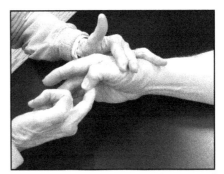

Figure 10-62. Testing position for MMT of thumb IP flexion.

Figure 10-63 displays the start position for thumb IP extension. The client is seated with the arm resting on a table on the ulnar border, forearm in mid-position, wrist in neutral, fingers extended, and thumb flexed into the palm at the IP joint. The client moves the thumb IP in the direction of extension. The therapist stabilizes the thumb at the proximal phalanx, and resistance is applied at the distal phalanx in the direction of flexion. Figure 10-64 displays the testing position.

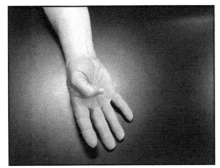

Figure 10-63. Start position for MMT of thumb IP extension.

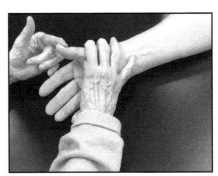

Figure 10-64. Testing position for MMT of thumb IP extension.

h. Thumb CMC palmar abduction
    i. Muscle palpation (if applicable)
    ii. Testing procedure: Figure 10-65 displays the start position for thumb palmar abduction. The client is seated with the arm resting on a table with forearm supinated, wrist in neutral, and the thumb relaxed in adduction against the volar aspect of the index finger. The client moves the thumb up in the direction of palmar abduction. The therapist stabilizes the metacarpals and wrist to avoid compensation. Resistance is applied at the lateral aspect of the proximal phalanx in the direction of adduction. Figure 10-66 displays the test position.

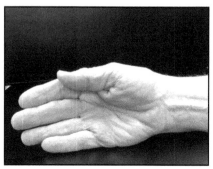

Figure 10-65. Start position for MMT of thumb CMC palmar abduction.

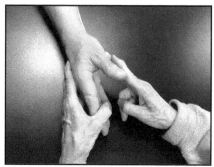

Figure 10-66. Testing position for MMT of thumb CMC palmar abduction.

i. Thumb CMC radial abduction (extension)
    i. Muscle palpation (if applicable)
    ii. Testing procedure: Figure 10-67 displays the start position for thumb radial abduction. The client is seated with the arm resting on a table on the ulnar border, forearm in mid-position, wrist in neutral, fingers extended, and the thumb adducted and flexed slightly across the palm. The client moves the thumb up or away from the fingers in the direction of radial abduction. The therapist stabilizes the wrist and metacarpals. Resistance is applied at the lateral aspect of the proximal phalanx in the direction of adduction. Figure 10-68 displays the test position.

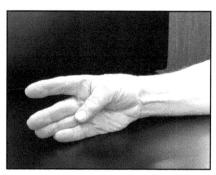

Figure 10-67. Start position for MMT of thumb CMC radial abduction.

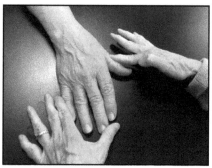

Figure 10-68. Testing position for MMT of thumb CMC radial abduction.

CHAPTER 11

Kinesiology and Therapeutic Exercise

Matthew J. Sabin, PhD, LAT, ATC, SMTC, CIDN and Carolyn L. Roller, OTR/L

Key Terms

activity limitations

arthrokinematic movement

balance

concentric contractions

eccentric contractions

fibroblastic phase

force–velocity curve

function

functional progression

healing process

impairment

individuality

inflammatory phase

intensity

isometric contractions

maturation phase

neuromuscular control

osteokinematic movement

overload

participation restrictions

progression

range of motion

safety

SAID principle

specificity

swelling and pain

therapeutic exercise

Wolff's law

Chapter Outline

Introduction

Occupational Profile

Therapeutic Exercise Across the Lifespan

    Benefits of Therapeutic Exercise

    Lifespan Implications

Foundations of Therapeutic Exercise

    Movement and the Healing Process

    Evaluation of Task as a Part of Therapeutic Exercise

    Basic Concepts of Therapeutic Exercise

    Components of a Therapeutic Exercise Program

    Integration of Healing, Assessment, and Therapeutic Exercise

Summary

References

Applications

Sain, S. J., & Roller, C. L. *Kinesiology for the Occupational Therapy Assistant: Essential Components of Function and Movement, Third Edition* (pp. 267-282). © 2024 Taylor & Francis Group.

Chapter Objectives

After completion of this chapter, students should be able to:

1. Define key terminology.
2. Explain the difference between an impairment, activity limitation, and participation restriction.
3. Describe the impact of the healing process on therapeutic exercise design.
4. Describe foundational concepts in therapeutic exercise program design.
5. Defend the use of movement as an essential aspect of the therapeutic experience.
6. Differentiate the appropriate movement considerations in respect to different evaluation findings.
7. Modify a prescribed therapeutic exercise program based on changes in a client's presentation (e.g., increased swelling and pain following return to work).
8. Construct a therapeutic exercise program that emphasizes various forms of movement aligned to the healing process for an optimal outcome.

Introduction

This chapter discusses the role of **therapeutic exercise** across the lifespan and the foundations of therapeutic exercise as it relates to kinesiology. The concept of **function**, which is the ability of an individual to move sufficiently and complete a task or goal to their satisfaction in any social context, will be explored. Current disablement models focus more on function rather than the injury or disability. This is a more holistic approach that requires an occupational therapist to assess both therapy- and client-rated outcomes at the same time. **Activity limitations** are described, for example, as decreased shoulder **range of motion** (ROM) which limits throwing. **Participation restrictions** are defined as how the activity limitations are impacting the client's occupational roles. For example, the inability to throw might have a minor impact on an older adult client but a major limitation on a high school baseball pitcher. The reader will learn how to take the knowledge learned in this text and apply it to the rehab setting in order to restore maintain and even improve physical function. Therapeutic exercise is defined as the application of movement to create structural and functional improvements in a client's occupational roles. Assessment of function and an understanding of the client's goals are important to the success of a therapeutic exercise program. The reader will learn how the three stages of the **healing process** must coordinate with progression to eliminate setbacks. The long-term goal of the therapeutic exercise program is to return the client to their desired function. The key to the process being successful is for the occupational therapy practitioner to utilize reassessment and observation skills to monitor progress and make the appropriate adjustments as needed.

Occupational Profile

Steve, a 42-year-old man, presents to therapy with a medical diagnosis from a local physician of biceps brachii tendinitis. Initial onset is unknown; however, discomfort increased recently following a weekend race. He is an avid adventure racer, which is an endurance event that combines many disciplines including, but not limited to, canoeing or kayaking (a paddling component), mountain biking, and hiking/orienteering. Most of Steve's races are between 12 to 24 hours in length. Outside of his training and racing, he is a self-employed contractor who works various construction jobs with a small crew of one to two other employees. He enjoys his work and specializes in carpentry. He is the father of three children between the ages of 6 and 12. Steve's chief complaint is generalized right anterior shoulder pain that increases with prolonged use and limits his strength during work, training, and racing. He reports that he experienced 4/10 pain hiking and swimming with the family last weekend, which limited his participation. He has also not been able to canoe for any extended periods of time. Minor chores around the house create minimal pain; however, using tools (e.g., a screwdriver) causes discomfort and decreases strength during the activity. He has also experienced discomfort while sleeping because he normally sleeps on his stomach with his arm above his head. At work, he has been unable to use tools overhead or extended his arm away from his body for prolonged periods and rarely without pain. Due to Steve's level of discomfort, he has been primarily supervising others at work. Unfortunately, he is unable to sustain this role for long without contributing to the manual work. He has also been unable to mountain bike or paddle a canoe due to the pain, but he has been able to run with no limitation and only minor discomfort. Goniometry measurements indicate limited active right shoulder flexion of 0 to 135 degrees with pain of 5/10 reported at end range (left active shoulder flexion is 0 to

BOX 11-1

MODEL	DESCRIPTION
Nagi Disablement Model	Developed in 1965, it was the first disability model. It expanded the understanding of disability beyond the physical limitations to include environmental and societal factors. This model separated disability into four levels: cellular, body system, person, and societal (the individual's inability to accomplish their roles).
National Center for Medical Rehabilitation Research Disablement Model	This model expands upon the Nagi model by adding the idea that disability can be impacted externally by societal limitations. These limitations can come in numerous forms but might include denials of service, loss of pay, and barriers to movement (e.g., lack of an elevator).
World Health Organization's (WHO) *International Classification of Functioning, Disability and Health*	This model is a universally applicable classification system created to standardize language around disability and function. It neutralizes the cause of the dysfunction (e.g., medical, societal) and focuses on the characteristics of function.

(Snyder et al., 2008; WHO, 2013)

165 degrees). Pain was also present in both shoulder abduction (4/10) and shoulder extension (3/10), though no ROM limitation was present. Pain (5/10) and weakness (4-/5) are present with right elbow flexion. His main concern at the time of the evaluation is the ability to function fully at work and ability to complete a race without pain, especially during the paddling leg of the race.

Therapeutic Exercise Across the Lifespan

The concept of function, health, and well-being is multidimensional, combining an individual's functional abilities, perceptions, and social interactions. Function is the ability of an individual to move sufficiently and complete a task or goal to their satisfaction in any social context; the ability to achieve occupation well and as desired. Current disablement models are implementing this concept of function more than previous models that focused on the specific injury or disability from a pure anatomical perspective.

As a result of these models, the evaluation process and therapeutic exercise programs are now geared toward addressing the functional abilities of the client holistically (Snyder et al., 2008). This occurs across multiple levels, such as the structural level, the biomechanical level, and the societal level, which focuses on the overall impact of the dysfunction on societal roles. This holistic approach requires the practitioner to assess and then address practitioner-rated outcomes across the whole kinetic chain and client-rated outcomes simultaneously. Box 11-1 briefly describes three common disablement models utilized by occupational therapy practitioners.

Upon initial presentation, a client's report may stem from an anatomical **impairment**. An impairment occurs at the structural level. Examples of impairments might include a sprained ligament, strained muscle, tissue contracture, hematoma, scar tissue restriction, or fracture. The practitioner must understand and treat what is occurring anatomically with regards to structure and the healing process. Additionally, the practitioner must consider how that impairment is impacting the individual's activity limitation. Activity limitations occur at the body system level and often result from structural damage or deficiency. Examples of activity limitations might be decreased ROM, strength, **balance**, or coordination. Activity limitations can also be expanded to include specific tasks, like squatting, walking, and throwing, and might describe the individual at the whole-body level. Participation restrictions reflect how these restrictions are impacting an individual's occupational roles and their interactions with society. The inability to sit and stand greatly impacts an individual who must sit and stand frequently throughout the day more so than an individual who sits consistently at work. The inability to throw might have minor impact on an older adult client but could greatly restrict a toddler or adolescent. Participation restrictions impact each client differently as they interact within sport, recreation, play, work, family, and hobbies. Participation restrictions must be considered across all aspects of an occupation as their impact on a client's life may have the greatest impact on perceived outcomes.

Upon initial presentation, Steve exhibits pain stemming from an anatomical impairment. Steve's tendinitis could be managed with immobilization, pain medication, ice, and general rest with positive outcomes on decreasing pain and inflammation. Prolonged immobilization, however, might contribute to further decreased structural mobility (i.e., impairment), resulting in decreased ROM (i.e., activity limitation), and an inability to participate in work and sport (i.e.,

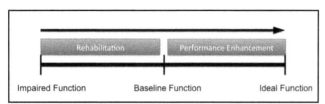

Figure 11-1. Continuum of function.

participation restrictions) to the desired level. Though decreased pain is a desired outcome of treatment, in this scenario, Steve's perception of the treatment efficacy will not be favorable as his perceived performance in sport and work may be subpar. This dissatisfaction will inherently influence the overall outcome; therefore, the evaluation and treatment of this injury must address all limitations, including appropriate client-response surveys that assess general health and function, joint-specific function, and client satisfaction. With this holistic approach the practitioner will better be able to treat all aspects of a client's individual limitations. Remember, within a client's treatment plan, including therapeutic exercise, the physician's orders and their protocols must be considered and discussed with the physician and the rehabilitation team.

Benefits of Therapeutic Exercise

Therapeutic exercise is the application of movement to create structural and functional improvements that decrease participation restrictions. It involves a continual process of evaluation and application of theory and skill to improve function. To benefit the client, therapeutic exercise must be applied within the appropriate context (healing phase or improvement) and in a manner that does not further inflammatory responses or anatomical restrictions. It will most often be applied in conjunction with other treatment methods, including the use of therapeutic modalities, manual techniques, and therapeutic activities. Though it is most often prescribed with these other treatments, therapeutic exercise is crucial in the establishment of proper mechanics and movement patterns, self-efficacy, and client satisfaction.

The greatest difference between therapeutic exercise and other treatments is movement. The benefits of movement extend to both those with and without a specific pathology or injury. The only difference between the injury and performance enhancement scenarios is whether the goal is to return to baseline performance or whether it is to improve past the baseline This is why the benefits of therapeutic exercise mimic the benefits of exercise, physical activity, and movement. These benefits have been clearly documented and extend beyond the musculoskeletal and cardiovascular systems. Therapeutic exercise decreases depression and improves health-related quality of life, sleep, and body composition (Physical Activity Guidelines Advisory Committee, 2008).

Lifespan Implications

Though it might seem reasonable to alter therapeutic exercise programs based on characteristics such as age and gender, practitioners must remember that function is the driving principle in program design. Two individuals of different ages with similar clinical presentation and functional goals may often have similar therapeutic exercise programs; however, when these external factors influence or alter the functional status or goals, the program must be altered as well to meet individual client needs. Therefore, though function remains the foundational principle dictating program design, other factors must be considered. Age, occupation, religion, mental status, and comorbidities must be considered to keep the program specific to the client. These factors will have an impact on client–practitioner interactions and communication. Terminology, vocabulary, and expression must be appropriate to the client and may need to be tailored to achieve the optimal outcome in treatment. Practitioners cannot effectively communicate to pediatric populations using the same language used to communicate to adults and vice versa.

Possible comorbidities might require the practitioner to be more flexible and creative in accomplishing the tasks needed to reach functional goals. In addition, different concerns about safety may arise and must be addressed to prevent injury during therapy. These conditions affect individuals of all ages but might be more prevalent in specific populations. For instance, a client with a restriction in shoulder movement that has difficulty with balancing may need to be placed in more stable positions (e.g., seated) while exercising the shoulder than an individual with normal balance. Another solution might be that the client wears a gait belt to increase safety during exercise.

Additionally, it is imperative that practitioners understand basic changes in anatomy and physiology throughout the lifespan in order to interpret findings during both the initial evaluation and re-evaluation in regard to program design. Pediatric clients present with open physeal plates skeletally, different physiological responses to resistance, and structural laxity (Best, 1995). Due to these differences, practitioners might need to consider the intensity of the exercise or the load to prevent unwarranted damage; however, it has been suggested that healing may occur more quickly in the pediatric population (Cohen & Sala, 2010). Ultimately, these considerations do not change the functional goals that drive program design, though they may change how these goals and the prognosis are being addressed.

As the assessment of function and an understanding of the client's goals are paramount to successful therapeutic exercise, practitioners should recognize that every client is represented along the continuum of function illustrated in Figure 11-1. Every client presents at the initial evaluation and subsequent evaluations with either a possible deficit from normal function or with a desire to improve function beyond the baseline presentation. Injury and pathology are mainly attributed to the decrease in function from the typical baseline. The move in function from baseline to a desired goal is often motivated internally and is termed *performance enhancement*. Performance enhancement may include increases in ROM, strength, endurance, power, skill level, accuracy, coordination, or a combination of these characteristics.

Clients with a desire to improve function can come from multiple settings and situations. Performance enhancement might include, for example, an exercise group for healthy older adults at a church or an athlete trying to get to the next level. Both groups are attempting to improve physical performance and move from the baseline to an ideal or desired level of function. The client's goals will be different based on required occupational function, recreational activity, priorities, family, play, and similar occupations, but goals will always be aimed at improving function from the current state. A client with Steve's exact work requirements might be satisfied with a full return to baseline function, whereas Steve may not be satisfied until he improves his endurance for his recreational activities. Practitioners must be able to apply their skills to any functional limitation across all populations, infant to older adult; sedentary to high-level athletes; and sick to well, to name a few. In all cases, the process is the same: evaluate the body structures, activity limitations, and participation restrictions and apply an appropriate intervention, depending on the rehabilitation setting.

Foundations of Therapeutic Exercise

Movement and the Healing Process

Both the assessment of a client's restrictions and the corresponding prescribed therapeutic exercise should be dictated by the client's progression through the healing process. The relationship between the healing process and progression continues throughout the entire therapy process; therefore, a basic understanding of the healing process is foundational in the design of a rehabilitation program.

The healing process is divided into three phases: inflammatory, fibroblastic, and maturation (Prentice, 2020). The **inflammatory phase** occurs directly after injury and can continue for several days in acute injuries with the duration depending on the severity of the injury and any potentially impeding factors. Though inflammation generally has a negative connotation, it is an essential component of the healing process. Without inflammation, healing will not occur.

This primary response serves to protect the area through an initial vasoconstriction response and then to transition chemical mediators that are essential to healing into the area. This phase consists of a very complex, physiologic interaction between the mediators and the injured tissue. Simplified, the chemical mediators prepare the area for tissue formation and vascularization. Inflammation during this period is often observed by five cardinal signs: pain, swelling, erythema, heat production and, consequently, loss of function.

Due to the initial injury, assessing movement during this phase may be challenging and will often be limited by pain. Assessment of ROM should include both active and passive measures to determine the limitations based on strength and tissue restrictions. The practitioner must assess ROM while considering client comfort as well as preventing further injury.

The **fibroblastic phase** is characterized by the development of scar tissue to strengthen the injured area. This process begins prior to the end of the inflammatory phase and can last upwards of 4 to 6 weeks, depending on the severity of tissue damage. During this phase, collagen and elastin are formed across the damaged area in a pattern resembling a haphazardly designed web. Fibers run in multiple directions, quickly increasing the strength of the injured area to resist forces acting in multiple directions. This increased strength helps to prevent further injury to the area and is essential to the healing process; however, when strength increases, mobility of the tissue initially decreases due to the restrictions along the tissue lines.

The client's activity limitations during this phase should decrease overall as the signs of inflammation decrease. As a result of these improved activity limitations, participation restrictions should decrease, leading to increased client satisfaction and better outcomes. Full function will not be achieved yet as the scar tissue has not achieved full mobility.

The final phase in the healing process is maturation. The **maturation phase** is characterized by the realignment of the scar tissue, which is achieved by progressively increasing movement and function to the preset ideal function. Movement helps to realign the fibers along the lines of physiologic tension. As these fibers realign, the area becomes more mobile while maintaining, and even increasing in, strength. This phase will generally continue past the time when individuals return to their occupation and can last upwards of 2 years.

Evaluation of Task as a Part of Therapeutic Exercise

A basic understanding of the healing process and the competency to evaluate signs and symptoms, activity limitations, and participation restrictions are impossible without assessment of movement. Whether the assessment is an initial evaluation, re-evaluation, or day-in day-out observation of a client, movement must be assessed. Individual movement of a single joint is important, but it may not translate to a specific task deficit, as multiple joint movements may be required to accomplish the task and may compensate.

Figure 11-2. Sit-to-Stand test.

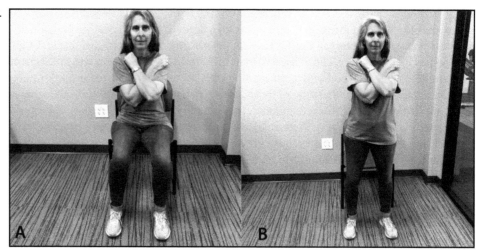

Figure 11-3. Timed Up and Go test.

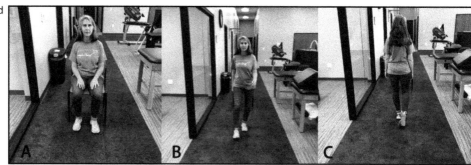

Therefore, practitioners must integrate task assessment into evaluations and be able to assess tasks as they are completed during therapeutic exercise. Task completion requires simultaneous use of multiple joints and muscles in a coordinated pattern with a specific, measurable outcome. Measurement of individual joint or muscle activity limitations may correlate to task completion but cannot be assessed alone to determine function. Measurements and gains of individual joints, however, may be necessary before assessment of multiple joint movements can begin.

In some instances, outcome measures have been created to assist the practitioner in task assessment. Figures 11-2 and 11-3 demonstrate two measures relating to bipedal tasks and function: the Sit-to-Stand test (Silva et al., 2014) and the Timed Up and Go test (Bennell et al., 2011). The Sit-to-Stand test counts the number of times a client can stand from a seated position without using their arms in 30 seconds. The Timed Up and Go task times clients as they start from a seated position, ambulate around a cone 3 meters away, and return to the starting seated position safely. These examples are measures of lower extremity function, endurance, and balance and do not address upper extremity function or shoulder ROM limitations as seen in the case of our occupational profile of Steve.

Basic Concepts of Therapeutic Exercise

In addition to understanding the injury evaluation process, the healing process, and what occurs in relation to injury, the practitioner must have a grasp on the basic principles of therapeutic exercise and exercise prescription. Practitioners who understand all of these aspects fully can match the required movement and exercise to accomplish the proper goal at the right time, culminating in the best possible outcome for the client. The concepts governing the design of a therapeutic exercise program are not incredibly complex, but it is paramount that practitioners consider them when designing an intervention. These basic principles include **specificity**, **individuality**, **intensity**, **overload/progression**, and **safety**.

Specificity

The first principle that is foundational to every exercise and rehabilitation program is the concept of specificity. Specificity refers to the ultimate goal of the program, which should mimic function at the desired level and combine both patient and clinician goals. All program design starts with the assessed deficits and uses exercises with parameters to accomplish a desired outcome. Steve presents to the clinic with increased pain as well as deficits in ROM, strength, and endurance. His program needs to start addressing these issues in a way that will allow him to return to adventure racing without restriction. Once pain is managed and ROM is returned, exercises will be developed to establish a foundation of strength, and then increase to focus on endurance.

Individuality

The second principle is the concept of individuality. Each client is unique with differing comorbidities, likes and dislikes, symptom presentations, pain tolerances, and past experiences. All of these distinctive characteristics require practitioners to design programs geared at meeting the client's individual needs. Clients will not be satisfied with, and often will not comply with, programs that do not meet their individual needs and desires.

An easy example is to consider an individual that presents with a desire to increase health through conditioning and weight loss with a goal to increase participation in activities with their grandchildren, particularly biking and hiking. This individual desires to become active outside and, therefore, will be more interested in meeting their goal through exercise outside. They may also prefer fewer stationary forms of activity and, if the exercise is more dynamic, may adhere to the program better. Individuals that hate stationary bike workouts and treadmill running will not adhere to programs that include these forms of exercise.

Intensity

The principle of matching the intensity of movement and exercise to the specificity can become confusing. Remember, intensity does not reflect motivation or desire. Intensity during exercise is reflected in a physiologic response to that exercise and not a mental response. For instance, cardiovascular exercise intensity can be measured by increased heart rate or perceived ratings of exertion, while resistance exercise intensity is often associated with increased external resistance as a percentage of a maximal effort.

Prescribed intensity is completely associated with the client's goals and baseline. In the case of injury, the initial therapeutic exercises will be designed to return the client to baseline levels. Steve will need the strength and endurance to meet the demands of his work as well as the endurance and ability to meet the demands of his race schedule. Working in construction, he requires varying levels of intensity based on the task; meaning the amount of force required or the length of use may not be consistent. If he is trying to use a hammer once, the demand in the intensity will be minimal, even though tasks like roofing might require this motion over a longer period, requiring endurance, intensity in force production will be low. During the same job, however, Steve may

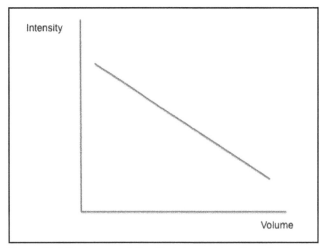

Figure 11-4. The inverse relationship between intensity and volume in terms of resistive training or cardiovascular training.

need to support and lift rafters, which would require a much greater intensity. Likewise, during a race, Steve will need endurance, less intensity, over a greater amount of time. To accomplish this, Steve must pace himself to survive the duration of the event.

Intensity and volume during training and conditioning must maintain an inverse relationship in order to maintain the safety of the client. With resistance training or strengthening exercises, volume refers to the number of repetitions and sets that are prescribed. With regards to cardiovascular training, *volume* refers to the duration or amount of time an exercise is being conducted. If the desired goal is high intensity, speed of movement, or heavy exertion, then therapeutic exercise must eventually mimic that with high intensity and low volume. If the goal is to return to a lower intensity level, then more volume is indicated in the therapeutic exercise program. Figure 11-4 illustrates the relationship between intensity and volume.

Overload/Progression

To see improvement from the initial clinical presentation, it is essential that the practitioner designs the program to progressively and safely overload the damaged structures in functional patterns. This principle is most often referred to as the **SAID principle**, which stands for Specific Adaptations to Imposed Demands (Wathen & Roll, 1994). In other words, if we want to change the function and structure of the body, it must be stressed beyond its typical baseline or current state in a way specific to the desired outcome. This principle is influenced by **Wolff's law** but is more generalized to fit the rehabilitation and training settings. Box 11-2 describes Wolff's law.

BOX 11-2

Wolff's law states that there is a relationship between the form and function of bone that is controlled by physical laws.

(Boyd & Nigg, 2007)

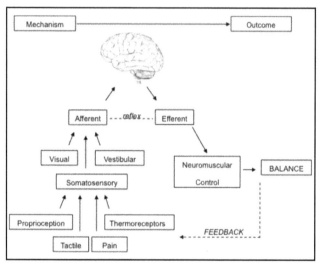

Figure 11-5. Rehabilitation progression graph.

Under the premise of this principle, progression must be intentional and appropriate to the level of tissue healing to see improvement toward client and practitioner goals. Progression should move from simplistic and general movement patterns to more client specific and complex patterns. The concept of program progression by varying movement parameters will be discussed later in the chapter. In general, however, this can be achieved by modifying resistance, speed, direction changes, simultaneous task completion, and any other exercise-specific parameters. These changes are often incremental and should be considered in turn rather than universally. In other words, too many changes at once limits the practitioner's ability to control the environment and monitor whether the changes stress the body adversely. Figure 11-5 outlines the stepwise process of progression from the initial restriction to the desired outcome.

The key to progression is to know the initial state of the client, activity limitations, and participation restrictions and to visualize the end goal or function. During therapeutic exercise, the long-term goal is to get the client from the current state to the end goal and, therefore, all progressions of exercise should be geared toward this outcome. Practitioners can adjust many different parameters during treatment, including resistance, speed, surface, sensory feedback, attention demands, movement, direction (uni- vs. multi-directional), and skill/coordination. All of these should be progressed in a systematic fashion to limit the overload to the body and

decrease inflammatory reaction to the increased stress. During treatment, the long-term goals should be adjusted in response to the client's progress or lack of progress.

Consider Steve again. The following is an example of a therapy program that would progress Steve gradually without a further setback. At the initial evaluation, his right shoulder was limited to 135 degrees of flexion. He would be educated on the importance of rest and home modalities of heat and cold. Using a warm heating pad for no more than 10 minutes before his ROM exercises may allow more ROM without increased pain. Then, after exercises or functional use, a cold pack to the shoulder to decrease pain and inflammation is helpful. Starting Steve on a program of controlled passive range of motion (PROM)/active assist range of motion (AAROM) in a decreased gravity position is the first exercise he will do at home. Lying in supine on the bed or floor, Steve will be instructed to use his left arm to lift the right arm overhead until he reaches a tight or slightly uncomfortable feeling in his right shoulder. He will hold that position for 10 to 20 seconds and then lower the arm. Steve will be reminded to only use the unaffected arm to move the injured arm. Gravity assists shoulder flexion after 90 degrees of flexion while in supine. He will perform 10 reps three times daily. His pain and ROM will be monitored at his therapy visits. As Steve progresses with more shoulder flexion and less pain he can progress to using a stick to help raise the injured arm into flexion while in the supine position. After he progresses to active range of motion (AROM) in supine with normal shoulder flexion and very little discomfort, he can perform AROM in shoulder flexion while seated or standing, which will be fully against gravity. Note that he may not have as much AROM standing as he had in supine, but this could be due to weakness in the shoulder muscles. Steve will continue with PROM, AAROM, and AROM in supine to warm up and then perform AROM while seated or standing. At this point, Steve may be ready to begin isometric shoulder exercises. Remember, isometric strengthening is resistance without movement. If he continues to progress while maintaining full ROM and less pain, he can move to TheraBand exercises. These strengthening exercises can be graded depending on the band resistance. Usually, Steve would begin with the easiest band resistance. He would walk while holding the end of the band, which is attached to a stationary object, keeping the shoulder stationary, which is another type of isometric exercise. As Steve continues to progress, he may be ready to move the band against gravity while moving his injured shoulder into 90 degrees of flexion. The next step, when he is ready, would be for him to begin lifting a 1- or 2-pound dumbbell with his healing shoulder, but only to 90 degrees initially. This step would only take place if performed without pain. This progress can continue by adding more complex overhead movements and more specific activities based on Steve's goals. This treatment plan is just an example as any number of adjustable variables that can be substituted along the axis in Figure 11-5.

Safety

The final principle revolves around the concept of doing no harm. Client safety can be ensured through various means, such as instruction in proper technique and being responsive to exercise precautions and contraindications. The biggest key to this principle is understanding and utilizing knowledge of the healing process and how movement can be used to impact the healing process in a positive manner.

Components of a Therapeutic Exercise Program

The long-term goal of the therapeutic exercise program is always to enhance the client's function (i.e., body function and structure, activity, and participation) to their desired level as quickly and safely as possible (WHO, 2013). To accomplish this, the process is divided into short-term goals aligned with the healing process that are both specific and individualized. Logical order allows for foundational improvements at the body systems level to be addressed prior to the focus on more physiologically complicated integration of systems. The typical sequence of rehabilitation will address **swelling and pain** first, followed by ROM, strength and endurance, **neuromuscular control** and balance, power, and, finally, some form of **functional progression**.

Swelling and Pain

The first goal of the rehabilitation process is to address swelling and pain. Both swelling and pain contribute to activity limitations and contribute heavily to client satisfaction with the overall outcome of the therapy; therefore, they must be addressed from the beginning. Decreasing pain and promoting swelling absorption can be accomplished using therapeutic modalities, manual techniques, and the use of therapeutic exercise and movement (Knygsand-Roenhoej & Maribo, 2011).

Range of Motion

The second major goal of therapeutic exercise is to increase ROM. Assessment techniques of individual ROM at each joint are covered in previous chapters and are linked to the movement that is utilized during therapeutic exercise. Movement at the joint occurs at two different levels: **arthrokinematic** and **osteokinematic**. Arthrokinematic movement occurs between joint surfaces and consists of three different patterns: roll, glide, and spin (Houglum, 2010). Roll describes movement like the runner of a rocking chair as it connects and moves against the floor during the rocking motion. One point of the runner connects to another point on the floor in a pattern that propagates across both surfaces in the same direction. Glide describes a movement pattern in which one point on the moving surface contacts multiple points on the stationary surface. This is represented by pushing the rocking chair across the floor. One constant point of contact of the chair contacts several points on the floor. Spin occurs in a joint when the moving surface is rotated around a stationary axis on the stationary surface. Reflected in the movement of a rocking chair, this might occur when the chair is maintained in the same location in the room but rotated to face the other direction. During joint movement, these arthrokinematic movements occur simultaneously with the express purpose of maintaining joint congruency.

If you were to hold a tennis ball in your hand to represent two joint surfaces contacting and created a rolling motion between the surfaces, the tennis ball would roll out of your hand. In the joint this would create instability, compression, and distraction of surrounding soft tissue, leading to functional limitations. Therefore, the surface must also glide to maintain the central position of the ball in the hand. Arthrokinematic movements are complicated but, in general, can be described with the following three rules:

1. Roll and glide occur simultaneously.
2. Roll always occurs in the direction of the osteokinematic movement.
3. The normal physiologic glide occurs in the direction of roll when the moving surface is concave and in the opposite direction when the moving surface is convex.

Once a practitioner understands the concepts of normal arthrokinematic movements, limitations can be assessed. Therapeutic movement will be utilized to address pain and ROM limitations by primarily focusing on restoring deficits in the glide. These deficits are addressed by gliding the joint in the direction of the normal arthrokinematic movement. Box 11-3 provides a quick guide to assessing arthrokinematic movement.

BOX 11-3

When assessing ROM, both osteokinematic and arthrokinematic movement must be assessed because they occur simultaneously and restrictions in either will create a deficit. Osteokinematic movement is assessed through measurement, while arthrokinematic movement is assessed through the feel of the joint. Clinicians replicate the arthrokinematic movement and assess for restrictions. As the joint moves it will reach an end feel. End feels are often described as absent, mushy, soft, or solid. The clinician must assess the quality of the end feel and the magnitude.

TABLE 11-1

Osteokinematic Movements

• Flexion	• Dorsiflexion	• Lateral flexion
• Extension	• Inversion	• Right rotation
• Abduction	• Eversion	• Left rotation
• Adduction	• Opposition	• Pronation
• Internal rotation	• Lateral deviation	• Supination
• External rotation	• Elevation	• Ulnar deviation
• Protraction	• Depression	• Radial deviation
• Retraction	• Upward rotation	
• Plantarflexion	• Downward rotation	

As arthrokinematic movement is restored, osteokinematic movement can be addressed. Osteokinematic movement is the movement of bones and is described in movement terms, such as *flexion* and *extension*, which are listed in Table 11-1. Osteokinematic movements create measurable angles that can be recorded with the use of goniometers, inclinometers, tape measures, and a variety of applications for mobile electronic devices. Deficits in osteokinematic movement can come not only from restrictions of static structures, such as ligaments and joint capsules, but they can also be the result of bone abnormalities, adipose tissue, decreased muscle elasticity, and/or neural restrictions. Some of these restrictions can be addressed in rehabilitation while others cannot be altered without surgical intervention.

Muscular restrictions can be addressed passively or actively with the practitioner using several different techniques. The simplest techniques utilize PROM and AROM in the osteokinematic directions. Static stretching is a form of PROM that is sustained near the pathophysiologic endpoint to affect tissue extensibility. This is what is typically perceived as stretching and requires a muscle to be put on stretch near the end range, while staying below the threshold of pain, and sustained for 20 to 30 seconds. Dynamic stretching is a form of AROM that can be utilized to enhance muscle extensibility and, therefore, increase ROM of a joint (Woods et al., 2007). Dynamic stretching is active and stretches the muscle while moving a joint through a full ROM. Another method utilized to increase ROM secondary to muscular

restriction is proprioceptive neuromuscular facilitation techniques. Proprioceptive neuromuscular facilitation stretching is a stretching method that can be performed in several ways that involves a series of muscle submaximal and maximal contractions and relaxation to theoretically override neural protective mechanisms within the muscles.

ROM deficits at a single joint must be measured and assessed to understand the impact of the limitation; however, the impact of the deficit on function and the whole kinematic chain is just as important, if not more so. Steve describes pain that affects shoulder ROM and movement. It is reasonable to understand the impact that biceps brachii tendinitis would have on the glenohumeral joint as the biceps brachii assists with shoulder flexion, but his function at work may not be affected beyond the increase in pain. He might be able to accomplish necessary tasks and movement through compensatory movement that allows essential shoulder flexion; therefore, without task assessment, the full extent of his participation restrictions will remain unknown and potentially unaddressed during the therapeutic exercise program.

Strength and Endurance

After addressing ROM, muscular function must be addressed in the therapeutic exercise program. In most cases, the focus on muscular function will overlap the emphasis on ROM because, in addition to potential deficits that result from decreased elasticity, strength or lack of strength can impact ROM. In later stages, muscular function might not impact ROM, but will influence a client's ability to accomplish a desired function.

Muscles are dynamic and create movement and provide force to overcome external resistance. To enhance muscular function, strength, endurance, and power must be addressed during the therapeutic exercise program. *Muscular strength* refers to the ability of a muscle to produce force against resistance. *Muscular endurance* requires different physiologic characteristics in the muscle and refers to the ability of the muscle to produce force over time. *Power* refers to the ability of the muscle to produce force quickly. Because power requires a foundation of muscular strength, it should not be directly addressed until that foundation has been established.

Muscle physiology adapts based on the stress placed on that structure during therapeutic exercise; therefore, program design must be aligned to the principles of specificity and intensity to prepare the individual to meet the desired goal. Adjusting the parameters of each exercise will allow the practitioner to adjust the exercise toward the intended goal. Intensity regarding muscular resistance exercise is gauged as a percentage of the maximum amount of resistance that can be overcome in a given number of repetitions. Generally, this is calculated off a 1 or 10 repetition max, the maximum amount of resistance that can be moved for 1 or 10 repetitions, respectively. As depicted in Figure 11-4, intensity and volume is inversely related to maintain safety of the client and proper progression. As intensity nears max, the number of repetitions performed must decrease. With regards to the overall goal, higher repetitions develop muscular endurance while fewer repetitions develop strength (American College of Sports Medicine, 2009).

Another consideration for the practitioner is how these contractions should be performed during therapeutic exercise. There are three main types of contractions that are used clinically to restore or gain strength: isometric, concentric, and eccentric. The decision to emphasize a particular contraction is based on several factors. The practitioner must consider specificity, the training level of the client, the healing process (if relevant), and the desired outcome and function of the client.

An **isometric contraction** is defined as a contraction of the muscle that does not create either arthrokinematic or osteokinematic joint movement. When a muscle is contracting in this way, the force generated by the muscle is equal to the external resistance. This might be as simple as holding a can of soup in your hand without raising or lowering it or could be as challenging as trying to push a car with all of your force while the brake is on. In either instance, the muscles being activated will produce force equal to the resistance and no movement is created.

Isometric contractions may strengthen a muscle but the change in the muscle has less functional application than contractions involving movement (American College of Sports Medicine, 2009). Therefore, this type of contraction has little functional implication, as function generally requires movement. Isometric contractions can play a role in therapeutic exercise, however, in that they can be utilized early in the rehabilitation process when muscle activation is acceptable but joint movement might need to be restricted. This might be relevant in a scenario where an acute ligamentous injury has occurred. Movement might be contraindicated in the healing process of the ligament, but muscle contraction could attenuate the loss of strength during the brief period of restricted movement.

Another instance of use for isometric contractions would be when we are trying to strengthen a movement pattern at a particular angle in the ROM. If the client has full ROM but struggles more at a specific angle, it is reasonable to try and strengthen the musculature at that specific angle by using isometric contractions. Strengthening the muscle at the point of weakness will allow increased resistance to be applied throughout the full ROM to enhance function.

Concentric contractions are a subset of isotonic contractions. *Isotonic* refers to contractions that maintain the same level of force during a movement. Concentric contractions occur as the muscle shortens, overcoming the resistance in a steady manner. Force generated internally is greater than the force of resistance. Physiologically, this occurs at the initiation of movement as a positive velocity. As concentric contractions are an essential component of activities of daily living (ADLs), as well as sport and recreational skill, their use in therapeutic exercise is imperative. Concentric contractions occur during many acceleration-type movements including grasping, pushing, and moving objects away from the body; writing; and many other movement patterns; however, it is almost impossible to separate the concentric contraction from the eccentric during function.

Eccentric contractions occur when the force generated by the muscle is less than the external resistance and, therefore, the muscle lengthens while it is contracting. Eccentric contractions are often utilized during function to slow and smoothly decelerate objects. Eccentric contractions can be fast or slow, but all are negative velocities. Examples of eccentric contractions include the follow-through of a pitcher, down phase of a squat, and resisting forces coming toward the body, such as a closing door.

The **force–velocity curve** outlines how different velocities in each of the isotonic contractions and isometric velocities impact force generation (Lieber, 2002). This graph, found in Figure 11-6, can be replicated by performing maximal contractions, with maximal muscle activation at different velocities on an isokinetic machine. The force–velocity curve demonstrates that as velocity increases with concentric activities, force decreases. Picture an individual trying to complete a bench press at maximal force. Pushing the bar away from the chest requires maximal effort and occurs slowly. If you speed the action up, maximal force can still be achieved only at the expense of resistance. If the weight is decreased, speed can increase.

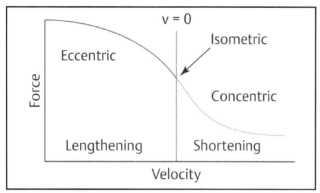

Figure 11-6. Force–velocity curve of a muscle.

The center of the force–velocity curve, where velocity is zero, signifies an isometric contraction. When the individual doing the bench press is not required to push the weight away from the body, more weight can be added, in which case, isometric force can be greater than concentric. However, maximal force generation occurs with eccentric contractions. As velocity increases eccentrically, more weight can be resisted. In resistance training, this is considered a negative exercise and is beneficial for overloading the muscle. Though this is important to consider with training and therapeutic exercise, keep in mind the safety considerations with negative training. Maximal force may be produced at high velocities, but when the force is greater than the capability of the muscle to resist, the result is injury.

When isolating the activity of one muscle, these contractions are easy to identify; however, normal movement consists of multiple types of muscle contractions occurring simultaneously or in series within different muscles and muscle groups. During resistance exercises alone, concentric and eccentric contractions are utilized to move resistance and return to the starting position, but do not correlate to typical functional movements perfectly. Functional movement is more synergistic and synergistic movements, where different muscles combine to produce a movement, need to be coordinated and often occur while opposing, or antagonist, muscles co-contract to decelerate and control the movement. Furthermore, isometric contractions occur simultaneously to stabilize moving segments and maintain postural equilibrium. One common mantra is that distal mobility requires proximal stability. This might be most easily reflected in movement of the shoulder girdle. The glenohumeral joint cannot effectively coordinate movement if the scapula is not stabilized.

Simple ADLs of eating, grooming, and playing require use of all forms of contractions. Work and recreational tasks are no different, integrating muscular functions to perform. Consider Steve's desire to row in a canoe. To pull the paddle, Steve must concentrically extend his shoulders. To produce the force needed to propel the canoe, he must also isometrically brace with his abdominals and, near the end of motion, eccentrically slow the shoulder movement. Simultaneously, he must stabilize with postural muscles while concentrically

and eccentrically producing force. This stabilization proximal or distal to the moving part allows for better energy transfer through the body, more efficient movement, and decreased likelihood of injury (Prentice, 2020).

The final concept required to understand muscle function during evaluation and resistance exercises relates to gravity. Gravity is a constant force pulling toward the ground that must be considered in client positioning, movement direction, and force generation. For example, a client extending the knee while sidelying exerts different amounts of force across several muscles than when they are supine. While supine, gravity is fully resisted with the quadriceps. While sidelying, the quadriceps do not need to produce as much force to produce movement, but hip abductors might be activated more to support the limb.

During the evaluation process, client positioning must be considered during muscle testing to consider the effect of gravity and accurately evaluate the muscular function. In addition, therapeutic exercise can increase in difficulty based on the additional resistance of gravity. If Steve's shoulder function limits his ability to lift overhead, the practitioner can focus on strengthening in a gravity-minimized position first. Then Steve can progress to AROM in a full-gravity position, and then into the same position with increased resistance.

Integrating knowledge of contraction types, coordination, positioning, and careful examination of movement into therapeutic exercise choice is important for the practitioner.

Neuromuscular Control and Balance

Emphasis on pain reduction, decreasing swelling, increasing ROM, and increasing muscular function are essential and foundational to function; however, these do not initially involve multi-joint coordination and movement patterns. Both neuromuscular control and the client's ability to balance require integration of multiple body systems across several regions and are more functional. Neuromuscular control is the unconscious efferent response to an afferent signal (Lephart et al., 2000). Balance is the ability to maintain a center of gravity within a base of support (i.e., the ability to not fall). Figure 11-7 demonstrates how neuromuscular control is a part of the postural control system and balance is an outcome.

Coordinated movement and complex skill completion require a system that not only initiates an appropriate movement, but also provides sensory feedback to produce necessary adjustments to fine-tune the movement pattern. Once a movement is initiated, sensory feedback is received through various mechanoreceptors, thermoreceptors, and nociceptors to provide somatosensory feedback. This feedback is integrated with visual and vestibular sensory signals to provide the brain with enough information to make an appropriate correction or response. Neuromuscular control is then observed through the coordination of movement and balance, which is the ability to keep the center of gravity within the

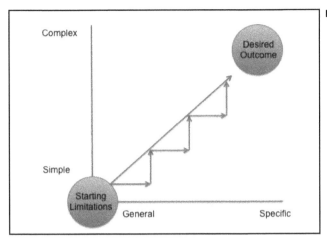

Figure 11-7. Postural control mechanism.

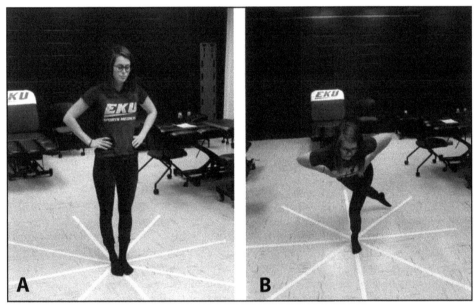

Figure 11-8. Star Excursion Balance test.

limit of stability and not fall. Based on these definitions and descriptions, neuromuscular control is required to balance; however, because the terms are not synonymous and there are numerous situations where movement does not require balance, balance is not required for neuromuscular control.

Techniques to assess neuromuscular control and balance are varied and vastly depend on available resources. Simple tests like Romberg's test and the Balance Error Scoring System can be utilized along with observation of tasks, such as transfer from a seated to a standing position, gait, reaching tasks, or the Star Excursion Balance test (Gribble et al., 2012; Murray et al., 2014). Figure 11-8 depicts the starting position and one reach direction of the Star Excursion Balance test. These listed measures and tests are only examples of possible tests that could be used and are not all that are available. These tests do, however, quantify performance during tasks that require multi-joint coordination, postural control, and neuromuscular control.

Repetition and use of the postural control system is key to improving neuromuscular control; however, there are some specific techniques that can help. One treatment technique would be to allow feedback during movement. Clients can perform a task while watching themselves in a mirror to provide visual sensory input in addition to somatosensory. Another technique is to create feedback from an external or, even sometimes, internal resistance. Clients can use resistance bands as a stabilizer to provide feedback. For instance, a client suffering from a lower extremity injury might be able to do single-leg squats with the band pulling them from the lateral side. Internal resistance through isometric contractions can also provide needed feedback when performed simultaneously as with clients diagnosed with a stroke. These exercises provide more sensory feedback that can be used by the brain to confirm or deny the inputs from the somatosensory afferent signals.

Functional Progression

The final component to the rehabilitation process is the connection between traditional therapeutic exercises to functional skill. A client at this point in the therapeutic exercise progression needs to take the ROM, strength, endurance,

BOX 11-4

POSSIBLE FUNCTIONAL PROGRESSIONS

Starting	End Goal
Slow	Fast
Anticipated	Unanticipated
Unidirectional	Multidirectional
Low force	High force
Stable	Unstable

(Prentice, 2020)

and neuromuscular control they have gained and start utilizing it in functional patterns. Functional progression moves the client from the basic ability to function toward the ability to complete ADLs to a desired standard. Steve might start taking the strength he has worked on and his neuromuscular control exercises, which might involve diagonal patterns, and start lifting and raising a hammer in a pattern exactly like his work function. He might start training for his adventure races by mimicking skills essential to race completion. These functional tasks will not only serve to prepare the body for the demands of the client's occupation, but they also will serve to mentally prepare the individual for the transition back to full participation.

Progression and exercise modification during this phase require more creativity from the practitioner. Within the confines of safety, progression, and specificity, the goal is to replicate reality as much as possible. Recall the basic principle of progression discussed earlier in the chapter and the model of how to progress towards the desired outcome (see Figure 11-7). For an athlete, this might mean use of sport-specific drills. For the industrial worker, this might require replication of task, intensity, and duration as much as possible. For the older adult client, this might require the practice of transfers using any assistive devices they would normally use. Though many possibilities exist, the practitioner must progress appropriately. The progression from simple to complex and from general to specific has already been addressed. Several other progressions exist. As function is improved, exercises should move from slow to fast, anticipated to unanticipated, unidirectional to multidirectional, low to high

force, and stable to unstable. Ideally, upon discharge, each client should be able to handle the unpredictable world at the desired level of function by creating movements that are optimal in direction, magnitude, speed, reaction, coordination, and force. Box 11-4 reiterates progressions that can be considered in the application of therapeutic exercises (Prentice, 2020).

Integration of Healing, Assessment, and Therapeutic Exercise

Once the practitioner understands the healing process, methods to assess function, progression of goals for therapeutic exercise, and techniques to address those goals, they must be able to integrate them into one program (Table 11-2). The long-term goal of this program is to return the client to their desired function. The key to the process is to continually utilize evaluation, assessment, and observation skills to monitor progress and adjust as needed.

Summary

The process of therapeutic exercise, whether enhancing function to return to baseline or beyond, requires the practitioner to understand kinesiology and how it impacts assessment and program development. Though specific techniques may vary, all therapeutic exercise should be focused on the assessed deficits and should utilize techniques linked to the specificity of the deficit and desired goals of the client. When applied in alignment to the healing process, the client will experience fewer setbacks and will progress more smoothly though the program.

Therapeutic exercises must be progressed sequentially and logically to move the client toward function. Integrating various components to address the basics of function, such as ROM, strength, neuromuscular control, and balance, is essential prior to functional progressions; however, each step should incorporate movement as a form of therapy in some capacity. Furthermore, all exercise prescription should address the client's activity and participation restrictions to keep the program specific to the individual and directed at the client's goals.

TABLE 11-2
Therapeutic Exercise and Healing Process Integration

HEALING PHASE	ASSESSMENT TECHNIQUE	THERAPEUTIC EXERCISE GOAL	THERAPEUTIC EXERCISE TECHNIQUE
Inflammatory phase	• Activity limitations (ROM, strength, swelling, pain) • Participation limitations (task)	• Control swelling and pain • ROM • Early strength	• Modalities, manual, movement • PROM, AAROM, pain-free AROM • Isometrics, pain-free strengthening
Fibroblastic phase	• Activity limitations (ROM, strength, swelling, pain), • Participation limitations (task)	• Full ROM • Full strength • Neuromuscular control/ balance • Functional	• Aggressive ROM • Advanced strengthening (isotonic) • Multi-joint, advanced • Simple and general
Maturation/repair	• Participation limitations (task)	• Neuromuscular control/ balance • Functional	• Specific to desired function

References

American College of Sports Medicine. (2009). American College of Sports Medicine position stand. Progression models in resistance training for healthy adults. *Medicine & Science in Sports & Exercise, 41*(3), 687-708.

Bennell, K., Dobson, F., & Hinman, R. (2011). Measures of physical performance assessments: Self-Paced Walk Test (SPWT), Stair Climb Test (SCT), Six-Minute Walk Test (6MWT), Chair Stand Test (CST), Timed Up & Go (TUG), Sock Test, Lift and Carry Test (LCT), and Car Task. *Arthritis Care and Research (Hoboken), 63*(Suppl. 11), S350-370.

Best, T. (1995). Muscle-tendon injuries in young athletes. *Clinics in Sports Medicine, 14*(3), 669-686.

Boyd, S. K., & Nigg, B. M. (2007). Bone. In B. M. Nigg & W. Herzog (Eds.), *Biomechanics of the musculoskeletal system* (3rd ed., pp. 73-80). Wiley.

Cohen, E., & Sala., DA. (2010). Rehabilitation of pediatric musculoskeletal sport-related injuries: A review of the literature. *European Journal of Physical and Rehabilitation Medicine, 46*(2), 133-146.

Gribble, P. A., Hertel, J., & Plisky, P. (2012). Using the Star Excursion Balance test to assess dynamic postural-control deficits and outcomes in lower extremity injury: A literature and systematic review. *Journal of Athletic Training, 47*(3), 339-357.

Houglum, P. (2010). *Therapeutic exercise for musculoskeletal injuries* (3rd ed.). Human Kinetics.

Knygsand-Roenhoej, K., & Maribo, T. (2011). A randomized clinical controlled study comparing the effect of modified manual edema mobilization treatment with traditional edema technique in patients with a fracture of the distal radius. *Journal of Hand Therapy, 24*(3), 184-193; quiz 194.

Lephart, S., Riemann, B., & Fu, F. (2000). Introduction to the sensorimotor system. In S. Lephart & F. Fu (Eds.), *Proprioception and neuromuscular control in joint stability*. Human Kinetics.

Lieber, R. (2002). *Skeletal muscle physiology: Skeletal muscle structure, function, and plasticity* (2nd ed.). Lippincott Williams & Wilkins.

Murray, N., Salvatore, A., Powell, D., & Reed-Jones, R. (2014). Reliability and validity evidence of multiple balance assessments in athletes with a concussion. *Journal of Athletic Training, 49*(4), 540-549.

Physical Activity Guidelines Advisory Committee. (2008). *Physical Activity Guidelines Advisory Committee Report, 2008*. U.S. Department of Health and Human Services.

Prentice, W. E. (2020). *Rehabilitation techniques for sports medicine and athletic training* (7th ed.). SLACK Incorporated.

Silva, P. F., Quintino, L. F., Franco, J., & Faria, C. D. (2014). Measurement properties and feasibility of clinical tests to assess sit-to-stand/stand-to-sit tasks in subjects with neurological disease: A systematic review. *Brazilian Journal of Physical Therapy, 18*(2), 99-110. Retrieved from Snyder, A. R., Parsons, J. T., Valovich McLeod, T. C., Curtis Bay, R., Michener, L. A., & Sauers, E. L. (2008). Using disablement models and clinical outcomes assessment to enable evidence-based athletic training practice, part I: disablement models. *Journal of Athletic Training, 43*(4), 428-436.

Wathen, D., & Roll, F. (1994). Training methods and modes. In T. Baechle (Ed.), *Essentials of strength training and conditioning* (pp. 403-415). Human Kinetics.

Woods, K., Bishop, P., & Jones, E. (2007). Warm-up and stretching in the prevention of muscular injury. *Sports Medicine, 37*(12), 1089-1099.

World Health Organization. (2013). *How to use the ICF: A practical manual for using the International Classification of Functioning, Disability and Health*. Author.

Applications

The following activities will help you apply knowledge of kinesiology and therapeutic exercise in real-life applications. Activities can be completed individually or in small groups to enhance learning.

1. Describe the difference between impairments, activity limitations, and participation restrictions.

2. What role does evaluation play in the design of a therapeutic exercise program?

3. Describe the three phases of the healing process. Be sure to describe the time frames of the phases as well as the main emphasis of each.

4. Partner with someone and assess the quality and magnitude of the arthrokinematic movement around a joint. (Hint: Start with an easier joint like the metacarpophalangeal joints. Grab the bones on either side of the joint, provide some distraction and glide them.) Demonstrate this on one joint in which the roll and glide occur in the same direction and on one in which they occur in opposite directions.

5. Using the force–velocity curve, create a list of four true statements about resistance exercise choice during a therapeutic exercise program design.

6. Generate a therapeutic exercise program for Steve based on his current activity restrictions and participation restrictions as outlined throughout the chapter.

7. Generate three different outlines of a therapeutic exercise program for Steve at three different time points within the healing process: mid-inflammatory phase, mid-fibroblastic, and mid-maturation.

CHAPTER 12

Functional Mobility in the Home and Community

Dana M. Howell, PhD, OTD, OTR/L, FAOTA and Susan J. Sain, MS, OTR/L, FAOTA

Key Terms

assistive technology	open environment
bed mobility	orthotics
body mechanics	physical environment
bridging	preparatory methods
closed environment	pressure relief
dependent transfers	prosthetic
diagonal lift	rolling
dynamic splints	space demands
energy conservation	squat pivot transfer
functional mobility	stand pivot transfer
golfer's lift	static splints
long sitting	transfer board
motor skills	transfers
occupation and activity demands	tripod lift
	wheeled mobility

Sain, S. J., & Roller, C. L. *Kinesiology for the Occupational Therapy Assistant: Essential Components of Function and Movement, Third Edition* (pp. 283-312). © 2024 Taylor & Francis Group.

Chapter Outline

Introduction

Occupational Profile

Functional Mobility in the Home and Community

    Home Versus Community Environments

    Body Mechanics

Functional Mobility in the Home

    Bed Mobility

    Transfers

    Bathroom Mobility

    Activities of Daily Living and Functional Mobility

    Instrumental Activities of Daily Living and Functional Mobility

    Energy Conservation

Functional Mobility in the Community

    Adaptive Mobility

    Prosthetics

    Orthotics

    Splinting

    Wheeled Mobility

    Driving

    Adaptive Mobility for Leisure

Summary

References

Applications

Chapter Objectives

After completion of this chapter, students should be able to:

1. Define key terminology.
2. Analyze client factors and motor skills, as well as activity, occupational, and space demands, required for the functional mobility tasks of bed mobility, transfers, and wheeled mobility.
3. Explain how the physical environment impacts functional mobility performance.
4. Apply body mechanics principles during lifting and activities of daily living and instrumental activities of daily living.
5. Identify assistive technology that will improve functional mobility tasks.
6. Understand the kinesiological principles of splinting.

Introduction

This chapter describes how various movement components combine to enable **functional mobility** in the home and other environments. The *Occupational Therapy Practice Framework: Domain and Process, Fourth Edition* (OTPF-4) categorizes functional mobility as an activity of daily living (ADL; American Occupational Therapy Association [AOTA], 2020). Principles of **body mechanics** are discussed in relation to enhancing safety. Functional mobility in the home leads to engagement in occupations. Home mobility addressed includes **bed mobility**, **transfers**, bathroom mobility, mobility needed for ADLs and instrumental activities of daily living (IADLs). **Bridging**, **rolling**, and **long sitting** are aspects of bed mobility that enable functional mobility. Stand pivot, squat pivot, **transfer board** and **dependent transfers** are defined. The importance of **energy conservation** is emphasized. Functional mobility in the community is explored encompassing adaptive mobility, use of **prosthetic** devices, **orthotics**, and splinting. Furthermore, approaches to mobility that enable a client to maneuver through space are considered. In this section, **wheeled mobility**, driving, mobility for leisure activities, and the importance of managing **pressure relief** are covered. Types of wheelchairs, cushions, wheelchair fit, and pressure relief are briefly discussed.

Occupational Profile

The following occupational profile is provided to demonstrate how limitations in body functions, body structures, and **motor skills** impact functional mobility in home and community settings. This profile will show how occupational therapy intervention can help to compensate for deficits in functional mobility and will be referred to throughout the chapter.

Rachel is a 40-year-old university marketing specialist who has spastic diplegia cerebral palsy (CP). She began occupational therapy services after experiencing a recent decline in functional mobility, including an increase in falls.

Medical history: Rachel was born 8 weeks prematurely in a breech delivery and was significantly underweight at birth. Her parents did not notice any developmental delays until she was 18 months old and was having difficulty learning to walk. Most of her major motor developmental milestones (rolling, crawling, and sitting) were significantly delayed. At 2 years old, she was formally diagnosed with CP. Although Rachel was able to ambulate independently by age 3, she underwent several surgeries as a preteen to improve her hip and knee alignment. These surgeries included bilateral intertrochanteric derotational femoral osteotomies, multiple muscle lengthening surgeries, and bilateral transfers of the distal ends of the rectus femoris to the sartorius. Following the surgeries, Rachel received physical therapy for lower extremity (LE) strengthening and lengthening, gait training, and balance. Ultimately, she returned to walking independently with no assistive devices. She has never used medication for spasticity management. Rachel has not received physical therapy services since childhood and she has never received occupational therapy services.

Subjective: Rachel reports that over the past few years she has noticed a decline in her ability to ambulate in the community. She has difficulty stepping up a curb without support and is only able to navigate steps if there is a railing. Her office recently moved to a new campus building, and she found that walking from the parking lot to her office was more challenging due to having to negotiate more curbs and stairs. She reports difficulty standing for long periods of time and feelings of instability when she has to walk while carrying something. She reports falling more frequently and stiffness after sitting for long periods, such as on a plane for an overseas flight, which is debilitating when she attempts to stand. She has calf and hip pain and has been told by her physician that she may require a hip replacement in the future. She reports an unclear understanding of her medical history, what surgeries were performed, and why.

Rachel lives independently in a one-story home with one step to enter. She enjoys going to movies, swimming, and caring for her home. She also enjoys yoga and international traveling, but has not engaged in either for several years due to her decline in mobility. In general, she has been slowly decreasing her activity level due to her declining mobility. Her goals are to improve her functional mobility and return to previous leisure activities.

Objective: Upon evaluation, Rachel demonstrated the following:

- ADL function: Rachel is independent in all basic ADLs, including dressing, toileting, grooming, self-feeding, and bathing.
- IADL function: Rachel requires assistance with heavy home maintenance, such as shoveling snow and lawn mowing, but is otherwise independent.
- Cognition, vision, and perception: Rachel demonstrates no deficits in these areas.
- Upper extremity (UE): Bilateral UE strength, range of motion (ROM), sensation, and coordination are within normal limits.
- LE ROM and strength: See Table 12-1.
- Muscle tone: 2/4 on the modified Ashworth scale for tone in bilateral hamstrings (more marked increase in muscle tone through most of the ROM, but affected part easily moved).
- Balance: 39/56 on the Berg Balance Scale (a score of 21 to 40 indicates a medium fall risk).
- Mobility: Rachel is independent in bed mobility. She requires moderate assistance to transfer into her bathtub but is independent in all other transfers. She is independent in ambulation but is slow and unstable. She requires moderate assistance to step up or down a curb without a handrail.

TABLE 12-1

Rachel's Lower Extremity Muscle Strength and Range of Motion Upon Evaluation

LEFT			EVALUATION	RIGHT		
Manual Muscle Testing	Passive Range of Motion	Active Range of Motion	Hip (Norms)	Active Range of Motion	Passive Range of Motion	Manual Muscle Testing
3/5	0 to 88 degrees	0 to 46 degrees	Flexion (0 to 120 degrees)	0 to 113 degrees	0 to 120 degrees	3/5
3-/5	0 to 25 degrees	0 to 9 degrees	Extension (0 to 30 degrees)	0 to 11 degrees	0 to 25 degrees	2+/5
2+/5	0 to 40 degrees	0 to 13 degrees	Abduction (0 to 45 degrees)	0 to 17 degrees	0 to 45 degrees	2+/5
2+/5	0 to 30 degrees	0 to 30 degrees	Adduction (0 to 30 degrees)	0 to 30 degrees	0 to 30 degrees	2+/5
2+/5	0 to 30 degrees	0 to 8 degrees	Internal rotation (0 to 45 degrees)	0 to 8 degrees	0 to 30 degrees	2+/5
2/5	0 to 30 degrees	0 to 8 degrees	External rotation (0 to 45 degrees)	0 to 17 degrees	0 to 30 degrees	2+/5
			Knee			
2+/5	15 to 94 degrees	22 to 94 degrees	Flexion (0 to 135 degrees)	20 to 92 degrees	10 to 100 degrees	2+/5
5/5			Extension			5/5
			Ankle			
*NT	*0 degrees	*0 degrees	Dorsiflexion (0 to 20 degrees)	0 to 4 degrees	0 to 8 degrees	5/5
2+/5	0 to 34 degrees	0 to 24 degrees	Plantarflexion (0 to 50 degrees)	0 to 14 degrees	0 to 14 degrees	5/5
*NT	*0 to 2 degrees	*0 to 2 degrees	Inversion (0 to 35 degrees)	0 to 35 degrees	0 to 35 degrees	5/5
*NT	*0 degrees	*0 degrees	Eversion (0 to 15 degrees)	0 to 8 degrees	0 to 8 degrees	5/5

NT=not tested.

*Rachel reports her left ankle was fused during a surgery as a child.

Goals: At the start of therapy, Rachel participated in the Canadian Occupational Performance Measure (COPM; Law et al., 2000), which is a reliable and valid client-centered outcome measure that assesses a person's perception of their own occupational performance (Carswell et al., 2004). This measure allows the client to identify problem areas in self-care, productivity, and leisure that are important to them and then rate their satisfaction with their current ability to perform those occupations. The measure is used to collaboratively set goals with the client and is administered again at discharge to demonstrate occupational therapy intervention outcomes.

On the COPM, Rachel identified stepping up onto curbs, participating in yoga, traveling independently, walking across campus, and climbing a pool ladder as her five most important problems. She rated her performance in these areas as a 3.8/10 and her satisfaction with her ability to perform these activities as a 2.4/10. Based on the COPM scores and objective evaluation, the following occupational therapy goals were established by the occupational therapist in collaboration with Rachel.

Short-Term Goals:

1. Client will independently access a swimming pool via ladder, ramp, or stairs in 4 weeks to perform an exercise program.

2. Client will independently perform a home exercise program in the swimming pool in 4 weeks to increase LE strength.

3. Client will demonstrate independence in three energy conservation techniques during an IADL task in 4 weeks.

4. Client will increase bilateral hip flexion strength to 3+/5 in 4 weeks to facilitate stepping up a curb.

Long-Term Goals:

1. Client will demonstrate increased occupational participation in valued leisure activities of yoga and swimming in 6 weeks.

2. Client will be independent in home exercise program in 6 weeks.

3. Client will be independent in energy conservation and work simplification techniques for all valued ADL, IADL, work, and leisure tasks in 6 weeks.

4. Client will walk from her parking space to her office without falling or loss of balance in 6 weeks.

The outcome of Rachel's occupational therapy intervention, along with the treatment techniques and goals achieved, can be found in Appendix C.

Functional Mobility in the Home and Community

Functional mobility is crucial for performance of valued occupations. *Basic mobility* refers to movements such as rolling from side to side in bed, transitioning from supine to seated, transferring from one surface to another, and ambulating. Mobility skills are the basis for engaging in functional mobility in the home and community. Functional mobility is much more than the ability to walk, it enables people to participate in activities such as self-care, leisure, work, and education. Examples of functional mobility include propelling a wheelchair, getting out of bed, pushing a shopping cart, riding a bike, driving a car, or transferring into the shower.

Functional mobility begins with an understanding of typical movement. What muscles are engaged when moving from sit to stand? How many degrees of freedom are normal in a hip or knee? What is the expected amount of active ROM in hip flexion? What is the best position of the pelvis for stable movement? Successful, safe functional mobility relies on more than just the LE. Pain may limit the available degrees of freedom in back motion, resulting in a decreased ability to bend over. A person with decreased ROM in their UEs may not be able to reach for their walker. A person with poor UE strength may not be able to push up from their arm rests to stand. A person with poor abdominal strength may struggle to move from supine to sitting in bed. Functional mobility may be limited or strengthened by any number of deficits related to kinesiology.

The OTPF-4 describes the domains and process of occupational therapy and provides a framework for functional mobility (AOTA, 2020). The OTPF-4 categorizes functional mobility under the domain of occupation as an ADL, which is an activity that is focused on personal care. Although functional mobility is categorized as an area of self-care in the OTPF-4, it is also strongly related to several other areas of occupation. For example, the ADLs of bathing, toileting, dressing, and sexual activity all require some level of mobility. A person with deficits in the ability to transfer from one surface to another may struggle to use the toilet independently. A person with deficits in bed mobility may require assistance to sit up from bed to get dressed. Similarly, many IADLs, which are more complex activities that help people to participate in home and community occupations, rely on functional mobility. Driving and community mobility may be the clearest example in the OTPF-4, but meal preparation, shopping, and home management tasks, such as house and yard work, also involve functional mobility. A person with paraplegia may require a wheelchair as their primary means of mobility and may need to drive using hand controls. A person who ambulates with a cane may need assistance to mow their lawn. Sleep, participation in education, work, play, leisure, and social events are also areas of occupation that may be affected by limitations in functional mobility. A person's ability to independently move through their home and community has a tremendous impact on their ability to engage in occupation.

A variety of client factors, which are structures of the body and their related functions, are necessary for safe and effective functional mobility (AOTA, 2020). For example, amputation of an LE (body structure) will have an impact on a person's ability to maintain standing balance and to walk. Back pain (body function) could prevent a person from participating in bed mobility or ambulation. Limited active or passive hip ROM (body function) could impair the ability to sit on a chair of standard height. An unstable LE joint, such as knee with a torn ligament (body structure), may prevent a person from placing full weight on the extremity without it buckling or causing pain, potentially resulting in a fall. All of these examples of deficits in client factors would limit a person's ability to engage in functional mobility and other valued occupations.

Functional mobility also relies on performance skills. Performance skills are a grouping of multiple observable and goal-directed actions and capacities that combine to create a basis for participation in functional tasks (AOTA, 2020). The type of performance skills most related to functional mobility are motor skills, which are defined in the OTPF-4 as a "group of performance skills that represent small, observable actions related to moving oneself or moving and interacting with tangible task objects" (AOTA, 2020, p. 79; Fisher & Marterella, 2019, p. 331). Examples of motor skills include stabilizing by holding on to a countertop to prevent loss of balance, positioning the body correctly to perform a task, reaching for an object, coordinating the use of both hands to accomplish a task, and lifting or carrying an object. A person with limitations in motor skills may be unable to independently complete a task requiring functional mobility, such as carrying clothing from the dresser to the bathroom in order to dress. This task is seemingly simple, but in actuality it involves the motor skills of positioning the body in front of the dresser, bending over, moving the dresser drawer, reaching for the clothing, gripping the clothing, stabilizing to stand, lifting the clothing, walking to the bathroom, and transporting the clothing. A deficit in any one of these motor skills may impact completion of the task.

It is important to note that many other intrinsic factors contribute to a person's ability to engage in functional mobility beyond the motor skills and client factors discussed previously. Impaired vision may create decreased standing balance; impaired visual perception (the brain's ability to interpret what it is seeing) may result in a person bumping into walls and furniture; impaired cognition may impede a person's ability to remember the correct sequence of an occupation requiring functional mobility; and impaired sensation in the feet may lead to tripping during ambulation. Each diagnosis, whether it be orthopedic (e.g., a hip replacement), neurologic (e.g., a stroke), or cardiopulmonary (e.g., chronic obstructive pulmonary disease), may result in deficits in functional mobility. Losses in joint mobility, abnormal muscle tone, decreased motor control, abnormal motor reflexes, impaired proprioception, impaired cardiovascular function (endurance, fatigue, stamina), and deficits in balance all have the potential to limit a person's ability to carry out functional mobility. Likewise, deficits in the performance skills of social interaction may limit functional mobility. For example, a person with severe speech and swallow deficits may refuse to visit a social event, thereby missing an opportunity to walk. Limitations in a process skill, such as initiation, may also prevent a person from carrying out a valued occupation. It is essential for the occupational therapist to conduct a thorough evaluation and to create clear goals that demonstrate the relationship between functional mobility and occupation for this reason. The occupational therapy assistant can then incorporate functional mobility in occupation-based treatment. Deficits in any client factor, performance skill, or any combination may impact functional mobility.

In addition to factors that are internal to the client, factors that are external to the client may also have a tremendous impact on the ability to engage in functional mobility. The OTPF-4 considers the **physical environment** under the domain of contexts, as the natural environment and human-made changes to the environment. In the OTPF-4, the area of environmental factors also addresses products and technology, support and relationships, attitudes, and services, systems, and policies (AOTA, 2020, p. 10). The natural environment consists of terrain, vegetation, and animals, while the built environment (human-made changes) includes places, objects, and tools constructed by humans. These contexts were more thoroughly discussed in Chapter 3. Humans interact with the physical environment in some way at all times. Whether it is in the home or the community, the environment provides a backdrop for occupational performance and, therefore, functional mobility. The height of a toilet, texture of the floor surface, distance to walk, steps to enter, size of a crowd, or a small dog underfoot are all environmental elements that may support or impede a person's ability to move from one location to another. Aspects of the physical environment that limit a person's functional mobility may be manipulated to improve occupational performance through the provision of adaptive equipment, techniques, or positioning of the person or tools. The OTPF-4 refers to knowledge of **occupation and activity demands** (AOTA, 2020, p. 57), which means that occupational therapy practitioners should carefully examine each occupation or task in relation to the context it is performed in. For instance, an understanding of the **space demands** of functional mobility may be essential for the client's success. A person with low vision and impaired gait may have difficulty navigating a path from the kitchen to the living room if there is clutter and dim lighting. Occupational therapy practitioners must also consider what body functions, body structures, and performance skills are necessary to perform the occupation to determine if compensation is needed for the person to be successful. In terms of functional mobility, this may mean providing a wheelchair in the absence of the ability to ambulate or providing a walker basket to transport items during ambulation. As the environment is such a crucial and ever-present aspect of functional mobility, it must be considered during intervention with just as much importance as intrinsic aspects.

Table 12-2 summarizes all the domains of the OTPF-4 described here that relate specifically to functional mobility.

Home Versus Community Environments

A person's quality of movement is impacted by their environment. When moving about in their home, a place that is comfortable and well known to them, movement tends to be smooth. When moving in a new, unfamiliar environment, such as exploring a park or going for a hike, movement may be more cautious. One reason for this difference in the quality of movement is that the home is considered a **closed environment**, while the community is an **open environment** (Schmidt, 1975). Closed environments have less variability and more structure, while open environments are less predictable. Open environments tend to have more variability and place greater demands on the person. Take the example of doing laundry. At home, someone may decide to do laundry and take the dirty clothes to their laundry room. Once

TABLE 12-2

Domains of the *Occupational Therapy Practice Framework: Domain and Process, Fourth Edition* as Related to Functional Mobility

DOMAIN	CATEGORY	DESCRIPTION
ADLs	Functional mobility	"Moving from one position or place to another (during performance of everyday activities), such as in-bed mobility, wheelchair mobility, and transfers (e.g. wheelchair, bed, car, tub, toilet, chair, floor). Includes functional ambulation and transporting objects" (AOTA, 2020, p. 30).
IADLs	Driving and community mobility	"Planning and moving around in the community and using public or private transportation, such as driving, walking, bicycling, or accessing and riding in buses, taxi cabs, or other transportation systems" (AOTA, 2020, p. 31).
Client factors	Body functions	Body functions are physiological functions of body systems, including "neuromuscular and movement related functions of joint mobility, joint stability, muscle strength, muscle tone, muscle endurance, motor reflexes, voluntary or involuntary movement, and gait pattern" (AOTA, 2020, p. 53).
Performance skills	Body structures	"Anatomical parts of the body, such as organs, limbs and their components" that support body function (World Health Organization, 2001, p. 10). Examples include legs, feet, abdominals, and pelvis.
	Motor skills	"Group of performance skills that represent small, observable actions related to moving oneself or moving and interacting with tangible task objects" (Fisher & Marterella, 2019, p. 331). Examples include move, walk, transport, endure, pace, and bend.
Occupation and activity demands	Space demands	"Physical environmental requirements of the activity (e.g., size, arrangement, surface, lighting, temperature, noise, humidity, ventilation)" (AOTA, 2020, p. 57).
Interventions to support occupations	Preparatory methods	"Methods and tasks that prepare the client for occupational performance…" (AOTA, 2020, p. 59), including splints, assistive technology and environmental modification, and wheeled mobility.

there, they probably perform the task in a similar way to how they have performed it in the past. There is little variability. If, however, they move to a new apartment and no longer have a washer or dryer in their own home, they may have to do laundry at a public laundry facility. Now, initiating laundry may be determined by the availability of washing machines, or their ability to get to the laundry facility. Their capability to launder clothes at the public facility may vary from time to time due to broken machines, not having enough money, or a crowded facility. The laundry facility is an open environment where each trial of doing laundry may differ from the last. The home is often considered a closed environment due to the familiarity of the context and well-established routines and habits within the space; however, this is not always the case. For example, after a recent move, or if the home is chaotic with multiple people or animals moving throughout, it becomes more open. In a similar respect, the community

tends to be more of an open environment with unexpected or variable people, actions, barriers, and supports that may influence the person's movement within the environment.

This concept can also be applied to occupational performance. When performing a closed skill, the person is in control of initiating the action and the environment remains essentially the same from one trial to the next. An example of this related to a motor skill would be walking from the bed to the bathroom at home. Many of us can accomplish this task in the dark because (generally) the number of steps and the path we take remains the same every time. When performing an open skill, however, the person must be more reactive to the skill itself because the skill and the environment are less familiar. Imagine walking from the bathroom to get into bed after breaking a leg. The motor skill of walking is now performed using crutches, so the number of steps, the method used, and even the pathway taken may be different. You now

Figure 12-1. Rachel ascending steps with support. (GBALLGIGGSPHOTO/ shutterstock.com)

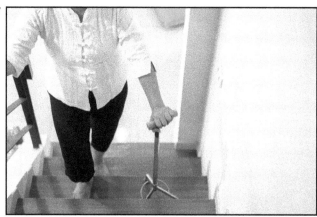

BOX 12-1

Ergonomics is "an applied science concerned with designing and arranging things people use so that the people and things interact most efficiently and safely."

(Merriam-Webster, n.d.)

must consider if there is enough space for the crutches to pass by the dresser or if you will be able to make it there without resting.

Recognizing if a skill or environment is open or closed is important for the occupational therapy practitioner to grade tasks for someone with impaired motor skills. When a person is first learning (or relearning) a motor skill, it is best to begin with a closed skill or environment for the client. This allows the person to learn the task and practice with little changes between each attempt, increasing the chances of success with each try. But as the person masters the skill, the occupational therapy practitioner must advance the client to an open skill or environment. This will increase the level of challenge and force problem solving and adaptation in new situations.

Rachel, from the occupational profile, has noticed that her decline in functional mobility is related more to the community than her home. This is in part due to the community being an open environment. For example, she finds that she is sometimes reluctant to go to dinner or to a movie with friends if she is not already familiar with the environment because she may face unexpected steps or curbs. Figure 12-1 shows Rachel ascending steps in a friend's home with a handrail and cane for support.

Body Mechanics

An understanding of basic body mechanics is essential for safe functional mobility. Body mechanics is an understanding of how the body moves in safe and efficient ways,

throughout all daily activities, in order to reduce the risk of injury. With poor body mechanics, the spine undergoes stress that can cause unnecessary wear and tear, leading to degeneration of spinal disks and joints. Stresses on the body may come in the form of force, pressure, gravity, friction, repetition, or torque.

Occupational therapy assistants should be able to observe a person's body mechanics and understand what is needed to help them to move more effectively and efficiently. Box 12-1 gives the definition of ergonomics, which is a guide for occupational therapy assistants to aid their clients. Poor body mechanics often lead to back injuries, such as herniated disks and lumbosacral sprains. Common causes of back problems include poor body mechanics during lifting as well as during common ADLs and IADLs. For example, bending incorrectly to pick up a mop bucket full of water may lead to back injury. Even sleeping on a mattress that is too soft or too hard may push the spine out of good alignment. Clients need to be trained to perform activities with proper body mechanics to prevent injury or to avoid reinjury.

There are several principles of body mechanics (Box 12-2). A primary foundation of body mechanics is good posture. Good posture consists of standing or sitting with the spine in neutral alignment, which means maintaining the four natural curves in the spine: cervical, thoracic, lumbar, and sacral. The cervical and lumbar curves are both convex, while the thoracic and sacral curves are concave (see Chapter 5 for more description of the spinal curves). These natural curves should be maintained during all postures and activities without overly arching the back. The pelvis should be kept in a neutral position. An anterior tilt of the pelvis creates an abnormal rounding of the lumbar spine known

BOX 12-2

PRINCIPLES OF BODY MECHANICS

- Be aware of the load before lifting or carrying.
- Move close to the client or to an object being lifted or carried.
- Maintain a wide BOS.
- Maintain the normal spinal curves.
- Bend the hips and knees.
- Stabilize the trunk before moving the extremities.
- Use larger muscles to perform work.
- Exhale during exertion.
- Avoid twisting the trunk, especially when the trunk is flexed.
- Push rather than pull an object when possible.
- Get help when needed.

(Johansson & Chinworth, 2012)

as lordosis of the back. Posterior pelvic tilt results in an abnormal rounding of the thoracic spine referred to as *kyphosis*. Sitting in a slouched position causes posterior pelvic tilt, lordosis, and forward head. In standing, poor posture results in rounded shoulders, forward head, and kyphosis. Long periods of standing or sitting can lead to poor posture with exaggerated spinal curves that may cause back strain.

Some activities require twisting. Twisting motions create more pressure on the nucleus of the intervertebral disks. The nucleus helps to distribute pressure evenly across the disk, but during twisting the rotational motion increases the pressure on one side of the nucleus more than the other. When bending is combined with twisting, the likelihood of injury is even greater. Twisting cannot always be avoided but bending and twisting motions together should be minimized. For example, standing at the sink and loading the lower shelf of a dishwasher may lead a person to bend and twist as they load each dish. To maintain good body mechanics, a better approach would be to take small steps to face the dishwasher and bend the legs into a squat to load each dish. This technique may feel awkward at first but will avoid twisting and bending.

Another source of injury is lifting because the added weight can add additional force to the spinal column. A common cause of back injury is lifting with poor body mechanics. Wilke et al. (1999) found that lifting with a bent waist and straight legs resulted in a 4.5-fold increase of pressure on the back, while lifting with a straight back and bent knees reduced the pressure on the back by 25%. Bending at the waist puts all of the force on the smaller and weaker back muscles instead of the large leg and buttock muscles and is likely to lead to back injury. When at all possible, avoid heaving lifting and instead push or slide an object rather than picking it

up or pulling it. Box 12-3 describes the National Institute for Occupational Safety and Health (NIOSH) lifting equation, which helps a therapist understand the risks of lifting.

The best technique to lift something heavy from the floor is to squat down with the legs at least hip width apart with one foot slightly in front of the other to provide a wide base of support (BOS) for stability. Keep the chin level with the floor and maintain the normal arches in the spine. Bring the object in close to the body to decrease the amount of force on the lower back (Wilke et al., 1999). This use of short lever arms will also provide better control. To stand, engage the large muscles in the quadriceps and buttocks, as well as the abdominal muscles. This lifting technique, called **diagonal lifting**, uses the largest and strongest muscles possible for the task (quadriceps and gluteus), to protect the more fragile back muscles. Another option for lifting is called the **tripod lift**, which is a good option for loads that may shift, such as a bag of dog food. To perform a tripod lift, slowly lower the body to kneel with one knee on the ground. Slide the object that needs to be lifted close to the body and lift it onto the knee opposite the one resting on the ground. Put the arms around the object and hug it into the chest. Extend the legs into standing while keeping the head lifted and the back straight. This technique is not appropriate for those with knee injuries. For lifting light objects, a **golfer's lift** may be more appropriate. This is commonly used on the golf course to pick up golf balls by using the golf club for support. The golfer's lift may be used to pick up small, light objects while stabilizing on a counter or chair. The back remains straight, and one leg extends behind the body to act as a counterbalance as the body bends forward. This is a good technique for those with knee pain. It can be used for daily activities, such as taking clothing out of a dryer or picking up an object from the floor. Figure 12-2 shows the golfer's lift. Lifting

BOX 12-3

"NIOSH Lifting Equation: LC (51) x HM x VM x DM x AM x FM x CM = RWL

The NIOSH lifting equation always uses a load constant (LC) of 51 pounds, which represents the maximum recommended load weight to be lifted under ideal conditions. From that starting point, the equation uses several task variables expressed as coefficients or multipliers (In the equation, M = multiplier) that serve to decrease the load constant and calculate the recommended weight limit (RWL) for that particular lifting task.

Task variables needed to calculate the RWL:

- H = Horizontal location of the object relative to the body
- V = Vertical location of the object relative to the floor
- D = Distance the object is moved vertically
- A = Asymmetry angle or twisting requirement
- F = Frequency and duration of lifting, activity
- C = Coupling or quality of the workers grip on the object

The NIOSH Lifting Equation is used to answer the questions:

- Is this weight too heavy for the task?
- How significant is the risk of lifting?"

(Middlesworth, 2012, para. 17-24)

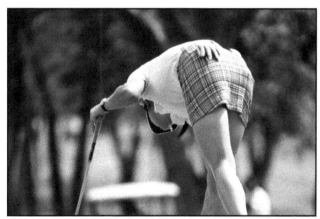

Figure 12-2. Golfer's lift. (Mai Groves/shutterstock.com)

overhead is especially dangerous as it creates a longer lever arm and creates additional force on the back. To lift overhead, begin by holding the object close to the body. Keep the feet shoulder width apart, with one foot slightly ahead of the other. Raise the object to the overhead shelf, keeping it close to the plane of the body. Breathe out while lifting. To place the object on the shelf, shift the weight from the back foot to the front foot and, keeping the back straight, push the object onto the shelf.

Learning to perform occupations while using good posture and body mechanics can be challenging for many clients, as it involves creating new habits and routines. Occupational therapy practitioners should cultivate the ability to recognize good and bad posture and body mechanics during all activities in order to cue a client to change their behavior.

Body mechanics can first be taught as individual skills in a simulated environment, such as lifting using weighted boxes. Ultimately, the skills must be transferred to ADLs and IADLs because participation in these life activities with poor body mechanics are likely to lead to injury. Lifting a weighted box in a clinical environment is different than lifting a bag of dry cement or a laundry basket full of wet towels during real-life activities. Clients need opportunities to practice and to apply skills learned in the clinic. Clients should be instructed on how to maintain body mechanics during all daily activities, such as showering, making a bed, yard work, and grocery shopping. This will involve application of the skills into a realistic situation.

Additionally, it is essential that therapists learn to monitor their own postural and body mechanic habits. One study found that occupational therapists had an annual injury rate similar to that of workers in heavy manufacturing jobs (Darragh et al., 2009). Good body mechanics will enable the occupational therapy practitioner to position their own body to avoid or minimize stress on the spine or other joints while helping clients. Over time, performing transfers, pushing wheelchairs, and assisting people in bed can increase the risk for injury, particularly if the therapist uses poor body mechanics. There are many ways to decrease the risk to the therapist. For example, during a maximum assist transfer of a client, the therapist should maintain a wide BOS by keeping their feet staggered and slightly wider than hip width apart, with their knees bent and their back straight. An even better way to reduce therapist injury would be to have another person assist with transfers when needed, or to use a transfer board.

Functional Mobility in the Home

In the home, people have a need to carry out basic self-care tasks, as well as IADLs related to home management and caring for others. Limitations in functional mobility may interfere with a person's ability to safely perform occupations in the home, such as getting out of bed, showering, dressing, preparing a meal, or performing yard work.

Bed Mobility

Bed mobility is the ability to move the body from one position to another in bed, and to move to and from a supine position. Bed mobility may be decreased due to neuromuscular or musculoskeletal impairments. For example, a person with hemiparesis following a stroke may struggle to independently get out of bed due to one-sided weakness and abnormal muscle tone. There are two basic skills that are foundational to bed mobility: bridging and rolling. These skills are the basis for other bed mobility movements, including scooting while in supine and moving from side-lying to sitting.

Bridging is useful for donning pants while in bed, placing a bed pan, or repositioning in bed. To bridge, the knees and hips are flexed, with the feet on the bed or mat surface. The hips are moved into extension to lift the pelvis and lower back off the surface. Figure 12-3 shows a person bridging. Occupational therapy practitioners may need to assist during any portion of this movement in the event of muscle weakness or limited ROM. An occupational therapy assistant can assist a person to bridge by stabilizing the LEs in the position to bridge and then placing their hands underneath, toward the top of the pelvis, to lift the client's hips up. A cue for the person to raise their hips can also be given by providing downward and forward pressure at the top of the knees. Bridging is the starting point for scooting in supine to reposition the body in bed. The person bridges, lifting the hips up and over to one side, or pushes the feet into the bed to scoot the body up. If a person is unable to bridge, rolling to one side may be another option for positioning.

Rolling is important for positioning in bed, comfort, and pressure relief. Rolling may be used as a technique for dressing in bed and can also be a precursor for moving from side-lying to sitting. To roll independently to one side, a person turns their head that direction and engages the core muscles. The LE opposite the direction of the roll may be used to push the body into the roll by flexing the knee and pushing the foot into the bed. The client should reach across their body with the UE opposite the direction of the roll; reaching for a bed rail may provide assistance to complete the roll. The occupational therapy assistant can also provide physical assistance by providing pressure at the client's shoulder and hip to pull them into the roll.

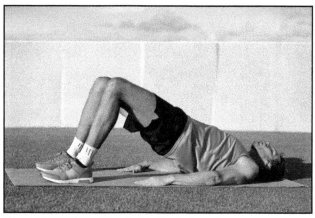

Figure 12-3. Bridging. (Maridav/shutterstock.com)

To move from supine to sitting at the edge of the bed independently, most people use abdominal strength and momentum to raise the upper body and swing the legs off the bed in one smooth movement. Clients with limited strength will benefit from breaking the movement down into segments by first rolling to one side and then moving from side-lying to sitting. To move from side-lying to sitting independently, the client first moves their legs off the edge of the bed. The UEs are used to push the upper body into an upright position: the arm that is on the bed will move into shoulder abduction, pushing the elbow into the bed as the elbow extends, while pushing the other hand into the bed and also moving that arm into extension. Figure 12-4 demonstrates using the arms to push up from side-lying to sitting. To assist a client with this movement, the occupational therapy assistant should help them to move their legs off the bed while the client is lying on their side. Then, the occupational therapy assistant places one hand under the client's shoulder that is on the bed and the other hand on the client's opposite hip. Applying pressure on the opposite shoulder and hip will help to raise the client into sitting at the edge of the bed. The occupational therapy assistant should take care to bend their knees and keep their back neutral while performing this assist to avoid personal injury.

There are other options for moving a client into a seated position. The head of the bed may be raised so the client is long sitting, which is sitting upright with the legs fully extended. Long sitting is used by some clients with spinal cord injuries (SCIs) to perform dressing and other self-care because the position provides support in the absence of abdominal innervation. From long sitting, the legs can be moved off the edge of the bed. Another option is to have the client use an overhead trapeze or a bed ladder to pull themselves into sitting. Frail older adults may benefit more from adaptive techniques than from trunk strengthening to improve their ability to move from supine to sitting (Alexander et al., 2000). Occupational therapy practitioners need to determine which method is best suited for each individual based on their available client factors and performance skills.

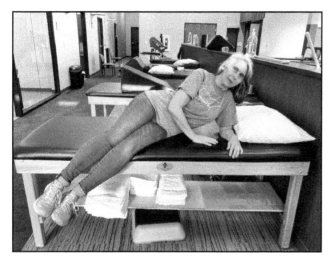

Figure 12-4. Using the arms to push up from side-lying to sitting.

Transfers

Transfers are defined as moving from one place to another, such as moving from a wheelchair to the toilet, or from the bed to a bedside commode. Clients with deficits in functional mobility often require assistance to transfer and training to increase independence in transfers. Occupational therapy practitioners must consider the client's available strength, ROM, muscle tone, balance, and endurance to determine the best transfer to use. Client factors such as cognition and vision may also impact the transfer. Other things to consider are if the client uses any assistive devices (e.g., walker, cane) or if they have any precautions (e.g., a weight-bearing restriction, hip precautions following hip replacement). Some clients will have intravenous (IV) lines, oxygen tubing, or catheters that will need to be managed during the transfer. Overall, the occupational therapy assistant should have a good understanding of the client's diagnosis and precautions before transferring them for the first time. If there is any doubt about the client's abilities, it is best to ask another person to help with the transfer rather than risk the safety of the client or injury to the therapist.

All transfers begin with preparation of the environment. Clear the environment of any obstacles and think through the transfer before beginning, in order to avoid starting a transfer only to realize midway that it is not going to be successful. Preparation of the environment may involve actions such as moving a hospital bed to the fully horizontal position, lowering a guard rail, moving an IV pole, or positioning a wheelchair. The client should be positioned at a 90-degree angle to the surface they will be moving to. Prepare the wheelchair by removing the arm and leg rests and locking the brakes.

The client should also be prepared for the transfer. Apply a safety belt to the client, instruct them in the transfer sequence, and explain to them what to expect. The client should be told what actions they should take during the transfer. Even if it is a completely dependent transfer, the client may have a role to perform, such as counting to three, holding on to their affected arm for safety, or looking toward the surface they are transferring to. Transfers can be frightening and even feel demeaning for some clients, so it is essential that the therapist take steps to prepare the client for the experience.

For many transfers, moving from sitting to standing is the first step. To move from sitting to standing, a person performs the following steps: scoot forward to the edge of the seat, move feet posteriorly under knees, lean forward, engage quadriceps and core muscles, and stand. This sit-to-stand movement requires moving the center of gravity (COG) forward and then upward (Roebroeck et al., 1994). Additional steps may be part of the transfer sequence, such as using arms to push up from the arm rests or reaching for a walker upon standing. Variations in the sit-to-stand sequence may be necessary, such as keeping the hip and knee extended as a precaution against possible hip dislocations. Moving from standing to sitting is the opposite. Beginning with the client backing up until the back of their legs touch the chair, reaching back for the seat, and sitting. Avoid letting the client "plop down," or sit down hard without control of the descent.

Assistance may be provided by standing in front of or next to the client, with hands on the safety belt or at the pelvis, depending on the type of transfer and how much assistance the client requires. If a person only requires minimal assistance to transfer, the therapist can stand to the side to provide minimal cuing. If a person requires moderate to maximum assistance to transfer, the therapist should stand in front of the client with bent knees and a wide BOS, and hands on the safety belt at the client's waist. The therapist must be aware of their own body mechanics during the transfer to avoid injury. Therapists are also at risk for injury during transfers (Andersen et al., 2014), so therapists must have a clear understanding of the principles of transfers.

Transfers, if done properly, do not involve brute force. A common mistake is to attempt to lift the client straight up and over to the other surface, which requires the considerable strength on the part of the therapist and can lead to therapist injury. Instead, good transfers rely on leverage and momentum. As the person leans forward, with their head past their knees, they take weight off the back of the body, making it easier to raise the client's bottom off the surface. The feet serve as a fulcrum as the therapist uses leverage to rock the person forward and over to the other surface. Adding a rocking motion, sometimes with a count of three to cue the client when it is time to move, may provide additional momentum. Keir and MacDonell (2004) found that more experienced therapists demonstrated increased trapezius and latissimus dorsi activity and lower erector spinae activity than novice therapists, possibly indicating that experienced therapists have learned to protect their spine by distributing the load from the back to the shoulder.

There are several types of transfers. **Stand pivot transfers** involve the client standing and pivoting the feet toward the new surface or standing and taking small steps toward the new surface. Stand pivot transfers may be performed with a walker or other mobility device. The stand pivot transfer works best with clients who are able to stand completely, at least for a short time. In the event of decreased standing balance and LE weakness, the therapist will provide support during the transfer. In some cases of LE weakness or hemiparesis, the therapist may need to guard the client's knees with their own knees to prevent buckling.

In a **squat pivot transfer**, the client does not rise into a full standing position. Instead, the client is positioned in sitting as though preparing to stand, moved forward to the edge of the seat, with feet on floor moved posteriorly under knees. If able, the client is cued to push up from the arm rests. The therapist stands in front of the client and, holding the safety belt, uses momentum and leverage to rock the client's COG forward and over to the new surface. The squat pivot transfer is best for clients who require moderate to maximum assist, have limitations in knee or hip extension strength, lack the ability to stand, or have poor trunk control.

A variation of the squat pivot transfer is known as a transfer board. A transfer board bridges the two transfer surfaces, to allow multiple squat pivot transfers to reach the other surface. Figure 12-5 shows several kinds of transfer boards. This is useful for clients who are learning to transfer independently but cannot make it the full distance, such as a client with an SCI. Clients with bilateral LE amputation also benefit from a transfer board, as well as clients with very low muscle tone in the LEs that prohibits them from bearing weight during the transfer. Transfer boards may also serve to aid the therapist in cases of a dependent transfer where a second person is not available to assist. To use the transfer board, the client leans away to place the board under the buttocks and upper thigh. It may help to have the client cross one leg over the other to provide a space to place the board underneath. Once the board has been placed, the client sits upright again. The client should be positioned as though preparing to stand, with feet under knees, and leaning forward. To perform the transfer independently, the client requires good triceps strength and shoulder depression to perform a series of push-ups, leaning forward to redistribute weight from the bottom to move toward the new surface. Multiple mini–squat pivot transfers should be used to complete the transfer, repositioning the hands and feet for each mini-transfer. The client should try to raise their bottom off the board each time, because sliding creates shearing friction on the skin and increases the risk of skin breakdown. To assist with the transfer, the therapist stands in front of the client with bent knees, a wide BOS, and both hands on the safety belt. Once the transfer is complete, the board should be removed. Figure 12-6 shows an independent lateral transfer using a sliding board from a wheelchair to a raised therapy mat.

Maximum assist transfers, or dependent transfers, are indicated when the client is unable to physically assist with the transfer. There are several methods for performing a dependent transfer. One possibility is a squat pivot transfer, but

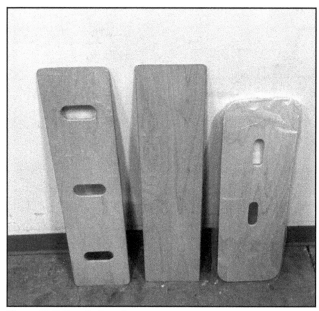

Figure 12-5. Transfer boards.

with the assistance of two people instead of one. One therapist stands in front and carries out the majority of the transfer while a second person stands behind and aids in moving the client's hips over to the new surface. The therapist in front leads the transfer and the person in the back provides support as needed. Dependent transfers may also be carried out through use of a mechanical lift, a sheet transfer, or a transfer board.

Transfers are influenced by the environment as well as client factors. A person with hemiparesis may transfer more independently toward their unimpaired side because they can rely on the strength and motor skills of the unaffected side. If a person transfers better to one side, the environment may be modified to encourage transfers to that side and, thus, encourage independence. Other times, the therapy practitioner may choose to force transfers to the weaker side in order to improve the skill. Chair height and arm rests may affect a person's ability to move from sitting to standing independently. One systematic review (Janssen et al., 2002) found that moving from sitting to standing is strongly influenced by the height of the chair seat, the use of arm rests, and foot position. A lower chair height requires greater momentum to rise from the chair. Transferring with a transfer board is more difficult if the two transfer surfaces are not of equal height. Therapists should determine how the environment should be adjusted to allow for more independence in transferring.

Bathroom Mobility

The bathroom presents unique challenges for many individuals with deficits in functional mobility. Rising from a low toilet, stepping into a bathtub, standing to shower, or

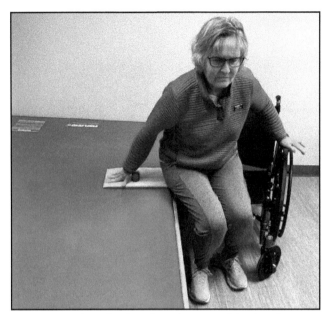

Figure 12-6. Independent lateral transfer using a sliding board.

standing to groom at the sink may not be safe or feasible for those with weak LEs, poor balance, or decreased endurance. Toilet transfers may be aided by adding a raised toilet seat and safety bars. Shower transfers may be made safer by adding a shower chair with adjustable legs, a tub bench, safety bars, and a non-skid mat. Many bathrooms have limited space and may not accommodate walkers or wheelchairs. Each bathroom environment will require problem solving to ensure the safety and independence of the user.

Transferring to a bathtub may be best achieved with a tub transfer bench or chair because it removes the possibility of tripping while stepping into the tub. The transfer is accomplished by first transferring to sit on the short edge of the tub bench. The client then turns toward the tub and lifts each leg into the tub while repositioning the body further onto the bench. The client bathes in sitting, using a handheld shower head or other adaptive equipment, such as a long-handled sponge, as needed. Some benches have an opening with a bucket underneath that allows the client to toilet and then shower. This option is especially good for those with SCIs because it reduces the number of daily transfers and conserves energy. Use of a tub transfer bench or chair is also a good option for those with limited balance or endurance.

Activities of Daily Living and Functional Mobility

Most ADLs require elements of functional mobility. Consider your own morning routine, which may consist of getting out of bed, moving to and from the bedroom and bathroom to toilet, shower, dress, and groom, and moving to and from the kitchen to prepare and eat breakfast. Each of these activities requires elements of bed mobility, transfers, and ambulation. Limitations in client factors will change the method used, require adaptive equipment, or require the client to improve in some way.

Bathing is a full body task. The OTPF-4 (AOTA, 2020) describes bathing and showering as "obtaining and using supplies; soaping, rinsing, and drying body parts; maintaining bathing position; and transferring to and from bathing positions" (p. 30). Breaking this down further, to shower a person must first perform a transfer into the shower, which may involve stepping into a bathtub or shower or sitting on a tub bench and swinging the legs in (depending on ability). Standing to shower may involve weight shifting to reach for shampoo, bending over to wash feet, or maintaining standing balance with arms overhead to wash hair.

Likewise, the functional mobility required for dressing will depend on the available client factors of the person. A person with paraplegia may don their pants while long sitting in bed. This requires bed mobility to move into long sitting, and then rocking from side to side to pull pants on. Once the pants are on, the person may transfer from long sitting to transfer into the wheelchair using a transfer board where they can don their shirt while in supported sitting due to poor sitting balance. Socks and shoes may also be donned while in supported sitting. Contrast this method of dressing with someone who has recently had a hip replacement and has hip precautions to avoid bending forward past 90 degrees, internal rotation of the hip, and hip abduction. This client will require adaptive equipment to don their pants to maintain the hip precautions. Sitting at the edge of the bed or in a supportive chair, they will use a reacher or dressing stick to start their pants over their feet, and then reach forward with their hand to pull their pants on the rest of the way, up to their thighs, at which point, they will need to stand to pull their pants on. To avoid bending too far forward at the hip, the best method is to extend the affected knee in front before pushing to stand. This keeps the hip angle greater than 90 degrees even as the person leans forward to stand.

Instrumental Activities of Daily Living and Functional Mobility

IADLs are activities that are beyond self-care. In the home, the focus of IADLs is on caring for the home and other people. Many IADLs that are performed in the home require extensive functional mobility, such as doing the laundry, making a meal, and doing yard work.

Functional mobility may be more challenging if there is a need to carry items. Carrying items with both hands may prevent someone from catching themselves if they fall or change the COG enough to cause a fall. Imagine carrying a heavy laundry basket: with a heavy load in front of the body, the COG shifts forward. Rachel reports feeling less stable when ambulating while carrying an item. She gave an example of being asked by her mother to help bring food to the table for Thanksgiving dinner, and declining due to the fear of falling or dropping the food. Rachel would benefit from using a small cart to transport items from the kitchen to the dining room. This would help with her stability, as well as conserve her energy for other tasks.

Energy Conservation

Energy conservation is a technique to use movements as efficiently as possible with the goal of saving energy for other tasks. There are several main principles of energy conservation that a person can use to pace their activities throughout the day, such as alternating heavy and light tasks. To determine if a task is light or heavy, the client and therapist should consider how much resistance the task requires, what position the task is performed in, how long it takes to perform the task, and if there is any muscle weakness or other deficits that will make the task harder to perform. For example, as Rachel plans her day, she should consider that she has more difficulty with laundry because it requires lifting a heavy basket of clothes and carrying the basket through the house. She may want to do one load of laundry in the morning and save the second load for the afternoon once she has rested, or she may want to be sure she only does laundry on days she does not have other heavy tasks scheduled, like snow shoveling.

Alternating heavy and light tasks will require planning ahead and even scheduling IADLs. This may mean performing only one heavy task, or it may mean spreading heavy tasks throughout the day, with one in the morning and one in the evening. Tasks may be broken into smaller parts or spread out over several days. For example, laundry can be broken into sorting in the evening, washing the next morning, and folding in the evening. Meal preparation can be accomplished by cutting all vegetables ahead of time, or buying pre-cut vegetables, so that when the meal is cooked that step is already done. Another principle is to ensure that there is enough time to do activities without rushing. Rushing may cause poor body mechanics. Periods of work should be balanced with periods of rest. Preventing fatigue will increase endurance over the long run.

Organization of workspaces such as the kitchen and laundry room can also conserve energy. Organization helps you find tools and supplies quickly and easily to reduce steps, bending, stooping, and lifting. To organize, place tools and supplies where they are most used. This may be counterintuitive for some. For instance, place a pot most often used in the kitchen directly on the countertop, rather than putting in a low cupboard that requires bending. Some people may be uncomfortable at first with having their kitchen "out of order," but ultimately the saved energy will enable the person to spend more time doing valued occupations. Gather all supplies before starting a task to avoid extra moves, transfers,

and ambulation. Using a wheeled cart may be a good way to do this. For instance, loading a cart with all items needed to set the table rather than making multiple trips back and forth between the kitchen and dining room.

Functional Mobility in the Community

In the community, functional mobility enables people to access valued social activities, leisure, work, and education, as well as the ability to perform some IADLs, such as shopping. Functional mobility in the community includes the ability to move from one place to another, whether that be through ambulation, propulsion, driving, or riding. Functional mobility in the community may require navigating the elements, such as snow, and other variables, such as crowds and narrow spaces.

The work setting may present unique challenges for functional mobility. A person with a deficit in functional mobility may have special needs to consider, such as bathroom ease of access and transfers, pressure relief, and wheelchair accessibility. Employers are required to provide reasonable workplace accommodations for people with disabilities via the Americans with Disabilities Act (1990). Reasonable accommodations are defined in Box 12-4. Examples of workplace accommodations for deficits in functional mobility include keeping a path clear in the workspace for a wheelchair or walker, providing a safety bar next to the toilet, installing a ramp, and providing an accessible parking space. Accommodations enable workers to perform their essential job functions. Occupational therapists may be asked to evaluate a client's ability to perform their work function, and occupational therapy assistants may be involved in training the client to carry out their work functions with or without accommodations.

The workplace presented unique challenges for Rachel, who expressed difficulty moving across campus and from the parking lot to her workplace. Rachel may request reasonable accommodations from her employer, such as a rail on the curb between her parking space and the building entrance, or use of a golf cart to aid her in moving across campus for meetings.

Like the workplace, educational settings may provide unique challenges for people with functional mobility deficits. A deficit in functional mobility may prevent a student from stepping onto a school bus, accessing the bathroom, moving through a cafeteria line independently, or going outside for recess. There are laws that help students with disabilities access educational environments (Individuals with Disabilities Education Improvement Act [IDEIA], 2004). Occupational therapy practitioners may work with students in the school system to address any mobility concerns that impact their education.

BOX 12-4

Reasonable accommodation is defined as "any change or adjustment to a job, the work environment, or the way things usually are done that would allow one to apply for a job, perform job function, or enjoy equal access to benefits available to other individuals in the workplace."

(Americans with Disabilities Act, 1990; Pub. L. No. 101-336)

Adaptive Mobility

As people age or experience limited mobility due to disease, injury, or disability, special equipment may be necessary in order to compensate for any missing client factors. Compensatory techniques or **assistive technology** may be necessary in the event that remediation of the deficits is not feasible, or to provide increased independence while the deficit is being remediated. For example, a client with a bilateral LE amputation will benefit from a wheelchair to promote increased independence in functional mobility to compensate for the absent body structure. A person with only one LE amputation, however, may require a wheelchair only while learning to walk on a prosthetic; thus, the compensatory technique is only temporary. Practitioners have to decide what assistive technology is necessary, at what point to provide it, and at what point to remove it, as appropriate. A systematic review of factors affecting older adult's use of adaptive equipment found that a variety of factors contributed to use or nonuse of the prescribed equipment (Kraskowsky & Finlayson, 2001). The authors found that therapists must consider client factors, factors related to the device itself, and the fit of the equipment with the client's environment. Nonuse is more likely if a client is not motivated to use the equipment, does not understand the reason for its use, finds it too complicated or inconvenient to use, is embarrassed to use the equipment, or is not properly trained (Kraskowsky & Finlayson, 2001; Wielandt & Strong, 2000).

There is a vast variety of assistive technology available to aid individuals with functional mobility. Table 12-3 lists some examples of adaptive equipment that may aid individuals to move around the home and community. Figure 12-7 shows a rolling walker with seat and basket.

The OTPF-4 categorizes assistive technology and environmental modification, along with splints and wheeled mobility devices, as **interventions to support occupations**. Interventions to support occupations are used to "prepare the client for occupational performance" (AOTA, 2020, p. 59). Interventions to support occupations should not be used in isolation, but rather as part of a full intervention approach designed to return a client to valued occupations. In many instances, interventions to support occupations are essential for client independence or improved function, but if not combined with other therapeutic approaches (occupations and activities), may fall short of full effectiveness and may not qualify as skilled therapy. For example, providing a client with a wheelchair and basic wheelchair training will not be as effective for improved function as providing the wheelchair and training the client to use it to safely perform a valued occupation in the natural context.

Prosthetics

A prosthetic is a device that compensates for a missing body part or a body part that is not working efficiently. Prosthetics may be used for both LE and UE amputations. After LE amputation, a prosthetic limb enables independent functional mobility. Likewise, a UE prosthetic may increase functional mobility as it may be used to operate a cane or walker, or to carry items for occupational engagement. Prosthetics may also be created to carry out specific occupational demands, such as customized prosthetic feet for running, climbing, or horse riding.

Lower Extremity Prosthetics

Following amputation, the residual limb must undergo a process of wound healing and shaping. Shaping is essential to ensure that the limb will fit into a prosthetic and is accomplished via wrapping and a progression of smaller shaping socks. The wound must also be desensitized in order to tolerate weight bearing and any pressure within the prosthetic. Physical therapists instruct in gait training with the prosthetic LE, but occupational therapists may be involved in facilitating the limb shaping and desensitization, teaching the client how to care for their residual limb, and engaging the client in functional mobility while wearing the prosthetic limb.

Prosthetics are constructed by prosthetists from plastic or a carbon graphite composite material. Prosthetic limbs have several parts. The socket is the connection between the prosthetic and the residual limb. The fit of the socket must be perfect to avoid creating pressure points or shearing of rotational forces as the client dons and doffs the limb. Generally, a liner fits inside the socket, (one or more layers of prosthetic socks may be worn as well), to create a snug fit and prevent

TABLE 12-3
Examples of Adaptive Equipment for Deficits in Functional Mobility

FUNCTIONAL MOBILITY PROBLEM	ADAPTIVE EQUIPMENT
Decreased bed mobility	• Bed ladder • Bed rails • Leg lifter • Trapeze • Slider sheets • Adjustable hospital bed
Impaired sit to stand	• Raised toilet seat • Electric lift chair • Safety bar
Impaired transfer	• Transfer board • Pivot disk
Impaired or absent gait	• Walker: Standard, rolling, or with seat • Cane: Single tip or quad cane • Crutches: Standard or loft-strand (forearm)
Absent gait	• Wheelchair: Manual or motorized • Motorized scooter
Decreased balance	• Safety bars • Mobility device • Tub bench or tub chair • Reacher or dressing stick
Low endurance and/or fatigue	• Tub bench or tub chair • Motorized wheelchair or scooter
Decreased grip or coordination	• Walker basket • Doorknob extender
Edema or hemiplegia	• Wheelchair lap tray
Impaired community mobility	• Motorized grocery cart • Driving adaptations • Motorized scooter

the residual limb from moving around inside the socket. The frame of the prosthetic limb is called a *pylon*. The pylon is generally a metal tube, but some pylons are covered to look like an actual limb, including skin color. Finally, a suspension system is used to keep the prosthetic limb attached to the body. There are several types of suspension systems, such as a vacuum seal and suction. A vacuum seal may be created with a seal around the top edge of the socket, and a pump-and-valve system to remove air between the prosthetic and the body. A suction system has a one-way valve in a sleeve. When the residual limb is placed into the sleeve, body weight expels the air through the valve, creating suction to hold the limb in the socket. Both of these systems help reduce friction and shear and provide stability during ambulation.

People with an above-the-knee amputation (transfemoral) require a prosthetic limb with a knee, either mechanical or computerized. Mechanical knees use a hinge to replace the knee joint. The simplest knee has a single axis and uses friction to keep the leg from swinging forward too quickly as it moves through to the next step. A locking mechanism provides stability when standing by preventing buckling. The lock may be manual or may lock upon weight bearing. Another option is a polycentric knee, which allows multiple axes of rotation. These knees are more complex but allow greater ease when moving from stand to sit and less risk of balance loss during gait. Many polycentric knees use pneumatic or hydraulic fluid to control the leg swing to allow variable walking speeds. Finally, a knee that is controlled by a microprocessor is able to monitor the entire gait cycle

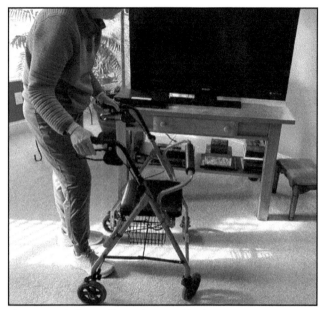

Figure 12-7. Rolling walker with seat and basket.

(when the leg is on the ground and when the leg is swinging through), and then automatically adjust a fluid or air control cylinder as needed to provide support and stability.

All prosthetic legs require a foot. There are many varieties of prosthetic feet. The foot must be durable enough to repeatedly tolerate full body weight, while also being lightweight and energy efficient. The foot needs to tolerate strong force and torque during ambulation, mimicking an actual foot and ankle structure, and the foot needs to act as a shock-absorber. Some prosthetic feet have an articulating ankle structure that allows the foot to move in multiple planes. This is a useful feature for walking on uneven terrain because it allows the foot to accommodate for the varying angles of the ground. Some carbon fiber feet store energy within them, compressing and releasing energy like a spring during each step. This feature is great for running or other athletics. The foot is often encased in a cosmetic shell that looks like an actual foot. This is cosmetic but also functional as the shape fits better into a shoe, allowing for more functional ambulation.

Upper Extremity Prosthetics

Just as with LE amputation, the residual limb following UE amputation must undergo limb shaping and desensitization to prepare for a prosthetic. Occupational therapists train clients to use their UE prosthetic in functional tasks, as well as how to don and doff the prosthetic and care for their residual limb. There are many physical and psychological reasons why a client may opt to go without a prosthetic, such as having poor training in how to use it, poor fit and discomfort while wearing it, or feeling self-conscious (Biddiss & Chau, 2007). An occupational therapy practitioner can train the client and address the client's other concerns as well (Resnik et al., 2012).

The UE prosthetic is comprised of a socket for the residual limb, a wrist joint, and a hand. Above-the-elbow (transhumeral) amputations also include an elbow joint. UE prosthetics may be body powered or myoelectric. Body powered prosthetics use a cable that is connected to a harness worn by the client. The client uses upper body movements, such as shoulder protraction, to control opening or closing the hand and bending (extending) the elbow. The wrist angle is generally moved manually with a body powered prosthetic. A myoelectric prosthetic is controlled by contracting muscles in the residual limb to generate electromyography signals that activate the motor in the elbow, wrist, and hand. The myoelectric prosthetic does not require a harness and may look more natural than a body powered prosthetic. People with high-level UE amputations (transhumeral or shoulder disarticulation) may benefit from targeted muscle reinnervation, a surgery that transfers intact residual peripheral nerves to the other areas (Stubblefield et al., 2009). This allows the client to use targeted muscle contractions to move the prosthetic with enough electromyography signals to simultaneously control the elbow, wrist, and hand.

The hand of a prosthetic is called a *terminal device*. Terminal devices may be body powered or myoelectric. Body powered devices are typically a hook and may be designed to be voluntary open (close at rest) or voluntary close (open at rest), depending on client preference. Grip strength is modulated via the addition or removal of rubber bands, and wrist position is manually changed as needed. Myoelectric hands look more natural and may have individual finger movement and the ability to automatically modulate grip strength; however, myoelectric hands have some limitations with durability and water proofing. Body powered terminal devices may be activity-specific, allowing the person to hold fishing poles, knives, hammers, or other tools.

Orthotics

An orthotic is a device that is designed to support or correct the alignment of a limb or to restrict movement. Many orthotics are constructed by a medical professional, called an *orthotist*, using high-temperature plastics, carbon fiber, or other materials. An example of this is an ankle-foot orthosis (AFO). An AFO is used to provide support to the ankle and foot after a stroke or other neurological conditions or orthopedic conditions, such as fractures. The AFO is used when weakness in ankle and toe muscles prevents the foot from maintaining dorsiflexion during gait, a condition called *foot drop*. An AFO can be made with or without ankle motion and can also include the knee (knee-ankle-foot orthosis). Another example of an orthotic is a thoracolumbosacral orthosis (TLSO; sometimes called a *turtle shell*). A thoracolumbosacral orthosis is designed to restrict trunk movement following spinal cord and/or vertebral column damage. It has two pieces that are custom molded to fit the anterior and posterior portions of the client's trunk and is secured with straps.

In occupational therapy, an orthotic for the hand is frequently called a *splint*. Occupational therapy assistants may be responsible for constructing or modifying splints, as well as teaching clients to care for the splint and to incorporate it into occupational performance.

Splinting

The OTPF-4 categorizes splints as preparatory to occupational performance. Splints are often used to remediate a client factor, such as immobilization following tendonitis, and may also be used to facilitate function. Splints may aid functional mobility by enabling a person to do things such as transport items, grip a baby carriage handle, or propel a wheelchair. See Table 12-4 for a list of reasons an orthotic may be prescribed.

According to the American Society of Hand Therapists (1992), splints are categorized according to six different criteria. The first is whether the splint is articular or nonarticular. *Articular* refers to a splint that crosses at least one joint (as opposed to a nonarticular splint immobilizing a humeral fracture, for instance). Most splints that are dealt with in occupational therapy are articular, so typically that term is left out of the splint name. The second criterion is a description of the primary joint addressed by the splint. Third is direction, explaining the position of the primary joint affected (e.g., flexion, extension). Fourth is the main purpose of the splint (e.g., immobilization, mobilization). Fifth is the number of secondary joints included in the splint, and sixth is the total number of joints included in the splint (these numbers are not always included when referring to the splint). So, using this system, one might refer to a splint as a "thumb abduction immobilization splint" or a "volar wrist immobilization splint." However, splints have many additional, more common names used by occupational therapists and other health care providers. Some splints are labeled using descriptors that refer to the anatomy upon which the splint originates and primarily functions. Examples of this are hand-based, which means that the splint involves only the hand and most likely allows wrist ROM, or ulnar gutter, which means that the splint encompasses only the ulnar part of the hand. Table 12-5 provides a list of common static immobilization splints and their purposes.

Immobilization is one of the most common indications for a splint. A joint may need to be immobilized for many reasons, and this is generally accomplished by using a **static splint**. A static splint does not allow motion at the affected joint. A joint may need to be immobilized to rest an overused muscle, protect a wound or surgical incision, or maintain the alignment of an anatomical structure. Immobilization splints can hold a limb in a position that limits soft tissue shortening, thereby preventing contracture. A static immobilization splint may help to reduce pain and edema or to protect a hypersensitive limb. Perhaps one of the most important reasons for an immobilization splint is to position the hand in a way that enables occupational performance.

TABLE 12-4
Purposes of Orthotics

- Maintain or restore joint alignment
- Protect soft tissue
- Correct or prevent deformities
- Substitute for weak or absent muscles
- Provide rest or support
- Increase ROM
- Limit or block joint motion
- Increase function
- Provide resistance to strengthen muscles
- Modify abnormal muscle tone

Immobilization splints are sometimes used to reduce spasticity, although some studies have found there is not enough evidence to support or refute the effectiveness of splints after stroke (Lannin & Herbert, 2003). Another study found that clients poststroke who wore a volar wrist/hand immobilization splint for several hours per day for up to 3 months had less elbow spasticity and greater wrist passive ROM (Pizzi et al., 2005). A systematic review focused on adults with UE spasticity who received a stretching intervention (including immobilization splinting), found low strength of evidence regarding the effectiveness of static splinting to reduce spasticity. They also found moderate strength of evidence supporting the effect of static splinting on hand function (Kerr et al., 2020).

Mobilization splints have a movable element that applies some force to the affected structure. A **dynamic splint** is a mobilization splint. A dynamic splint typically has a static splint as the base, with outriggers, pulleys, and rubber bands to provide force. Splints may be used to increase passive ROM, substitute for weak or absent muscle motion, or provide resistance to a muscle motion for strengthening. Figure 12-8 shows a dynamic splint.

Splints are made from low-temperature plastic, which is heated in water until malleable enough to cut and form in the desired shape. There are many different types of splinting materials, so it is important to understand the characteristics of the material and match it to the type of splint being constructed as well as the experience of the therapist. Each material has a different feel and quality and there are a variety of brands available. Splint material may be purchased in variable thicknesses, but the most common thickness is 1/8 inch. Splint material also has options for perforations, color, design, and other unique features. Splint materials vary in heating time and working time. Heating time is the amount of time it takes for the material to become soft enough to work with. This is an important characteristic in a busy clinic where the occupational therapy assistant may not have time to wait for the material to soften. Working time is the amount of time before the material loses its malleability. Therapists who are new to splinting often

TABLE 12-5
Names and Purposes of Common Immobilization Splints

ASHT SPLINT NAME	COMMON NAMES	PRIMARY PURPOSES
Digit-Based Splints		
Distal interphalangeal (DIP) immobilization splint	DIP extension splint Gutter splint	Immobilize or rest DIP joint
Proximal interphalangeal (PIP) immobilization splint	PIP extension splint Gutter splint	Immobilize or rest PIP joint
Hand-Based Splints		
Thumb metacarpal (MP) immobilization splint	Short opponens splint Gamekeeper's thumb splint	Immobilize or rest thumb MP joint
Thumb carpometacarpal (CMC) immobilization splint	CMC palmar abduction splint Short thumb spica splint Short opponens splint	Immobilize or rest thumb CMC and MP joints
Forearm-Based Splints		
Volar wrist immobilization splint	Wrist cock-up splint Thumb hole wrist splint	Immobilize or rest wrist joint Improve grasp in the event of weak wrist extensors
Ulnar wrist immobilization splint	Ulnar gutter splint	Immobilize or rest wrist
Radial wrist/thumb immobilization splint	Radial gutter splint	Immobilize or rest wrist and thumb joint
Volar wrist/thumb immobilization splint	Thumb spica splint Long opponens splint	Immobilize or rest wrist and thumb joint
Volar wrist/hand immobilization splint	Resting hand splint Resting pan splint	Immobilize or rest wrist and hand (and thumb if desired) Reduce abnormal muscle tone Prevent joint contracture

Data source: Jacobs, M., & Austin, N. (2003). *Splinting the hand and upper extremity: Principles and process.* Lippincott Williams & Wilkins.
ASHT = American Society of Hand Therapists.

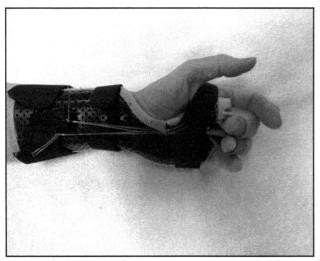

Figure 12-8. Dynamic splint with pulleys.

prefer a long working time, while experienced splinters only need a short working time. Some materials are strong and durable, which may be necessary for a client with spasticity who provides constant pressure against the material. Other materials are more flexible and lightweight, which may be good for a hand-based thumb immobilization splint that will be worn by a client all day during functional activities. Memory is the ability of the material to return to its original preheated size and shape; a great quality for new splinters who may need to start over frequently. Drapability means the material conforms to the underlying shape of the hand easily. Drapability is useful when making small, lightweight splints but may be less effective for a more durable splint like a volar wrist and hand immobilization splint. Elasticity of material allows for stretching to extend a portion of the splint and bonding and allows the splint material to adhere to itself. It is up to the occupational therapy assistant to determine what qualities are needed for any given splint and then carefully select the best material.

BOX 12-5

Collaboration between the client and the occupational therapy practitioner is an essential part of orthotics. Here are six essential characteristics to consider when providing an orthotic to a client:

1. Client centeredness: Address the client's occupational performance needs, personal needs, and goals.
2. Comfort: The orthotic should cause no pain.
3. Cosmesis: The orthotic should be aesthetically pleasing.
4. Convenience: The orthotic should fit into the client's lifestyle.
5. Less is more: Use of minimalism in orthotic design.
6. Follow-up: Identify reasons for nonuse of the orthotic.

(McKee & Rivard, 2004)

Splints are attached to the hand using hook and loop straps. An adhesive-backed hook strip is attached to the splint and loop strips wrap around the client's limb. Another option is to attach one end of the strap to the splint using a rivet and the other end using adhesive-backed hook. This ensures that the strap does not get lost. Wider straps help to distribute pressure, and foam straps provide comfort. Splints may also be padded for comfort, but this can prevent splints from being thoroughly cleaned and may limit airflow. Outrigger components for dynamic splints are commercially available. Prefabricated splints are also available for purchase. These splints are off the shelf and ordered in small, medium, and large.

Prepare the client for the splinting process by educating them about the splinting process and the purpose of the splint. It is important that clients know what to expect and clearly understand the reasons for wearing the splint (McKee & Rivard, 2004). Position the client comfortably by resting the arm and hand on a padded surface. In some cases, a second therapist may be needed to help to position the hand, wrist, or forearm during splinting; this is especially true in cases of severe spasticity. Remove any jewelry that may be affected by the splint. Apply a stockinet over the arm to provide a barrier between the splint material and the skin; this is especially important in when splinting older adults, as they have fragile skin. Plan ahead for the splinting process by gathering all materials prior to the client's arrival. Splinting may be broken into multiple sessions for pattern making, splint making, and education or training. Box 12-5 identifies six essential characteristics to consider when providing an orthotic to a client.

Knowledge of anatomy is essential to construct a splint. Splint material over a bony prominence (e.g., the radial and ulnar styloids), may cause a pressure point because bony prominences tend to have little soft tissue covering them. Splints should be contoured over pressure points rather than adding padding. Padding may actually increase the pressure because it is adding more material into an area that is already under pressure. Creases in the hand and wrist are used as guides to maintain full ROM of the joints outside of the splint edges. For example, a hand-based splint should not extend proximally up the arm past the wrist crease because this will limit wrist active ROM. The therapist should use the creases as landmarks when making a splint pattern. The natural arches of the hand are also used to ensure the splint is functional and does not inadvertently cause deformity. Splints should never position the hand so that it is flat. The three arches (longitudinal, proximal transverse, and distal transverse; see Chapter 10 for a full description) must be maintained within the design of the splint. The therapist should also know what muscles, nerves, and joints may be impacted by the splint. For example, a splint could prevent compression of the median nerve at the wrist, or the same splint could inadvertently cause pressure on the median nerve if made incorrectly. Nerve compression results in symptoms of numbness, pain, and tingling sensations, and may result in long-term damage.

Principles of Splinting

There are several mechanical principles that must be respected to create a splint that is safe and effective for the client. By their very nature, splints apply force. The force that the splint places on soft tissue and bony prominences should be dispersed as much as possible to prevent excessive pressure. Increasing the area of force serves to decrease the pressure on the client's limb. From a splint design standpoint, this means that a wide and long splint is generally preferred over one that is short and narrow (Fess et al., 2004). Functionally, this means that the length of the forearm trough should be two-thirds the length and half the width of the forearm. However, allow for optimum function by not immobilizing or restricting joints without reason. The splint should not extend past a joint if is not necessary to restrict that joint's motion. Construct the splint so that it fits as close as possible to the arm and hand in order to provide the largest surface area possible and, thereby, dispersing the force from any one area. Finally, it is better to have a splint that applies a small amount of force over a long period of time instead of one that a client can only tolerate for short periods because the force is too strong.

Splints are considered first class levers (see Figures 3-3 and 3-4). Most splints have three distinct points of pressure in which the middle force is directed in an opposite direction from the other two forces (Fess et al., 2004). For the best mechanical advantage, splints should have a long lever arm. Consider the weight of the hand to be a steady force on the surface of a volar wrist immobilization splint. If the forearm trough is too short, more pressure will occur at the end of the splint. If the forearm trough is lengthened (providing a longer lever arm), there will be less force at the end of the splint. This principle of increasing mechanical advantage also helps to direct the placement of the splint straps on the opposite side of the splint itself. The straps must be placed as far distally and proximally on the splint as possible in order to maintain the mechanical advantage of the lever.

Force is also a factor in mobilization splints with dynamic components. When attaching an outrigger to the splint, making it longer where it attaches will create less force and make it more likely to stay bonded to the splint. Use of an outrigger with digit pulleys adds a layer of complexity. The direction of the force must be perpendicular to avoid pushing or pulling (rotational) forces on the joint. Construction of dynamic splints may involve consideration of multiple rotational forces across multiple joints.

Clients must be trained to look for potential skin breakdown associated with their splint. After the splint is constructed, ask them to wait 30 minutes before leaving so that they can be monitored for pain, redness, swelling, numbness, skin indentations, or blue fingers. The client should be instructed to remove the splint and call the therapist if any of these signs are seen once they leave the clinic. Ensure the client has a number to reach a therapist at the clinic in the event of any problems. Education should be provided both orally and in written form. Teach the client the purpose of the splint, how to don and doff it, and the wearing schedule. Provide the client with a wearing schedule that tells them exactly when the splint should be worn, during which activities, and for how many hours. Some splints are considered nonfunctional and, as such, should be worn only at night or at rest, while other splints are designed to facilitate occupation performance and so should be worn during specific activities. Other splints may need to be worn at all times and only removed for cleaning. If the splint will be given to someone in a long-term care or assisted living facility, particularly if the client has cognitive or communication deficits, take extra care to ensure the splint is labeled with the client's name, and whether it should be on the right or left hand. Provide the client and staff with pictures illustrating how the splint should look when it is applied correctly. Teach clients and staff how to clean the splint. Splints may be washed in cold or lukewarm water or wiped with rubbing alcohol if the splint is not padded. Splints should not be washed in hot water, put through the dishwasher, or left in a hot car, which may cause them to lose their shape.

Wheeled Mobility

The OTPF-4 defines wheeled mobility as the use of "products and technologies that facilitate a client's ability to maneuver through space, including seating and positioning; improve mobility to enhance participation in desired daily occupations; and reduce risk for complications such as skin breakdown or limb contractures" (AOTA, 2020, p. 60). The occupational therapy assistant needs to understand how wheeled mobility may be used for occupational performance and must have the ability to train clients to use the wheelchair in different environments and situations. The occupational therapy assistant should also have a firm knowledge of proper wheelchair fit, pressure relief techniques, and concepts of correct and safe positioning with the goals of preventing skin breakdown and improving functional mobility.

There are two primary types of wheelchairs: manual and power. A manual wheelchair is physically propelled by the individual, typically by using both UEs. Manual wheelchairs may also be propelled by the individual using one or both feet, one arm in a modified manual wheelchair, or pushed by a caregiver. To manually propel with both arms, the client first uses shoulder extension, elbow flexion, wrist extension, and finger flexion to reach back and grip the hand rims. Pushing the wheel forward requires primarily shoulder flexion with some shoulder internal rotation and adduction. Shoulder pain and injury are well-documented results of the repetitive movement patterns required to manually propel a wheelchair, along with frequent shoulder use during transfers (Jain et al., 2010; Samuelsson et al., 2004).

A standard wheelchair is typically 16 or 18 inches wide with a nonadjustable backrest, detachable or fixed arm rests, and fixed or movable leg rests. It is a heavy chair weighing approximately 36 pounds and is not particularly customizable. The frame may be foldable or rigid. The standard chair is typically used for someone who will only use the wheelchair for short periods. A hemi chair is a standard wheelchair that is lower to the ground so the user can propel using one or both feet. Ultralightweight chairs generally weigh less than 30 pounds. The lighter weight means there is less resistance when rolling. These chairs often have low profile backrests, removable or no arm rests, and a fixed footplate; these specifications make transferring quicker and easier. Ultralightweight chairs are fully customizable for the client's needs and are good for long-term manual wheelchair users. Reclining wheelchairs have a manual or power recline feature that changes the angle of the backrest. Tilt-in-space wheelchairs tip backward while keeping the 90-degree seat-to-back angle. Recline and tilt are both useful for providing pressure relief; some wheelchairs have both options. Figures 12-9 through 12-11 show an ultralightweight wheelchair, a manual chair with head support, and a wheelchair with tilt-in-space.

A power wheelchair is used by someone who is unable to manually propel or who can only manually propel for short distances. Power chairs are controlled by the individual

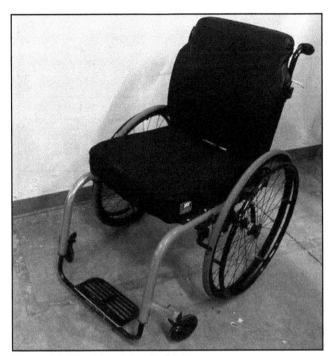

Figure 12-9. Ultralightweight wheelchair.

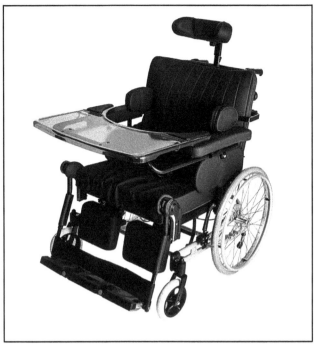

Figure 12-10. Manual wheelchair with head support and lap tray. (Risal Khan/shutterstock.com)

using a controller. There are many different controllers available depending on the client's available active movement. Power chairs can be driven by a hand operated joystick or a switch that is accessed by movements like shoulder elevation or a head turn. Power chairs can also be driven with breath control via a sip-and-puff mechanism.

When determining the appropriate wheelchair for a client, many factors must be considered. Manual wheelchairs are lighter weight and may be transported in a regular automobile. They are less expensive than electric chairs and are simpler to fix and maintain. Manual chairs are likely to fit through standard door frames and are often a good height for independent transfers. Using a manual chair provides the client with a level of physical fitness; although, over time this can lead to overuse syndromes of the shoulder and wrist that may ultimately require surgery and limit independence (Samuelsson et al., 2004). Users may also find it difficult to manually propel the wheelchair over long distances, uneven terrain, and hills. Power chairs, on the other hand, are heavy, expensive, and require a modified van for transportation. The seat height of the power chair may be higher than many other transfer surfaces, such as a bed or toilet, and the overall footprint of the chair may be too large for some doorways, sharp turns, and elevators. The length of battery charge may dictate participation in some occupations. Repairs may be expensive, and batteries need to be replaced. But the benefits may far outweigh these negatives. If a client is unable to manually propel, a power chair provides the greatest range of mobility with the least amount of muscle use. Power chairs may also allow for independence in pressure relief, with power tilt, power recline, or both.

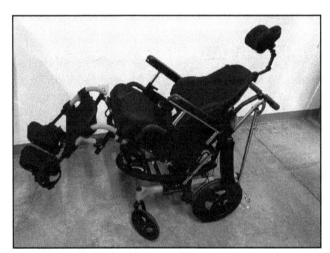

Figure 12-11. Child's wheelchair with tilt-in-space.

Wheelchair fit is an essential part of wheeled mobility. Poorly fit wheelchairs will lead to pain and injury, so clients must be carefully matched with their wheelchair (Vegter et al., 2010). The width of the wheelchair influences the person's ability to reach the hand rims. Generally, the frame should be snug to the body to help the shoulders align over the hand rim to improve propulsion. The seat height should allow the user to reach the back of the wheel for propulsion. The depth of the seat should allow 2 to 3 inches of clearance between the back of the knee and the seat. Seat angle may also be adjusted from a standard 90-degree hip angle. Hip flexion of less than 90 degrees can help a client with poor or absent abdominal muscles to be more stable in the chair and propel more easily. The backrest should be low enough that it does not interfere with arm movement during propulsion or

TABLE 12-6
Potential Problems Resulting From Poor Wheelchair Fit

WHEELCHAIR FEATURE	POTENTIAL PROBLEM
Seat width (hips should not come into contact with wheels or arm rests)	• Seat too wide: Difficulty with wheelchair propulsion, limited access through doorways • Seat too narrow: Skin breakdown over greater trochanters
Seat depth (there should be 1 to 2 inches from the back of the knee to the edge of the seat)	• Seat too long: Impaired circulation below knees • Seat too short: Increased pressure on back of thighs could result in pressure injury
Seat height (measure with cushion in place)	• Seat too low: Footrests scrape ground • Seat too high: Elevated COG increases risk for tipping chair, chair may not fit into van, transfers more difficult
Backrest height (measure with cushion in place)	• Backrest too high: Impedes shoulder motion for propulsion • Backrest too low: Poor trunk support

Adapted from Somers, M. F. (2010). *Spinal cord injury: Functional rehabilitation* (3rd ed.). Pearson.

high enough to provide trunk support for those who will not manually propel the chair. In some cases, lateral supports, head rests, and elevating leg rests will need to be included. Other measurements that should be taken include arm rest height and leg rest length. Wheelchair measurement guides should be used to ensure correct fit. The client should be measured when seated in a standard height chair with hips, knees, and ankles at 90 degrees, if possible. Table 12-6 shows potential problems resulting from poor wheelchair fit.

Seat cushions are an essential part of the wheelchair. The human body is not designed to sit for long periods of time. Many individuals who use a wheelchair have decreased sensation in their lower body and may not sense when they need to shift or change position. This can cause skin breakdown if not addressed through a good seat cushion. Wheelchair cushions help with comfort, stability, and pressure management, and may also improve the position of the client in the chair. Foam cushions are the cheapest and most basic form of cushion. Foam cushions may not provide much in the way of positioning, but generally provide a comfortable seat with some pressure relief. Gel cushions consist of a gel pack on a stable contoured base, which may aid in positioning. Gel cushions are designed to distribute the pressure, so they are a good option for long-term wheelchair use. Air cushions have air-filled chambers that may be adjusted for firmness and positioning. Air cushions are lighter weight than gel cushions and are good for users with limited upper body strength. Some cushions provide combinations of foam, gel, and air. Cushion covers should be used in case of incontinence. Cushions should be considered when ordering a wheelchair because the height of the cushion will impact the overall height of the wheelchair as well as other measurements like back height and leg rest length. Pressure mapping may be used to determine pressure distribution of a given

cushion. The client is seated on a sensor pad that relays a map of pressure points displayed in colors and numbers to the computer screen. This is a useful tool to determine if the client's cushion is suitable for their needs.

Pressure Relief

Even if a client has an excellent cushion, pressure relief must be performed at minimum every 15 to 20 minutes in sitting or every 2 hours when lying down to prevent skin breakdown (Sprigle & Sonenblum, 2011). Pressure injuries can occur with high loads for short periods and low loads for long periods (Sprigle & Sonenblum, 2011). Pressure relief in the form of weight shifting restores blood flow to areas of skin that have been bearing weight. This is especially important over bony prominences, such as the ischial tuberosities. There are many ways to relieve pressure when sitting in a wheelchair. Wheelchair push-ups are effective for those with triceps and shoulder depression strong enough to lift their own body weight. The person uses their arms to push off the arm rests and raise their buttocks off the cushion. Another option is a lateral lean to shift weight off of one side of the buttocks, leaning to each side for at least 1 minute. For stability in those with limited trunk control, it may help to hook the arm on the unweighted side over the push handle. The forward lean involves laying the trunk forward over the thighs and reaching hands to the floor. This method removes weight from the back of the buttocks; some individuals may need to hook one arm over the push handle for stability. Finally, tilt-in-space and reclining wheelchairs may be used to shift weight. When a client first begins to use a wheelchair, it is important to teach them a regular schedule for performing pressure relief. Weight shifts should be performed every 15 to 20 minutes for at least 1 minute, using one or more techniques. Using a timer will help to establish a routine. Pressure relief should also be performed in bed by shifting position every 2 hours and using pillows to prevent bony prominences, like ankle bones, from touching. Skin should be examined daily for areas of redness or skin breakdown.

Wheelchair Skills for Occupational Performance

Clients must first be taught how to prepare a wheelchair for a transfer, which is considered part of independence in transferring to and from a wheelchair. Therapists must educate clients about each step, including locking the brakes, removing leg and arm rests as appropriate, and positioning the wheelchair correctly.

Always lock the brakes before transferring into or out of a wheelchair. Some clients with decreased UE strength may benefit from extended brake handles to increase the lever arm and make it easier to lock and unlock. This adaptation is also useful for people with unilateral weakness or a missing UE, allowing them to reach across their body to lock and unlock the brake.

Leg rests should be lowered, and the footrests should be folded. Swing the leg rests to the side and remove entirely for the greatest clearance space in preparation for the transfer. If the leg rests are fixed and cannot be moved, the client should scoot forward and place their feet on the floor in front of the leg rests, or, if it is a dependent transfer, they may leave their feet on the leg rests. It may also help the wheelchair to be more stable if the front casters are pointed forward.

Some wheelchairs have removable arm rests. Removing the arm rest on the side the client is transferring toward is useful during a moderate or maximum assist transfer, and essential when using a transfer board. For clients who are performing a minimum assist or independent stand pivot transfer, leaving the arm rest in place may be more beneficial so they can use it as leverage to push themselves into a standing position.

Wheelchair users must master a variety of skills. Those using a manual chair should know how to propel forward and backward, turn, ascend and descend an incline, perform a wheelie, and ascend and descend a curb. Some may need to be able to move from the floor to the wheelchair in the event of a fall. For occupational performance, wheelchair users should practice opening and going through doors, reaching for items from the floor and high surfaces, and carrying items. For manual wheelchair users who plan on independent driving, it may be important to be able to fold the wheelchair, remove the wheels, and lift the frame into a car. Figure 12-12 shows a wheelchair and cushion ready for transport. Power chair users should also know how to turn the power on and off, move the controller, select speed, stop, and operate the battery charger. Good cognitive and safety skills are needed for power chair users.

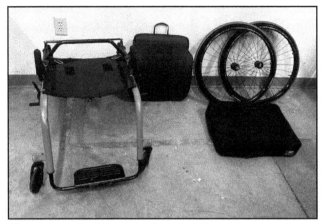
Figure 12-12. Wheelchair and cushion ready for transport.

Community wheelchair use presents many challenges for the individual. Curbs, ramps, hills, stairs, elevators, uneven terrain, and poor accessibility all pose potential tests for the wheelchair user to master. Even in homes, tight corners can be difficult to turn, and bathrooms may be too small to position the wheelchair for a safe transfer. The occupational therapy assistant should be aware of training and equipment that will help the client handle issues such as these. For example, teaching a client in a manual chair to perform a wheelie is necessary to ascend a curb, as well as a step, speed bump, or even some high-profile doorway transitions. Grade Aid (Motion Composites) is a device that will keep the wheelchair from sliding backward on hills, allowing the client to rest without losing ground up a hill. Extended brake handles provide leverage to engage wheelchair brakes for those with muscle weakness; they also provide enough length for someone with only one functioning arm to reach the brake on their impaired side. Very active wheelchair users may prefer scissor brakes, which are found underneath the chair and do not interfere with transfers. Quick-release wheels are useful to disassemble the chair for transportation. Power assist is a battery-powered device for a manual wheelchair that provides extra propulsion, so the client uses less muscle power. Power assist has been shown to significantly decrease shoulder flexion, internal rotation, and adduction motions needed for propulsion, as well as to decrease the forces on the shoulder (Kloosterman et al., 2012). Camber means the top of the wheels are angled in toward the body, and the bottom of the wheels are angled away from the body. Camber creates more stability and allows tighter turns, so it is a good option for sports and athletics. One drawback is the wider wheelbase means the chair may not fit through standard doorways. The occupational therapy assistant should provide a variety of different functional scenarios for the client to practice, such as accessing a public restroom or baking cookies in the kitchen. Grade the tasks to begin with basic wheelchair skills to more advanced, with opportunities for the client to problem solve.

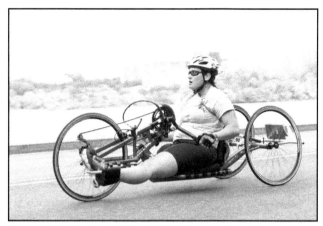

Figure 12-13. Hand cycle. (Rena Schild/shutterstock.com)

Driving

Driving is often an essential means of accessing the community, especially for people with limited functional mobility. Physical deficits such as decreased strength, decreased ROM, and abnormal muscle tone may impede the ability to drive. A variety of diagnoses may require driving accommodations. SCI, including both paraplegia and quadriplegia, CP, and amputation, are just some diagnoses that may benefit from driving accommodations and training.

People who use wheelchairs have specific needs related to driving and riding in vehicles and may require a custom car or van or a wheelchair lift to accommodate their needs. There are two types of wheelchair lifts. One kind lifts the driver and mobility aid together, and the other just lifts the mobility aid to store it during trips. A person who uses a manual wheelchair may be able to transfer from the wheelchair to the driver's seat, dismantle their wheelchair, place it in the seat next to them, and then drive using hand controls; or, they may use a power transfer seat, which is a car seat that electronically moves out of the vehicle to enable the driver to transfer from the wheelchair. The seat then returns into the position for driving. An option for both manual and power chair users is to use a van that has been specially modified with ramp and has the driver's seat removed. The person propels their wheelchair up the ramp and up to the steering wheel where they lock their wheelchair into place to drive.

Adaptations are also available for controlling the vehicle. For people with SCI or LE amputation, hand controls are used to operate the brakes and the accelerator with a single lever. Hand controls also allow the user to operate the headlights, turn signals, windshield wipers, and horn from the same central place and at the same time as the brakes and accelerator. Cars may also be controlled from a joystick or infrared control panel. Pedal extensions may be appropriate for clients with dwarfism or amputation and are inexpensive and easily installed. Steering wheel adaptations include smaller circumference, a steering knob for one hand use, and wrist support. The occupational therapy assistant may be involved in training an individual to use adapted driving equipment.

Adaptive Mobility for Leisure

Regaining leisure skills may be an important goal for many individuals who rely on wheeled mobility. Some people may require activity-specific wheelchairs. Individuals may have chairs specifically designed to engage in sports such as tennis, basketball, and wheelchair rugby. Hand-crank bicycles allow wheelchair users to power the bike by hand, while tricycles allow people with balance limitations to cycle. Figure 12-13 shows a hand cycle. There are also side-by-side and tandem bike options for people with mobility or visual deficits. Four-track skiing uses two skis with two outriggers for four points of control; it is ideal for people with balance deficits. Mono-skis with outriggers are another option. To access the wilderness, personal recreation vehicles, snow mobiles, and even horses are options for people with deficits in functional mobility. There are many resources available for people to participate in sports and leisure activities via wheeled mobility or other adaptations; the occupational therapy assistant should be aware of local resources for their clients.

Summary

This chapter explored how different aspects of movement contribute to functional mobility in the home and community. Functional mobility, which includes basic motions such as bed mobility, transfers, and ambulation, enables independence in valued occupations, such as propelling a wheelchair and driving a car. Functional mobility begins with an understanding of typical movement, which is impacted by client factors, motor skills, activity, occupation, and space demands, as well as the physical environment. Proper body mechanics during movement require an understanding of motion in a variety of conditions to reduce the risk of injury. Adaptive mobility, prosthetics, and orthotics are all ways to modify factors to improve safe movement and functional mobility. Occupational therapy practitioners need to incorporate client goals and interests to facilitate optimal functional mobility.

References

Alexander, N.B., Grunawalt, J. C., Carlos, S., & Augustine, J. (2000). Bed mobility task performance in older adults. *Journal of Rehabilitation Research & Development, 37*(5), 633-638.

American Occupational Therapy Association. (2020). Occupational therapy practice framework: Domain and process (4th ed.). *American Journal of Occupational Therapy, 74*(Suppl. 2), Article 7412410010. https://doi.org/10.5014/ajot.2020.74S2001

American Society of Hand Therapists. (1992). *Splint classification system*. Author.

Americans with Disabilities Act of 1990, 42 U.S.C. § 12101 *et seq.* (1990). https://www.ada.gov/pubs/adastatute08.htm

Andersen, L. L., Burdorf, A., Fallentin, N., Persson, R., Jakobsen, M.D., Mortensen, O.S, Clausen, T., & Holtermann, A. (2014). Patient transfers and assistive devices: Prospective cohort study on the risk for occupational back injury among healthcare workers. *Scandinavian Journal of Work, Environment, and Health, 40*(1), 74-81.

Biddiss, E. A., & Chau, T. T. (2007). Upper limb prosthesis use and abandonment: A survey of the last 25 years. *Prosthetics and Orthotics International, 31*, 236-257.

Carswell, A., McColl, M. A., Baptiste, S., Law, M., Polatajko, H., & Pollock, N. (2004). The Canadian Occupational Performance Measure: A research and clinical literature review. *Canadian Journal of Occupational Therapy, 71*(4), 210-222.

Darragh, A. R., Huddleston, W., & King, P. (2009). Work-related musculoskeletal injuries and disorders among occupational and physical therapists. *American Journal of Occupational Therapy, 63*, 351-362.

Fess, E. E., Gettle, K. S., Philips, C. A., & Janson, J. R. (2004). *Hand and upper extremity splinting: Principles and methods* (3rd ed.). Elsevier-Mosby.

Fisher, A. G., & Marterella, A. (2019) *Powerful practice: A model for authentic occupational therapy.* Center for Innovative OT Solutions.

Individuals with Disabilities Education Improvement Act of 2004, Pub L No. 108–446, 118 Stat 2647 (2004).

Jacobs, M., & Austin, N. (2003). *Splinting the hand and upper extremity: Principles and process.* Lippincott Williams & Wilkins.

Jain, N. B., Higgins, L. D., Katz, J. N., & Garshick, E. (2010). Association of shoulder pain with the use of mobility devices in persons with chronic spinal cord injury. *Physical Medicine and Rehabilitation, 2*(10), 896-900.

Janssen, W. G., Bussmann, H. B., & Stam, H. J. (2002). Determinants of the sit-to-stand movement: A review. *Physical Therapy, 82*(9), 866-879.

Johansson, C., & Chinworth, S. A. (2012). *Mobility in context: Principles of patient care skills.* F. A. Davis Company.

Keir, P. J., & MacDonell, C. W. (2004). Muscle activity during patient transfers: A preliminary study on the influence of lift assists and experience. *Ergonomics, 47*(3), 296-306.

Kerr, L., Jewell, V. D., & Jensen, L. (2020). Stretching and splinting interventions for poststroke spasticity, hand function, and functional tasks: A systematic review. *American Journal of Occupational Therapy, 74*, 7405205050. https://doi.org/10.5014/ajot.2020.029454

Kloosterman, M. G., Eising, H., Schaake, L., Buurke, J. H., & Rietman, J. S. (2012). Comparison of shoulderload during power-assisted and purely hand-rim wheelchair *propulsion. Clinical Biomechanics, 27*(5), 428-435.

Kraskowsky, L. H., & Finlayson, M. (2001). Factors affecting older adults' use of adaptive equipment: Review of the literature. *American Journal of Occupational Therapy, 55*, 303-310.

Lannin, N. A., & Herbert, R. D. (2003). Is hand splinting effective for adults following stroke? A systematic review and methodological critique of published research. *Clinical Rehabilitation, 17*(8), 807-816.

Law, S., Baptiste, S., Carswell, A., McColl, M. A., Polatajko, H., & Pollock, N. (2000). *Canadian Occupational Performance Measure.* Canadian Association of Occupational Therapists Publications ACE.

McKee, P., & Rivard, A. (2004). Orthoses as enablers of occupation: Client-centered splinting for better outcomes. *Canadian Journal of Occupational Therapy, 71*(5), 306-314.

Merriam-Webster. (n.d.). *Merriam-Webster.com dictionary.* http://www.merriam-webster.com/dictionary

Middlesworth, M. (2012). Step by step guide to the NIOSH lifting equation. *Ergonomics Plus.* http://ergo-plus.com/niosh-lifting-equation-single-task/

Pizzi, A., Carlucci, G., Falsini, C., Verdesca, S., & Grippo, A. (2005). Application of a volar static splint in poststroke spasticity of the upper limb. *Archives of Physical Medicine and Rehabilitation, 86*(9), 1855-1859.

Resnik, L., Meucci, M. R., Lieberman-Klinger, S., Fantini, C., Kelty, D. L., Disla, R., & Sasson, N. (2012). Advanced upper limb prosthetic devices: Implications for upper limb prosthetic rehabilitation. *Archives of Physical Medicine and Rehabilitation, 93*(4), 710-717.

Roebroeck, M. E., Doorenbosch, C. A., Harlaar, J., & Lankhorst, G. L. (1994). Biomechanics and muscular activity during sit-to-stand transfer. *Clinical Biomechanics, 9*, 235-244.

Samuelsson, K. A. M., Tropp, H., & Gerdle, B. (2004). Shoulder pain and its consequences in paraplegic spinal cord–injured, wheelchair users. *Spinal Cord, 42*(1), 41-46.

Schmidt, R. A. (1975). A schema theory of discrete motor skill learning. *Psychological Bulletin, 82*, 225-260.

Somers, M. F. (2010). *Spinal cord injury: Functional rehabilitation* (3rd ed.). Pearson Education.

Sprigle, S., & Sonenblum, S. (2011). Assessing evidence supporting redistribution of pressure for pressure ulcer prevention: A review. *Journal of Rehabilitation Research and Development, 48*(3), 203-214.

Stubblefield, K. A., Miller, L. A., Lipschutz, R. D., & Kuiken, T. A. (2009). Occupational therapy protocol for amputees with targeted muscle reinnervation. *Journal of Rehabilitation Research and Development, 46*(4), 481-488.

Vegter, R. J., De Groot, S., Hettinga, S. F. J., Veeger, D. H., & Van Der Woude, L. H. V. (2010). Wheelchair design of a manually propelled wheelchair: Optimizing a wheelchair-user combination). In J. H. Stone & M. Blouin (Eds.), *International encyclopedia of rehabilitation.* Center for International Rehabilitation Research Information & Exchange.

Wielandt, T., & Strong, J. (2000). Compliance with prescribed adaptive equipment: A literature review. *British Journal of Occupational Therapy, 63*(2), 65-75.

Wilke, H., Neef, P., Caimi, M., Hoogland, T., & Claes, L. E. (1999). New in vivo measurements of pressures in the intervertebral disc in daily life. *Spine, 24*(8), 755-762.

World Health Organization. (2001). *International classification of functioning, disability, and health.* Author.

Applications

The following activities will help you apply knowledge of functional mobility in the home and community and adaptive mobility. Activities can be completed individually or in small groups to enhance learning.

1. **Bed Mobility**: Watch a partner perform each of the following skills:
   a. Bridging
   b. Rolling
   c. Moving from supine to sit
   d. Moving from side-lying to sit

   Analyze what joint motions are required for each skill, considering trunk flexion and extension, hip flexion and extension, knee flexion and extension, ankle flexion and extension, arm and hand movements, and head and neck movements.

2. **Transfers**: With a partner, practice each type of transfer from one chair to another chair of equal height. Do each transfer first with minimum assistance and then with maximum assistance. Then do the same with transfer surfaces of different heights (e.g., a hospital bed to wheelchair). How do the transfers change when one surface is higher than the other?
   a. Stand pivot (with and without a mobility device)
   b. Squat pivot
   c. Transfer board

3. **Wheelchairs**: This activity will require access to several different wheelchairs.
   a. Wheelchair parts: Interact with as many wheelchairs as you can, performing each of the following actions on a different wheelchair (note that not every wheelchair has each of these features):
      i. Take the arm rests off and put them back on
      ii. Take the leg rests off and put them back on
      iii. Set the brakes
      iv. Recline the chair
      v. Elevate the leg rests
      vi. Remove the wheels (requires quick-release wheels)
      vii. Fold the chair
   b. Sit in each of the wheelchairs. Which wheelchair fits you best? Why? Locate a chair that does not fit you well. Identify the problems that may result if you stayed in this ill-fitting wheelchair all day.
   c. With a partner spotting you for safety, perform a wheelie (pop the front casters off the ground). How does this movement affect your COG? How do you compensate? What if you could not use your abdominal muscles or your legs as a counterbalance?
   d. Download a wheelchair measurement form. Sit on a chair or mat while a partner measures you for a wheelchair and completes the measurement form.
   e. Download a wheelchair order form. Consider what components you would order based on each of the cases below:
      i. Jane has a T3 SCI. She is a 43-year-old student at a university. She needs a wheelchair that she can load and unload into her car independently and that she can use to propel herself to all of her classes across campus independently.
      ii. Lee is a 74-year-old man who had a left cerebrovascular accident. He is able to propel his wheelchair independently using his right foot and hand. His sitting balance is fair. He tends to have edema in his left foot. He will primarily use his wheelchair in his home and in community settings such as church and the senior center. His wife helps him transfer, and she loads and unloads his wheelchair into the trunk of their car.
   f. Spend a full day using a wheelchair.

4. **Body Mechanics**: With a partner, practice each of the following activities with one person performing the skills and the other analyzing the body mechanics. Give feedback to improve body mechanics.

    a. Lifting: Using an empty crate, practice each type of lift from the floor to waist height. For each lift, discuss when it would be appropriate to use.

        i. Diagonal lift

        ii. Tripod lift

        iii. Golfer's lift

    b. Now, slowly add weight to the crate in 5- or 10-pound increments. Do not add more than you can safely lift. How do your body mechanics change? Consider the four arches in the spine. Which type of lift is most effective for increased weight?

    c. Practice the lift floor-to-waist heights using an object with an unstable load, like a large bag of dog food. How do your body mechanics change? Consider the four arches in the spine. Which type of lift is most effective for increased weight?

    d. Once you have mastered the different types of lifting, practice lifting an empty crate from floor to overhead. How do your body mechanics change as you lift to different heights? Slowly add weight. How do your body mechanics change as you lift heavier weights?

    e. Carrying: Carry an empty crate loaded with weights across the room with your partner observing. Slowly add weight until you are carrying a maximum load. How do your body mechanics change with heavier weights?

    f. Practice the following chores while maintaining proper body mechanics:

        i. Access oven

        ii. Wash dishes

        iii. Access bottom shelf in cabinet

        iv. Sweep

        v. Load and unload washing machine or dryer

What are specific techniques that could improve body mechanics during these tasks? Consider counter height, twisting motions, and bending. How could you change the tools or the task to improve body mechanics?

    g. Practice the following ADLs while maintaining proper body mechanics:

        i. Donning and doffing shoes

        ii. Donning and doffing pants

What are specific techniques that could improve body mechanics during these tasks? Consider adaptive equipment that could improve body mechanics.

5. **Splints**: This activity will require access to a lab with splint pans and splinting equipment.

    a. Gather a variety of types of splint material. Look for varying thickness, color, with and without perforation, and brands. Heat a small piece of each in a splint pan and evaluate each the following properties:

        i. Heating time

        ii. Working time

        iii. Flexibility

        iv. Memory

        v. Drape

        vi. Elasticity

        vii. Bonding

Compare the splint material to the splints listed in Table 12-5. Which material would be best suited for each splint? Why?

b. This activity will help you learn the landmarks needed during splint construction. Trace a partner's hand and forearm on a piece of paper or paper towel. Trace around each finger and the thumb. Before your partner lifts their hand, make a mark at each of the following landmarks:

   i. Radial styloid

   ii. Ulnar styloid

   iii. Distal wrist crease

   iv. CMC joint

   v. MP joint of the first finger (thumb)

   vi. Interphalangeal joint of the first finger (thumb)

   vii. MP joint of the second and fifth fingers (index and small fingers)

   viii. PIP joint of the second and fifth fingers (index and small fingers)

   ix. DIP joint of the second and fifth fingers (index and small fingers)

   x. Center of the web space

Why are these landmarks necessary for splinting? Compare these landmarks to the splints in Table 12-5. Which landmarks would you need to mark for each type of splint? What other measurements would you need to make?

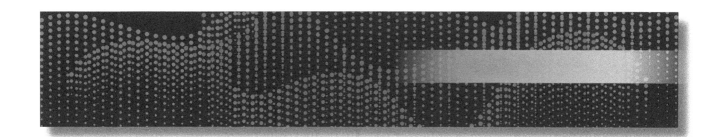

Glossary

A

abnormal atypical movement: Movement characterized by the inability to produce the desired movement strategy necessary to complete an activity within generally accepted parameters.

abnormal end feel: The feel experienced when the typical quality of feel is different.

acceleration: "The rate in change of velocity with respect to time" (Merriam-Webster, n.d.).

accessibility: "…removing barriers that prevent people with activity limitations from the use of services, products, and information" (Cronin & Mandich, 2005, p. 351).

accessory motion: Increases the pain-free movement available at a given joint. Accessory movements cannot be performed voluntarily. They occur between the articular surfaces of a joint in conjunction with voluntary movement. There are three types of accessory motions: roll, spin, and glide.

active assist range of motion (AAROM): Identifies that manual assistance is needed for the client to move the joint, but the client also activates some joint motion.

active insufficiency: Occurs when a muscle cannot shorten or contract any further and fails to shorten to the extent required for simultaneous full range of motion at all joints crossed.

active range of motion (AROM): Describes the joint movements as the client alone moves a joint through the available range of motion.

activities of daily living (ADLs): "Activities that are oriented toward taking care of one's own body (adapted from Rogers & Holm, 1994) and are completed on a daily basis.…These activities are 'fundamental to living in a social world, they enable basic survival and well-being'" (Christiansen & Hammecker, 2001, p. 156; see Table 2)" (American Occupational Therapy Association [AOTA], 2020).

activities: "Actions designed and selected to support the development of performance skills and performance patterns to enhance occupational engagement" (AOTA, 2020).

activity limitation: Level of dysfunction identified by the *International Classification of Functioning, Disability and Health*, including those that occur at the individual level (World Health Organization [WHO], 2001).

adaptive motor behaviors: Certain ways the body acts in a situation (Horak, 1987). Appropriate and efficient movement strategies used by the body (Horak, 1987). The body's ability to apply normal movement strategies to achieve functional goals (Landel & Fisher, 1993).

afferent neurons: Sensory neurons are afferent, or ascending to the central nervous system, and send sensory information to the cortex for interpretation. Afferent neurons are located dorsally; also referred to as *sensory neurons* (Solomon, 2009).

agonist: A muscle that is the prime mover.

ambulation: The process of moving from place to place by walking.

Sain, S. J., & Roller, C. L. *Kinesiology for the Occupational Therapy Assistant: Essential Components of Function and Movement, Third Edition* (pp. 313-325).

amphiarthrodial articulations: Allow for limited movement, as in the pubic symphysis. Sometimes called *cartilaginous joints*.

anatomical position: Reference position in which the subject is standing in an upright posture, eyes looking forward, feet parallel with toes pointed forward and the arms slightly abducted at the side of the body, and the palms facing forward (Solomon, 2009).

anatomical snuff box: A small depression formed where the thumb joins the wrist. The depression is formed when the abductor pollicis brevis, extensor pollicis longus, and extensor pollicis brevis tendons contract.

antagonists: Muscles that work against each other to equal or cancel out the movement and, therefore, gain stability.

anterior pelvic tilt: Characterized as the pelvis dipping forward. The anterior superior iliac spine landmarks move forward of the pubic symphysis.

anticipatory postural movements: "Reflect movements of the trunk or posture in response to changes in task or environmental demands" (Shumway-Cook & Woollacott, 2001).

appendicular skeleton: Composed of the shoulder girdle, pelvic girdle, upper extremities, and lower extremities.

areas of occupation: Areas of occupation include activities of daily living, instrumental activities of daily living, health management, rest and sleep, education, work, play, leisure, and social participation (AOTA, 2020). Areas of occupation include those individual daily activities that have meaning and purpose in our lives.

arthrokinematic: A movement that occurs between joint surfaces and consists of three different patterns: roll, glide, and spin.

arthroplasty: In Chapter 10, it refers to a wrist scope where the surgeon makes portal incisions and looks at the wrist joint structures with a tiny camera.

articulations: Connect bones. More commonly known as *joints*.

assistive technology: Compensatory techniques and devices used to provide increased independence when the remediation of deficits is not possible.

atlas: The first cervical vertebra; commonly called *C1* (Luijkx et al., 2014).

atrophy: Wasting of tissue, especially muscle, due to lack of use.

attrition rupture: Tendon rupture caused by movement across a roughened bone.

autonomic: The autonomic division is part of the peripheral nervous system and helps maintain an internal balance as it responds to internal stimuli, providing functions such as maintaining body temperature, regulating heart rate, and regulating blood pressure (Solomon, 2009).

avascular necrosis: Death of bone tissue due to lack of blood supply.

avulsion fracture: An injury to the bone at the attachment when the ligament or tendon tear and pull off a piece of the bone.

axial skeleton: Composed of the skull and trunk.

axis: The center or point around which the object rotates.

B

backward pelvic rotation: When the anterior superior iliac spine moves backward relative to the contralateral side

balance: The ability to maintain a center of gravity within a base of support; that is the ability not to fall.

ball-and-socket joint: Triaxial, able to move in all three planes including flexion and extension, abduction and adduction, horizontal abduction and horizontal adduction, internal and external rotation, and circumduction; consists of spherical head on one bone that fits into cup- or saucer-like cavity on adjoining bone; an example is the hip joint (Luttgens & Wells, 1982).

base of support (BOS): "The area beneath an object or person that includes every point of contact that the object or person makes with the supporting surface. These points of contact may be body parts (e.g., feet or hands) or they may include things like crutches or the chair a person is sitting in" (Physiopedia, 2023).

beliefs: A person's basic truth that remains, regardless of what another person might say, think, or believe.

biomechanical model: A restorative approach that attempts to isolate and remediate impairments in body structure and function with the end result of improving occupational performance (James, 2003).

body functions: Focus on the physiological functions of body systems, such as sensory, neuromuscular, psychological, respiratory, and cardiovascular.

body mechanics: An understanding of how the body moves in safe and efficient ways throughout any task in order to reduce risk of injury.

body structures: Anatomy and specific body parts, such as organs, skin, muscles, bones, and limbs.

brachial plexus: Relating to the arm, usually indicates nerve roots C5-T1.

bridging: A technique used in therapy to help a person reposition themselves in bed.

boutonniere deformity: Describes a finger with a flexed proximal interphalangeal joint and a hyperextended distal interphalangeal joint.

buoyancy: A phenomenon of water defined as an upward force equal to the weight of the displaced liquid.

C

carpal tunnel syndrome (CTS): A compression of the median nerve at the level of the wrist. It can lead to sensory loss and motor weakness of the intrinsic muscles of the hand and, consequently, in a loss of hand function.

carrying angle: Of the elbow, is described as the angle formed by the long axis of the humerus and forearm.

center of gravity (COG): Refers to the balance point of an object where all sides are equal (Lippert, 2006).

central nervous system (CNS): The CNS is commonly defined as the brain and spinal cord. The CNS ends at the point where nerve fibers exit the spinal cord. Motor neurons in the CNS are referred to as *upper motor neurons.*

cervical rotation: Turning the head to the left or the right (Jung et al., 2023).

circumduction: Defined in this context as when the leg advances in a circular motion during the swing phase of gait. This is an abnormal gait.

client factors: "Specific capacities, characteristics, or beliefs that reside within the person and that influence performance in occupations. Client factors include values, beliefs, and spirituality; body functions; and body structures (see Table 9)" (AOTA, 2020).

closed environment: Environment that is more predictable as there is more structure and less variability.

closed kinematic chain: The distal segment past a joint is fixed or stabilized so movement in one joint will automatically necessitate movement at connecting proximal joints.

close-pack position of joint: Most stable position of joint. The two articulating bones in this position have the greatest amount of contact between surface areas; the ligaments and joint capsule are taut. Often occurs at one extreme of the range of motion; in the knee the close-pack position is flexion (Lippert, 2006).

complex regional pain syndrome (CRPS): A posttraumatic neuropathic syndrome characterized by pain and vasomotor and pseudomotor changes in the involved extremity. Also called *reflex sympathetic dystrophy.*

compression: An external force causing two joint surfaces to be in closer contact with each other; the pushing together of the two bones in the joint. Also referred to as *joint approximation.*

concave: A concave curve is one that extends inward or anteriorly. The opening part of a curve.

concentric contractions: An isotonic contraction is considered concentric when the muscle shortens and the joint angle is decreased.

condyloid joint: Allows for biaxial movement occurring in two planes including flexion and extension as well as abduction and adduction. When movements occur concurrently, the movement is termed *circumduction*. This joint is usually oval-shaped with the end of one bone having a convex shape that fits into the concave surface on the articulating bone. An example is the metacarpophalangeal joints of the four lesser digits (Luttgens & Wells, 1982).

contact force: The force between two objects that are in physical contact (Science Facts, 2023).

context: "Construct that constitutes the complete makeup of a person's life as well as the common and divergent factors that characterize groups and populations. Context includes environmental factors and personal factors (see Tables 4 and 5)" (AOTA, 2020).

contractility: A muscle's ability to shorten in length. Not all contractions result in muscle shortening.

convex: A convex curve is one that extends outward or posteriorly; the closed part of a curve.

cranial nerve: Twelve pairs of nerves that transmit information directly to the brain.

cubital tunnel syndrome: Syndrome frequently involving pressure at the medial side of the elbow, which compresses the ulnar nerve.

cumulative trauma disorders: A group of signs and symptoms that, over time, affect the joints and soft tissues of the upper and lower extremities and back. Signs and symptoms may include pain, numbness, and tingling. Also known as *repetitive stress injuries*, *repetitive motion injuries*, or *repetitive strain injuries.*

crepitus: A crunching or grinding noise that accompanies moving the joint.

D

decubitus: Short for decubitus ulcer; a lesion on the surface of the skin caused by superficial tissue loss often with inflammation present. May be caused by excessive pressure, shearing pressure, or static postures over a period of time. Commonly referred to as a *bed sore* (Steadman, 1982).

degree of freedom: The number of axes a joint can rotate around and the number of planes the joint can move in.

de Quervain's disease: Tenosynovitis that causes pain and swelling of the thumb and wrist over the anatomical snuff box.

dermatome: The area of skin that is innervated by cutaneous (pertaining to the skin) branches form a single spinal nerve (Steadman, 1982).

diagonal lift: A technique used to lift heavy objects to increase safety and decrease stress on the body.

diarthrodial articulations: Considered freely moving. Joint movement is limited primarily by muscles, tendons, and ligaments rather than by the joint structure itself. Diarthrodial joints are enclosed within a joint capsule that secretes synovial fluid to lubricate the joint; thus, these joints are also referred to as *synovial joints*.

distal biceps tendon rupture: When the distal portion of the biceps tendon that attaches at the radial to tuberosity completely tears or ruptures.

distal radioulnar joint (DRUJ): This joint is an articulation between the radius and the ulna that enables the forearm to rotate into pronation and supination.

distraction: An external force causing slight separation between the two surfaces of a joint; slight pulling apart of a joint. Also referred to as *traction* or *tension*.

dorsal: Pertaining to the back of the body; synonymous with posterior (Steadman, 1982).

dorsal interossei: Muscles of the hand that abduct the metacarpophalangeal joints of the index, ring, and small fingers away from the long finger.

dorsiflexion: Occurs when the wrist is bent back as seen in weight bearing; also known as *wrist extension*.

double support: Position during walking when both feet are in contact with the ground.

drag: Resistance to forward motion.

Dupuytren's disease: A contracture of the palmar aponeurosis; named after French surgeon, Baron Guillaume Dupuytren, who first operated on it in 1831.

dynamic balance: "The ability to remain standing and stable while performing movements or actions that require displacing or moving oneself" (Rehametrics, 2023).

dynamic splint: Has moving parts, primarily used for increasing range of motion.

E

eccentric contraction: The muscle is actually lengthening under stress. Eccentric contractions work to decelerate the movement, as a brake would do for a car.

edema: The technical word for swelling; occurs frequently after injury and is especially problematic in the fingers, hands, and wrists.

efferent neurons: Motor neurons that terminate on muscle fibers causing a contraction are generally regarded as efferent, or exiting the central nervous system. Efferent neurons are located ventrally; interchangeable with the term *motor neurons* (Solomon, 2009).

elasticity: Describes the muscle's ability to return to its original length after it has been stretched.

elbow complex: Consists of the body structures that provide motion at the elbow and the forearm.

end feel: How the joint movement feels at the end of the range of motion. See **abnormal end feel, firm end feel, hard end feel**, and **soft end feel**.

energy conservation: A technique to use movements as efficiently as possible with the goal of saving energy for other tasks.

environmental factors: "Aspects of the physical, social, and attitudinal surroundings in which people live and conduct their lives" (AOTA, 2020).

equilibrium: A state of balance of opposing forces due to equal action.

Erb's palsy: Disorder characterized by weakness or paralysis of the arm by affecting nerve roots C5, C6, and C7.

ergonomics: The study of the interaction between human capabilities and the demands of their occupational roles. Occupational therapy and ergonomics are both concerned with an individual's adaptation to their physical environment (Hertfelder & Gwin, 1989).

excursion ratio: The difference between how long the muscle is when stretched as compared to its length when contracted. For most muscles, this ratio is 2:1, indicating that most muscles are capable of stretching twice as long as they can shorten (Gench et al., 1999).

extensibility: Depicts a muscle's capacity to be stretched or lengthened.

extrinsic muscles: "Originating from or on the outside; especially originating outside a part and acting upon the part as a whole" (Merriam-Webster, n.d.).

extrinsic muscles of the hand: Muscles that originate proximal to the wrist joint.

F

fall on an outstretched hand (FOOSH): Occurs when a person falls and they extend their wrist to catch their fall. Frequently results in the fracture of the distal portion of the radius.

fasciculus: Fascicle, a bundle or band, usually of muscle or nerve fibers (Steadman, 1982).

fasciotomy: A procedure involving removing the thickened fascia or connective tissue that releases the palmar contraction through a single, larger incision.

fibroblastic stage: Characterized by the development of scar tissue to strengthen the injured area. This process begins prior to the end of the inflammatory phase and can last upwards of 4 to 6 weeks depending on the severity of tissue damage. During this phase, collagen and elastin are formed across the damaged area in a pattern resembling a haphazardly designed web.

Finkelstein's test: A provocative test for diagnosis of de Quervain's disease. The movement invokes pain and is tested by extending the elbow with ulnar deviation of the wrist and the thumb held in the palm by the digits.

firm end feel: The end feel experienced when a normal joint or ligament is stretched.

flaccid paralysis: Loss of voluntary movement due to lack of muscle tone; tendon reflexes are also decreased or absent (Merriam-Webster, n.d.).

foot drop: A common disorder in neurological conditions where a person has an inability, or difficulty, in creating ankle dorsiflexion. The foot, toes, and ankle have difficulty pointing up in the air, procuring the name foot drop.

force: A push or pull upon an object resulting from the object's interaction with another object (The Physics Classroom, n.d.).

force couple: Muscles that act as synergists to one another to provide a stronger action on the joint, resulting in stronger functional movement for the client. The resulting movement must be rotary in nature, and the line of force and the pull or angle of muscle fibers of all muscles involved must be in opposing directions.

force–velocity curve: Outlines how different velocities in each of the isotonic contractions and isometric velocities impacts force generation.

forward pelvic rotation: When the anterior superior iliac spine moves forward relative to the contralateral side.

friction: Force acting in the opposite direction to the desired movement and occurring at the area of contact between the two surfaces.

frozen shoulder: See **primary adhesive capsulitis**.

function: The ability of an individual to move sufficiently and complete a task or goal to their satisfaction in any social context; the ability to achieve occupation well and as desired.

functional mobility: An activity of daily living focused on personal care.

functional position: This is most effective in terms of strength and precision during activities. In the functional position the wrist is slightly extended at approximately 20 degrees, the fingers are slightly flexed at all their joints, and the thumb is in opposition with the metacarpophalangeal joint moderately flexed.

functional progression: Moves the client from the basic ability to function toward the ability to complete activities of daily living to a desired standard.

fundamental position: Reference position where the subject is standing in an upright posture, eyes looking forward, feet parallel with toes pointed forward, the arms slightly abducted at the side of the body, and the palms facing the side of the body (Solomon, 2009).

G

gait: The way a person walks.

gait cycle: Describes the movement from the heel strike of one leg to the heel strike of the same leg on the ground.

gait patterns: "In the OTPF 4 gait patterns are found under neuromuscular and movement-related functions; gait patterns are gait and mobility in relation to engagement in daily life activities (e.g. walking patterns and impairments, asymmetric gait, stiff gait)" (AOTA, 2020).

glenohumeral joint: A ball-and-socket joint that includes a complex dynamic articulation between the glenoid of the scapula and the proximal humerus.

gliding joint: Considered nonaxial as the only movement permitted is gliding in nature, as in one bone over another. An example is the carpal joints. Also referred to as *irregular*, *arthrodial*, or *plane joints* (Luttgens & Wells, 1982).

golfer's lift: A technique used for picking an object up off of the ground when one is unable to flex a hip joint past 90 degrees; also decreases stress on lumbar spine.

H

handheld electronic devices: Communication devices such as cellphones, computer notepads, and electronic readers that require repetitive hand movements.

hard end feel: The feel experienced when two bones block motion.

healing process: Divided into three phases: inflammatory, fibroblastic, and maturation.

hemiparesis: Paralysis affecting only one side of the body (Thomas, 1989).

hemiplegia: Paralysis of one side of the body after a cerebrovascular accident or stroke.

hinge joint: Uniaxial, allowing movement in one plane to include flexion and extension; the end of one bone is spool-like, whereas the articulating bone is concave to fit around the spool. An example is the elbow joint (Luttgens & Wells, 1982).

humeral positioners: Muscles that position the humerus in space during or after actions of the scapular pivoters (Glinn, 2008).

humeral propellers: Muscles that propel or move the humerus (Glinn, 2008).

hypertonia: "Above or over tone"; extreme tension of the muscles.

hypertonic: An increase in tone in muscles that prevents normal movement.

hypothenar: The muscular portion of the palm of the hand on the small finger side.

hypotonia: "Under tone"; having a lesser degree of tension, diminished muscular tone.

I

impairment: Level of dysfunction identified by the *International Classification of Functioning, Disability and Health* that occurs at the body part level (WHO, 2001).

individuality: Qualities that make a person different from others. A principle that is foundational to the rehabilitation/exercise program.

inertia: "The state of a physical body in which it resists any force acting to move it from a position of rest or to change its uniform motion" (Steadman, 1982).

inflammatory phase: Occurs directly after injury and can continue for several days in acute injuries with the duration depending on the severity of the injury and any potentially impeding factors. Though inflammation generally has a negative connotation, it is an essential component of the healing process. Without inflammation healing will not occur.

insertion: The end point of a muscle attachment. The insertion is usually distal, or further away from the trunk and midline of the body, and is considered the most movable part.

instrumental activities of daily living (IADLs): "Activities that support daily life within the home and community and that often require more complex interactions than those used in activities of daily living (see Table 2)" (AOTA, 2020).

intensity: The principle of matching the intensity of movement and exercise to the specificity. It does not reflect motivation or desire and is reflected in a physiologic response to that exercise and not a mental response.

intervertebral disc: A cushion of fibrocartilage and the principal joint between two vertebrae in the spinal column (Physiopedia, 2023b).

intrinsic muscles: "Originating and included wholly within an organ or part" (Merriam-Webster, n.d.).

intrinsic muscles of the hand: Muscles that originate distal to the wrist joint.

irritability: Describes the property of the muscle to receive and respond to a stimulus, whether chemical, electrical, or mechanical (Hall, 1999; Thompson & Floyd, 2004).

isometric contraction: Muscle tension develops, but the muscle length does not change. This means that the joint angle or measurement does not change either.

isotonic: Isotonic contractions maintain the muscle at equal tension. This means that the length of the muscle changes, causing joint movement.

J

juncturae tendinae: Fibrous bands at the level of the metacarpophalangeal joints that impede individual finger extension; however, they provide stabilizing forces to the metacarpophalangeal joints while the fingers are flexed during forceful gripping.

K

kinematic chain: Linkage system of joints between bony segments in the body. In engineering terms a kinetic chain is a series of rigid links connected in a specific way to allow motion (Dail et al., 2011). In human bodies, the rigid links are bones and the motion occurs at joints. See **closed kinematic chain**, **open kinematic chain**. Also referred to as *kinetic chain*.

kinesiology: The study of the principles of mechanics and anatomy in relation to human movement (Merriam-Webster Collegiate Dictionary, 1991).

kinetic model: A model, or treatment approach, used in medicine and therapy to address deficiencies by focusing on forces that act on muscle strength and joint motions during movement.

kyphosis: A spinal deformity; an excessive curvature in the thoracic spine.

L

lateral epicondylitis: Signified by pain and inflammation caused by microscopic tears where the extensor carpi radialis brevis attaches to the lateral epicondyle of the humerus at the elbow; commonly called *tennis elbow*.

lateral pelvic tilt: When the pelvis shifts side to side so much that one hip is higher than the other (ISSA, 2023).

lever: A rigid bar resting on a pivot, used to help move a heavy or firmly fixed load with one end when pressure is applied to the other (Oxford Languages, n.d.).

lift: Refers to a change in fluid pressure as a result of differences in air or liquid flow velocities around an object.

line of gravity (LOG): The vertical line from the center of gravity to the earth; base of support is the area contained within the area of the body parts in contact with the ground (Lippert, 2006).

locus of control: Refers to whom, or what, has impact over outcomes. Can be external to a person or internal in nature.

long sitting: Sitting on a flat surface with a person's legs fully extended in front of them.

lordosis: An exacerbated curvature of the lumbar spine; also called *swayback*.

lower motor neurons (LMNs): Responsible for transmitting the signal from the upper motor neuron to the effector muscle to perform a movement. Begin in the spinal cord and go on to innervate muscles and glands throughout the body (Zayia & Tadi, 2023).

lumbosacral plexus: Relating to the lower back and lower extremity; usually refers to nerve roots L1-L5 (lumbar portion) and L5-S3 (sacral portion; Thompson & Floyd, 2004).

lumbricals: Muscles of the hand that flex the metacarpophalangeal joints as they extend the proximal interphalangeal and distal interphalangeal joints of all four fingers.

M

malunion: A deformity that can occur after a properly aligned fracture slips in the cast during healing.

manual muscle testing (MMT): A manual technique used for estimating the relative strength of specific muscles (Thomas, 1989).

maturation stage: Characterized by the realignment of the scar tissue, which is achieved by progressively increasing movement and function to the preset ideal function. Movement helps to realign the fibers along the lines of physiologic tension.

motivation: An internal factor that might create good feelings about oneself for reaching a goal. External or social motivators might include a high grade, parental approval, or retention of scholarship monies. Motivation can be intrinsic, coming from internal sources, or extrinsic, reinforced by external factors.

motor behavior: Observable and measurable movement (Spaulding, 2005).

motor control: The outcome of motor learning involving the ability to produce purposeful movements of the extremities and postural adjustments in response to activity and environment demands (Pendleton & Schultz-Krohn, 2006).

motor development: The changes in movement behavior that occur as the client progresses through the lifespan from infancy until death (Whiting & Rugg, 2006).

motor learning: The acquisition and/or modification of learned movement patterns over time (Pendleton & Schultz-Krohn, 2006).

motor neurons: See **efferent neurons**.

motor skills: Voluntary movements used to complete a desired task or achieve a specific goal (Whiting & Rugg, 2006).

muscle fiber architecture types: Refers to the direction of muscle fibers and includes pennate, unipennate, bipennate, flat, parallel, fusiform, strap, radiate, and sphincter.

muscle imbalance: "When a muscle (or muscles) on one side of your body is larger, smaller, stronger, or weaker than the corresponding muscle on the other side" (Frothingham, 2020).

musculotendinous junction: The area where the tendon and the muscle join.

N

negotiability: The ability of a person to interact with the environment and independently use common features, such as a toilet paper dispenser.

nerves: Transmit stimuli from the central nervous system to the periphery or vice versa; a microscopic bundle or one or more fascicles of either myelinated or unmyelinated fibers; can also be a mixture of both fiber types (Steadman, 1982).

neuromuscular control: Unconscious efferent response to an afferent signal.

neutral pelvic tilt: Characterized as equal weight distribution across the femurs in a sitting position.

nonstructural scoliosis: "This type of scoliosis isn't structural so can be addressed with treatment that doesn't have to impact it on a structural level. The causes can include chronic poor posture and/or other body irregularities" (Nalda, 2023). Also called *functional scoliosis*.

normal atypical movement: Reflects the motor behavior response when typical movement strategies are temporarily or no longer feasible.

normal enhanced typical movement: Highly trained motor skills and motor control that allow for high efficiency, adaptability, and consistency in performance of a task in a variety of environments.

normal typical movement: Movement characterized by smooth, coordinated, efficient, automatic movements that reflect a variety of movement options, high complexity, decreased time, high velocity, and high acceleration.

nursemaid's elbow: An injury that is seen involving the annular ligament known as *pulled elbow*. It is seen mainly in children less than 6 years of age and is caused by a traction force pulling the forearm distally from the elbow. This may occur by swinging or lifting a young child by the hands.

O

occupation and activity demands: "The components of occupations and activities that occupational therapy practitioners consider in their professional and clinical reasoning process. *Activity demands* are what is typically required to carry out the activity regardless of client and context. *Occupation demands* are what is required by the specific client (person, group, or population) to carry out an occupation" (AOTA, 2020).

occupational demands: "Aspects of an activity needed to carry it out, including relevance and importance to the client, objects used and their properties, space demands, social demands, sequencing and timing, required actions and performance skills, and required underlying body function and body structures (see Table 10)" (AOTA, 2020).

occupation: "Everyday personalized activities that people do as individuals, in families, and with communities to occupy time and bring meaning and purpose to life. Occupations can involve the execution of multiple activities for completion and can result in various outcomes. The broad range of occupations is categorized as activities of daily living, instrumental activities of daily living, health management, rest and sleep, education, work, play, leisure, and social participation (see Table 2)" (AOTA, 2020).

open environment: Environment that is less predictable as there is less structure and more variability.

open kinematic chain: The distal segment past a joint is freely moving and, therefore, one joint can move without impacting movement of the other proximal joints.

open-pack position of joint: Least amount of contact between the two articulating surfaces; ligaments and joint capsule are loose or lax. This position allows for normal accessory motions in the joint to occur, thus allowing for normal range of motion; considered to occur whenever the joint is not in a close-pack position. Also referred to as *loose-pack* (Lippert, 2006).

open reduction with internal fixation (ORIF): A plate and screws are utilized by the surgeon to stabilize the radius after fracture.

origin: Describes where a muscle begins or originates. This point is usually proximal or closer to the trunk or middle of the body and is often considered to be more stable.

orthopedic model: The orthopedic model took into consideration anatomy, physiology, pathology, and kinesiology in addressing client impairments and disabilities. Activities, or occupations, were selected depending on the desired movements. Greater care was also undertaken to record client information, number of treatments, results, and remarks (Haworth & Macdonald, 1940).

orthotics: A device that is designed to support or correct the alignment of a limb or to restrict movement.

osteoarthritis (OA): A condition of the joints causing pain and stiffness; caused by degenerative changes of the joints over time.

osteokinematic movement: The movement of bones; described in movement terms, such as flexion and extension. Osteokinematic movements create measurable angles that can be recorded with the use of goniometers, tape measures, and a variety of applications for mobile electronic devices.

overload: Part of the SAID principle, which states that it is essential that the practitioner design a program to overload the damaged structures of the body progressively and safely in functional patterns.

P

palmar aponeurosis: The thickened, central portion of the deep palmar fascia. Its main function is mechanical as it protects the flexor tendons of the palm and gives firm attachment to the skin of the palm to help with grip.

palmar interossei: Muscles of the hand that adduct the metacarpophalangeal joints of the index, ring, and small fingers to the long finger.

palpation: To medically examine by touch.

paralysis: Loss of voluntary movement; a complete or partial loss of function that may include movement and/or sensation; inability to move (Merriam-Webster, n.d.). See **flaccid paralysis** and **spastic paralysis**.

participation: "Involvement in a life situation" (WHO, 2002).

participation restriction: Level of dysfunction identified by the *International Classification of Function, Disability and Health* that occurs at the societal level (WHO, 2001).

passive insufficiency: Occurs when a muscle cannot be stretched any further, yet it has not stretched the amount required for full range of motion at all joints crossed at the same time.

passive range of motion (PROM): Refers to joint movement created by manual assistance only.

pelvic obliquity: The rotation of the pelvis within the coronal plane (Feger & Bell, 2021).

performance patterns: "Habits, routines, roles, and rituals that may be associated with different lifestyles and used in the process of engaging in occupations or activities. These patterns are influenced by context and time and can support or hinder occupational performance (see Table 6)" (AOTA, 2020).

performance skills: "Observable, goal directed actions that result in a clients' quality of performing desired occupations. Skills are supported by the context in which the performance occurred and by underlying client factors (Fisher & Marterella, 2019)" (AOTA, 2020).

peripheral nervous system (PNS): The motor neurons found in the PNS are called *lower motor neurons*. Cell bodies of the lower motor neurons are located in the anterior horn of the spinal cord and sometimes are referred to as *anterior horn cells*.

physical environment: "The part of the human environment that includes purely physical factors (as soil, climate, water supply)" (Merriam-Webster, n.d.).

pincher grasp: A developmental milestone at about 9 to 12 months of age. It enables a young child to pick up small objects using the thumb, index finger, and often the middle finger. It allows for a more refined, neater way of getting food to the mouth.

pivot joint: Movement allowed is uniaxial, occurs in only one plane, and consists of rotation; joint is a peg-like pivot where one bone can roll or rotate around another. An example is the atlantoaxial joint. Also termed *screw joint* (Luttgens & Wells, 1982).

plexus: Bundle or interconnection of nerves including the brachial plexus and lumbosacral plexus. Latin term for "braid"; network or interjoining of blood, nerve, or lymphatic vessels (Steadman, 1982). See **brachial plexus** and **lumbosacral plexus**.

pointing muscle: A common term for the extensor indicis proprius muscle because it is responsible for extending the index finger especially when the other fingers are flexed.

posterior pelvic tilt: Characterized by the tailbone tucking beneath the body on the posterior superior iliac spine shifting backward. The anterior superior iliac spine landmarks move posteriorly to the public symphysis.

postural control: "The regulation of the body's position in space for the dual purpose of stability and orientation" (Shumway-Cook & Woollacott, 2001).

posture: "State of the body in relationship to gravity, the ground and to its body parts or extremities" (Martin, 1977).

praxis: "The ability to plan and execute coordinated movement" (Venes, 2013).

preparatory methods: "Provided by the practitioner to help aid in occupational performance by preparing the client for their occupations and activities. These may be modalities and assistive technology devices supplied and fitted by the occupational therapist, such as orthotics and splints to deal with pain management and muscle placement, a wheelchair to assist in mobility, or a recommended change in environment to address activity demands" (Davies, 2022).

primary adhesive capsulitis: Condition of the shoulder involving progressive stiffness and diffuse pain that limits function. Also called *frozen shoulder*.

progression: Under the SAID principle, progression should move from simplistic and general movement patterns to more client specific and complex patterns and be appropriate to the level of tissue healing.

pronation: In Chapter 6, refers to the inward roll of the foot during normal motion.

proprioceptive: From the Latin terms for "to take" and "from one's own"; the ability to receive stimuli from within one's own body, such as from muscles, tendons, and other internal tissues (Steadman, 1982).

prosthetic: A device that compensates for a missing body part or body part that is not working efficiently.

qualitative: Includes information that may come from observation or interview.

quantitative: Identifies numerical data under standardized situations to gather information.

R

radiocarpal joint: A biaxial or condyloid joint; also known as the *wrist joint*.

range of motion (ROM): The arc of motion through which a joint moves.

reflex sympathetic dystrophy (RSD): See **complex regional pain syndrome**.

repetitive stress injuries (RSIs): A group of signs and symptoms that commonly affect the joints and the soft tissues of the arms, hands, knees, and back (Hertfelder & Gwin, 1989). Also known as *repetitive motion injuries, repetitive strain injuries*, or *cumulative trauma disorders*.

resistance: "The act or power of resisting, opposing, or withstanding; the opposition offered by one thing, force, etc., to another" (Dictionary.com, n.d.).

reversal of muscle function: Occurs when the muscle is used in such a way that the normally stable origin moves toward the insertion; in typical muscle function, the insertion moves toward the origin.

rheumatoid arthritis (RA): A systemic autoimmune disorder causing fatigue, joint pain, and inflammation that leads to deformity and joint destruction.

rotator cuff: Tendon connecting four muscles that cover the head of the humerus. The rotator cuff muscles together lift and rotate the humerus and maintain the humeral head in the glenoid fossa.

rotator cuff tendinitis: This most common cause of shoulder pain; occurs when there is impingement of an inflamed rotator cuff tendon between the humeral head, swollen bursa, and acromion process. Also called *shoulder impingement*.

S

saddle joint: Often considered a modified condyloid joint; the end surfaces of both bones are tipped up, somewhat like a western saddle for horses. This joint is also biaxial, allowing flexion and extension, abduction and adduction, and circumduction; the saddle joint has more mobility than a traditional condyloid joint. The only example in the human body is the carpometacarpal joint of the thumb (Luttgens & Wells, 1982).

safety: Under the SAID principle, it revolves around the concept of doing no harm. Client safety can be ensured through various means, such as the instruction of proper technique.

SAID principle: Stands for Specific Adaptations to Imposed Demands (Wathen & Roll, 1994). In other words, if we want to change the function and structure of the body, it must be stressed beyond its typical baseline or current state in a way specific to the desired outcome.

scaphoid fracture: A break in one of the carpal bones of the wrist after a fall on an outstretched hand.

scaption: A functional movement of the glenohumeral joint that occurs about midway between shoulder flexion and abduction.

scapular pivoters: Muscles that are involved with motion at the scapulothoracic joint (Glinn, 2008).

scapulohumeral joint: An articulation between the scapula and the head of the humerus.

scapulohumeral rhythm: Describes the movement relationship between the scapula in the shoulder girdle and the glenohumeral joint.

scoliosis: A spinal deformity in the frontal plane characterized by a lateral curvature of the vertebra.

sensory neurons: See **afferent neurons**.

shear force: A force that attempts to move one object against another.

shoulder complex: Includes all of the body structures that provide motion at the glenohumeral joint and scapula.

shoulder dystocia: Condition that may occur more often in births involving larger than average babies in which one of the infant's shoulders becomes stuck under a portion of the parent's pelvic bone during childbirth.

shoulder girdle: Part of the shoulder complex that makes up the scapula and the clavicle.

shoulder impingement: See **rotator cuff tendinitis**.

shoulder protectors: Muscles that act as a force couple with the humeral positioners to keep the structures of the shoulder complex safe. These include the rotator cuff muscles (Glinn, 2008).

shoulder subluxation: Partial dislocation of the humerus at the glenohumeral joint that is seen in many individuals after a stroke (Ohio Health, 1995).

single support: Position during walking when one foot is in contact with the ground.

sitting balance: The ability to maintain a seated posture without falling; refers to the ability to reach.

skier's thumb: An acute injury to the ulnar collateral ligament of the thumb.

soft end feel: The end feel experienced when two muscle groups are compressed.

somatic: The somatic division is part of the peripheral nervous system and is primarily responsible for responding to the external environment, or things happening outside of the body.

spastic paralysis: Loss of voluntary movement due to increase in muscle tone including spasms; tendon reflexes are increased or hyperexcitable (Merriam-Webster, n.d.).

spasticity: Unusual rigid or increase muscle tone.

specificity: Refers to the ultimate goal of the program, which should mimic function at the desired level and combine both patient and clinician goals.

spinal nerves: Nerves that link the spinal cord with sensory receptors and other parts of the body. The spinal nerves are all mixed nerves, transmitting sensory information to the spinal cord through afferent neurons, and also relaying motor information from the spinal cord to the various parts of the body using efferent neurons.

spirituality: The search for meaning in all that one does, which includes values and beliefs.

stability: Refers to the ability to maintain the body in equilibrium.

stand pivot transfer: "'Pivot' indicates that the person bears at least some weight on one or both legs and spins to move their bottom from one surface to another" (Shepherd Center, 2020).

static balance: "Refers to the ability of individuals to remain standing and stable without displacing their bodies. That is, static balance can be defined as the ability to remain standing on one's feet in a controlled manner without moving one's body" (Rehametrics, 2023).

static splint: Has no moving parts, primarily used for immobilization or support.

Stener lesion: Happens when the aponeurosis of the adductor pollicis muscle is interposed between the bones of the metacarpophalangeal joint and the torn ulnar collateral ligament.

stretch reflex: Slight stretching of a muscle lengthens fibers causing stimulation of sensory endings, which leads to contraction of the muscle. This is a protective reflex to avoid overstretching. One role of the muscle spindle is to detect stretch and respond to it via the stretch reflex; this phenomenon is in constant use and provides adjustment to muscle tone.

structural scoliosis: "A structural abnormality within the spine itself; structural scoliosis is far more complex to treat because it's a structural condition" (Nalda, 2023).

supination: Defined in this context as referring to the outward roll of the foot during normal motion.

swan neck deformity: A finger with a hyperextended proximal interphalangeal joint and a flexed distal interphalangeal joint.

swelling and pain: Contribute to activity limitations and contribute heavily to client satisfaction with the overall outcome of therapy.

synarthrodial articulations: Joints that are immovable, such as the suture joints of the skull.

syndesmosis: Articulation in which the bones are united by ligaments (Thomas, 1989).

synergist: Muscles that work together to increase the strength of a desired movement as they work in unison.

synovial joints: Refers to diarthrodial articulations.

synovitis: A thickening and inflammation of the synovial lining of the joints.

T

tendinitis: An irritation or inflammation of the tendons.

tendon rupture: A tendon weakened by disease or injury may rupture or separate. See also **attrition rupture**.

tenodesis: "Literally means tendon binding, or fixation of a tendon. Related to grasp, tenodesis is defined as 'flexing of the fingers through tendon action of the extrinsic finger flexor muscles…during wrist extension'" (Venes, 2013, p. 2293).

thenar: The thumb side of the hand. The thenar eminence is the musculature in the palm at the base of the thumb.

therapeutic exercise: The application of movement to create structural and functional improvements that decrease participation restrictions. It involves a continual process of evaluation and application of theory and skill to improve function.

thoracic kyphosis: Condition seen in older individuals that features forward head posture and rounded shoulders.

thumb spica splint: A wrist and thumb splint fabricated with the wrist in neutral to 15 degrees of extension, the thumb in radial abduction, and the thumb metacarpophalangeal and interphalangeal joints in extension.

transfer board: "Commonly rigid, flat boards made of wood or plastic. The board acts as a bridge to allow individuals to move from one seated surface to another such as moving from a wheelchair to a bed" (Physiopedia, 2023c). Also known as *sliding boards*.

trigger finger: A thickening of the flexor tendon sheath at the A1 pulley in the palm of the hand; can cause the finger to lock as a "trigger" while making a fist.

U

ulnar collateral ligament (UCL): A ligament that is on the medial side of the elbow and supports the humerus and ulna. It can be injured by being stretched or torn. The injury can cause pain, instability, and loss of function.

universal design: "The design of products and environments to be usable by all people, to the greatest extent possible, without the need for adaptation or specialized design" (The Center for Universal Design, 1997).

upper motor neurons (UMNs): The nerves in the central nervous system that carry the impulses for movement. First-order neurons that are responsible for carrying the electrical impulses that initiate and modulate movement (Emos & Agarwal, 2023). Originate in the cerebral cortex and travel down to the brain stem or spinal cord (Zayia & Tadi, 2023).

V

Valsalva maneuver: Attempt to forcibly exhale with the nose while the mouth closed. This causes increased intrathoracic pressure, slowing of the pulse, decreased return of blood to the heart, and increased venous pressure (Thomas, 1989).

values: Principles and standards that an individual considers to be essential to follow in order to lead a good life. A person might value honesty, integrity, hard work, or family relationships, to name a few.

ventral: Pertaining to the front of the body; synonymous with anterior (Steadman, 1982).

vertebral column: "The central axis of the skeleton in all vertebrates" (Kayalioglu, 2009). Also known as the *spinal column*.

vestibular: Related to the vestibule of the ear; the vestibule is a small space or region at the entrance of a canal; vestibular organ—the organ of equilibrium.

W

wheeled mobility: "Wheeled and seated mobility devices are medical devices that are intended to provide mobility and function for persons with restricted or no ability to ambulate without assistance from technology" (Flaubert et al., 2017).

winging of the scapula: Seen when the inferior angle of the scapula protrudes, or wings out, due to serratus anterior muscle weakness.

Wolff's law: States that there is a relationship between form and function of bone that is controlled by physical laws.

X

XIAFLEX: An enzyme drug that is injected into the contracture in the palm. The enzyme quickly dissolves a portion of the thickened fascia, making it possible for the surgeon to manipulate the contracture, straightening the finger the next day in the office.

References

American Occupational Therapy Association. (2020). Occupational therapy practice framework: Domain and process (4th ed.). *American Journal of Occupational Therapy, 74*(Suppl. 2), Article 7412410010. https://doi.org/10.5014/ajot.2020.74S2001

Cambridge Dictionary. (n.d.). Orthotics. https://dictionary.cambridge.org/us/dictionary/english/orthotics

The Center for Universal Design. (1997). Center for Universal Design. NC State. https://design.ncsu.edu/research/center-for-universal-design/

Cronin, A., & Mandich, M. (2005). *Human development and performance throughout the lifespan.* Thomson Delmar Learning.

Dail, N. W., Agnew, T. A., & Floyd, R. T. (2011). *Kinesiology for manual therapies.* McGraw-Hill.

Davies, L. (2020). What are the five types of interventions in occupational therapy? *Occupational & Behavioral Therapy.* https://resources.noodle.com/articles/occupational-therapy-intervention-methods/

Dictionary.com. (n.d.). *Resistance.* https://www.dictionary.com/browse/resistance

Emos, M. C., & Agarwal, S. (2023). Neuroanatomy, Upper Motor Neuron Lesion. *StatPearls.* https://www.ncbi.nlm.nih.gov/books/NBK537305/

Feger, J., & Bell, D. (2021). Pelvic obliquity. Reference article. *Radiopaedia.* https://doi.org/10.53347/rID-81050

Fisher, A. G., & Marterella, A. (2019) *Powerful practice. A model for authentic occupational therapy.* Center for Innovative OT Solutions

Flaubert, J. L., & Spicer, C. M., & Jette A. M. (Eds.). (2017). *The promise of assistive technology to enhance activity and work participation.* National Academies Press. https://www.ncbi.nlm.nih.gov/books/NBK453286/

Frothingham, S. (2020). What causes muscle imbalances and how to fix them. *Healthline.* https://www.healthline.com/health/muscle-imbalance

Gench, B. E., Hionson, M. M., & Harvey, P. T. (1999). *Anatomical kinesiology.* Eddie Bowers Publishing, Inc.

Glinn, J. E., Jr. (2008). Shoulder biomechanics. *Physical Therapy's Clinical Educator,* 49-53.

Hall, S. (1999). *Basic biomechanics* (3rd ed.). WCB/McGraw-Hill.

Haworth, N. A., & Macdonald, E. M. (1940). *The theory of occupational therapy.* Bailliere, Tindall, & Cox.

Hertfelder, S., & Gwin, C. (1989). *Work in progress: Occupational therapy in work programs.* American Occupational Therapy Association.

Horak, R. (1987). Clinical management of postural control in adults. *Physical Therapy, 67*(12), 1881-1885.

ISSA. (2023). Pelvic tilt: What is it and how do you correct it? https://www.issaonline.com/blog/post/pelvic-tilt-what-is-it-and-how-do-you-correct-it

James, A. B. (2003). Biomechanical frame of reference. In E. B. Crepeau, E. S. Cohn, & B. A. Boyt-Schell (Eds.), *Willard & Spackman's occupational therapy* (10th ed., pp. 240-242). Lippincott Williams & Wilkins.

Jung, B., Black, A. C., & Bhutta, B. S. (2023). Anatomy, head and neck, neck movements. *StatPearls.* https://www.ncbi.nlm.nih.gov/books/NBK557555/

Kayalioglu, G. (2009). The vertebral column and spinal meninges. In: C. Watson, G. Paxinos, & G. Kayalioglu. (Eds.), *The spinal cord* (pp. 17-36). Academic Press.

Landel, R., & Fisher, B. (1993). Musculoskeletal considerations in the neurologically impaired patient. *Orthopaedic Physical Therapy Clinics of North America, 2*(1), 15-24.

Lippert, L. S. (2006). *Clinical kinesiology for physical therapy assistants* (3rd ed.). F. A. Davis Company.

Luijkx, T., O'Shea, P., Murphy A. (2014). Atlas (C1). *Radiopaedia.* https://doi.org/10.53347/rID-30850

Luttgens, K., & Wells, K. F. (1982). *Kinesiology: Scientific basis of human motion* (7th ed.). Saunders College Publishing.

Martin, J. P. (1977). A short essay on posture and movement. *Journal of Neurology Neurosurgery and Psychiatry, 40,* 25-29.

Merriam-Webster. (n.d.). *Merriam-Webster.com dictionary.* http://www.merriam-webster.com/dictionary

Merriam-Webster's Collegiate Dictionary (9th ed.). (1991). Merriam-Webster.

Nalda, T. (2023). Functional scoliosis vs. structural scoliosis: The differences. https://drtonynalda.com/functional-scoliosis/

Ohio Health. (1995). Shoulder subluxation. www.ohiohealth.com

Oxford Languages. (n.d.). https://languages.oup.com/google-dictionary-en/

Pendleton, H. M., & Schultz-Krohn, W. (2006). *Pedretti's occupational therapy: Practice skills for physical dysfunction* (6th ed.). Elsevier-Mosby.

The Physics Classroom. (n.d.). The meaning of force. https://www.physicsclassroom.com/class/newtlaws/Lesson-2/The-Meaning-of-Force

Physiopedia. (2023a). Base of support. https://www.physio-pedia.com/Base_of_Support

Physiopedia. (2023b). Intevertebral disc. https://www.physio-pedia.com/Intervertebral_disc

Physiopedia. (2023c). Transfer boards. https://www.physio-pedia.com/Transfer_Boards

Rehametrics. (2023). Dynamic balance. https://rehametrics.com/en/dynamic-balance/

Scuebce Facts. (2023). Contact and non-contact forces. https://www.sciencefacts.net/contact-and-non-contact-forces.html

Shepherd Center. (2020). Pivot transfer. https://www.myshepherdconnection.org/sci/transfers/pivot-transfer

Shumway-Cook, A., & Woollacott, M. H. (2001). *Motor control: Theory and practical applications* (2nd ed.). Lippincott Williams & Wilkins.

Solomon, E. P. (2009). *Introduction to human anatomy and physiology*. Saunders-Elsevier.

Spaulding, S. J. (2005). *Meaningful motion: Biomechanics for occupational therapists*. Elsevier-Churchill Livingstone.

Steadman, T. (1982). *Steadman's medical dictionary* (24th ed.). Williams and Wilkins.

Thomas, C. L. (1989). *Taber's cyclopedia medical dictionary* (17th ed.). F. A. Davis Company.

Thompson, C. W., & Floyd, R. T. (2004). *Manual of structural kinesiology* (15th ed.). McGraw-Hill.

Venes, D. (2013). *Taber's cyclopedic medical dictionary* (22nd ed.). F. A. Davis Company

Wathen, D., & Roll, F. (1994). Training methods and modes. In T. Baechle (Ed.), *Essentials of strength training and conditioning* (pp. 403-415). Human Kinetics.

Whiting, W. C., & Rugg, S. (2006). *Dynatomy: Dynamic human anatomy*. Human Kinetics.

World Health Organization (2001). *International classification of functioning, disability and health*. WHO Press.

World Health Organization. (2002). *Towards a common language for functioning, disability and health* (ICF). https://www.who.int/publications/m/item/icf-beginner-s-guide-towards-a-common-language-for-functioning-disability-and-health

Zayia, L. C., & Tadi, P. (2023). Neuroanatomy, motor neuron. *StatPearls*. https://www.ncbi.nlm.nih.gov/books/NBK554616

Web Resources

Accessibility

Americans with Disabilities Act: Accessibility Guidelines (ADAAG) Checklist for Buildings and Facilities

https://www.access-board.gov/guidelines-and-standards/ buildings-and-sites/about-the-ada-standards/background/ adaag

Accessibility standards issued under the Americans with Disabilities Act (ADA) apply to places of public accommodation, commercial facilities, and state and local government facilities in new construction, alterations, and additions. The ADA Standards are based on minimum guidelines set by the Access Board.

Americans with Disabilities Act: Checklist for Readily Achievable Barrier Removal

http://www.ada.gov/checkweb.htm

Select PDF version for checklist. This checklist has been made available over the internet with permission of Adaptive Environments. This checklist may be copied for your own use as many times as desired but may not be reproduced in whole or in part and sold for commercial purposes by any entity without written permission of Adaptive Environments.

Checklist of Checkpoints for Web Content Accessibility Guidelines

https://www.w3.org/TR/WCAG21/

United States Access Board

https://www.access-board.gov

The Access Board is an independent federal agency that promotes equality for people with disabilities through leadership in accessible design and the development of accessibility guidelines and standards.

WebAIM

http://www.webaim.org/standards/508/checklist

Checklists for web content accessibility.

Anatomy and Physiology Tutorials

Duke Orthopedics: Wheeless' Textbook of Orthopedics

http://www.wheelessonline.com

Extensive links, pictures, diagrams, explanations; very thorough; easy to search.

Get Body Smart

http://www.getbodysmart.com/

An online exploration of human anatomy and physiology.

Gray's Anatomy

http://www.bartleby.com/107/

The Bartleby.com edition of *Gray's Anatomy of the Human Body*.

Sain, S. J., & Roller, C. L. *Kinesiology for the Occupational Therapy Assistant: Essential Components of Function and Movement, Third Edition* (pp. 327-328). © 2024 Taylor & Francis Group.

Inner Body: Anatomy Explorer
https://www.innerbody.com/htm/body.html
Interactive anatomy tutorial.

OrthoInfo
http://orthoinfo.aaos.org
American Academy of Orthopedic Surgeons.

Foot and Ankle

FootCareMD
http://www.footcaremd.org
American Orthopedic Foot and Ankle Society.

Hand

e-Hand
http://www.e-hand.com
Electronic textbook of hand surgery, diagrams, text, videos, other images; very thorough site.

Shoulder

Shoulderdoc
http://www.shoulderdoc.co.uk
Information, including online books, regarding every aspect of shoulder anatomy, physiology, function, illness, and treatment.

Study Aids

Quizlet
http://quizlet.com
Quizlet makes it easy to study things like vocabulary words with online study tools. You can make quizzes, use your friend's, or browse existing flashcards on the site. Answers are not verified.

SimpleNote
https://simplenote.com/
Take and store your notes online; edit and revise notes with peers.

Study Stack
http://www.studystack.com
Find flashcards to study or create your own. May need to create an account. Answers are not verified; however, you can find occupational therapy specific questions.

APPENDIX B

Available Range of Motion Norms

Table B-1 presents range of motion norms for the upper extremity.
Table B-2 presents range of motion norms for the lower extremity.

TABLE B-1		
Range of Motion Norms for the Upper Extremity		
JOINT	**JOINT MOTION**	**RANGE OF MOTION (DEGREES)**
Glenohumeral	Flexion	0 to 180
	Extension (also referred to as hyperextension)	0 to 50
	Abduction	0 to 180
	Adduction	180 to 0
	Internal rotation	0 to 90
	External rotation	0 to 90
	Horizontal abduction	0 to 45*
	Horizontal adduction	0 to 135*
Elbow	Flexion	0 to 40
	Extension	Extension is the return to 0
Forearm	Supination	0 to 80
	Pronation	0 to 80
		(continued)

Sain, S. J., & Roller, C. L. *Kinesiology for the Occupational Therapy Assistant: Essential Components of Function and Movement, Third Edition* (pp. 329-331).

TABLE B-1 (CONTINUED)
Range of Motion Norms for the Upper Extremity

JOINT	JOINT MOTION	RANGE OF MOTION (DEGREES)
Wrist	Flexion	0 to 60
	Extension (also referred to as hyperextension)	0 to 60
	Ulnar deviation	0 to 30
	Radial deviation	0 to 20
Finger digits 2 to 5 metacarpophalangeal	Flexion	0 to 90
	Extension	Extension is the return to 0
	Hyperextension	0 to 20
	Abduction	0 to 20*
	Adduction	Adduction is the return to 0 with fingers touching each other
Proximal interphalangeal	Flexion	0 to 100
	Extension	Extension is the return to 0
Distal interphalangeal	Flexion	0 to 70
	Extension	Extension is the return to 0
	Hyperextension	0 to 30
Thumb metacarpophalangeal	Flexion	0 to 60
	Extension	Extension is the return to 0
Interphalangeal	Flexion	0 to 80
	Extension	Extension is the return to 0
	Hyperextension	0 to 30

*Identified from Latella, D., & Meriano, C. (2003). *Occupational therapy manual for the evaluation of range of motion and muscle strength.* Delmar Carnage Learning.

Adapted from American Medical Association. (2008). *Guides to the evaluation of permanent impairment* (6th ed.). Author.

TABLE B-2

Range of Motion Norms for the Lower Extremity

JOINT	JOINT MOTION	RANGE OF MOTION (DEGREES)
Hip	Flexion	0 to 100
	Extension (also referred to as hyperextension)	0 to 30*
	Abduction	0 to 25
	Adduction	Adduction is the return to 0
	Internal rotation	0 to 20
	External rotation	0 to 30
Knee	Flexion	0 to 110
	Extension	Extension is the return to 0
Ankle	Plantarflexion	0 to 50
	Dorsiflexion	0 to 10
	Eversion	0 to 10
	Inversion	0 to 20
Lesser toes (2 to 5) metatarsophalangeal	Flexion	0 to 40*
	Extension	Extension is the return to 0*
	Adduction	Adduction is the return to 0
	Abduction	Compare to opposite side*
Lesser toes (2 to 5) proximal interphalangeal	Flexion	0 to 35
	Extension	Extension is the return to 0*
Lesser toes (2 to 5) distal interphalangeal	Flexion	0 to 60*
	Extension	Extension is the return to 0*
Great toe (1) metatarsophalangeal	Flexion	0 to 45
	Extension	Extension is the return to 0*
Great toe (1) interphalangeal	Flexion	0 to 20
	Extension	Extension is the return to 0*

*Identified from Latella, D., & Meriano, C. (2003). *Occupational therapy manual for the evaluation of range of motion and muscle strength*. Delmar Carnage Learning.

Adapted from American Medical Association. (2008). *Guides to the evaluation of permanent impairment* (6th ed.). Author.

Epilogues of Occupational Profiles

Chapter 5—Terrence

Occupational Therapy Plan of Care

Terrence was seen in outpatient occupational therapy five times per week for the first 2 weeks and then three times per week for the following 4 weeks. Terrence remained at the assisted-living facility while he was receiving occupational therapy. His discharge from occupational therapy was determined by his input, progress in occupational therapy, third-party payer approval of occupational therapy services, and report from staff at the assisted-living facility.

Terrence remained at the facility upon discharge with no further occupational therapy recommended. Occupational therapy recommended continued assistance as needed with activities of daily living (ADLs) and simple instrumental activities of daily living (IADLs) to facilitate safe functional ability. It was recommended that Terrence did not need 24-hour supervision and assistance. A summary of his goals and functional outcome follows.

Occupational Therapy Outcomes

Short-Term Goals:

1. Client will demonstrate safe and independent use of power seat functions of tilt, recline, elevator, and leg elevation by 2 weeks. **Goal met**—Terrence demonstrated appropriate use of a powered mobility wheelchair by 2 weeks.

2. Client will demonstrate safe and proficient use of power mobility device including on and off, steering, and navigating doorways and areas where furniture is in close proximity by 2 weeks. **Goal met**—Terrence demonstrated appropriate use of a powered mobility wheelchair by 2 weeks.

3. Client will be safe and independent in sit-to-stand transfers using the seat elevator to assist by 2 weeks. **Goal met**—Terrence demonstrated independence with seat elevator in sit-to-stand by 2 weeks.

4. Client will demonstrate improved endurance with use of power mobility device by 2 weeks in order to finish eating meal in dining area without need for breaks. **Goal met**—Terrence reports improved engagement in daily tasks of interest by 2 weeks.

5. Client will demonstrate improved sitting posture by 2 weeks in order to raise arms overhead for hair grooming. **Goal met**—Terrence reports independently brushing hair.

Sain, S. J., & Roller, C. L. *Kinesiology for the Occupational Therapy Assistant: Essential Components of Function and Movement, Third Edition* (pp. 333-341). © 2024 Taylor & Francis Group.

Long-Term Goals:

1. Client will prevent the development of pressure injuries and orthopedic deformities by discharge. **Goal met**—No pressure injury or orthopedic deformity developed.

2. Client will be independent in pressure relief with power wheelchair features after instruction by 4 weeks. **Goal met**—Terrence was able to demonstrate pressure relief techniques with power wheelchair by 4 weeks.

3. Client will be independent and safe in sit-to-stand transfers using appropriately placed grab bars in the bathroom by discharge. **Goal met**—Terrence was independently able to use grab bars in bathroom for upper extremity (UE) support during standing, dynamic standing, and stand pivot transfers.

4. Client will demonstrate improved respiration with appropriate use of tilt and recline position by 4 weeks in order to improve endurance for simple meal preparation. **Goal not met**—While Terrence was able to demonstrate appropriate use of the tilt and recline position on the wheelchair, he continues to present with impaired respiration upon exertion similar to nonuse of the tilt and recline position.

5. Client will demonstrate improved social interactions secondary to improved endurance and improved posture by 4 weeks in order to engage in groups at the university and assisted-living center. **Goal met**—Terrence was able to resume his prior patterns of activities at the assisted-living facility and was able to return to his prior level of ability in daily tasks.

6. Client will demonstrate decreased risk for falling during transfers by discharge. **Goal met**—No incidents while at facility.

Occupational Therapy Services Provided

Occupational therapy services provided included ADLs, simple IADL tasks, therapeutic activities, therapeutic exercise, safety, standing balance, functional transfers, activity tolerance, and graded functional tasks. Occupational therapy services provided for wheelchair seating and positioning follow.

The occupational therapy practitioner recommended a power mobility device for the client after taking linear and angular measurements and determining the client's needs, goals, functional skills, and activities. Terrence sits with a flexible posterior pelvic tilt, slight obliquity to the right, and minimal rotation on the right. He exhibits mild thoracic kyphosis and mild cervical hyperextension. Having a flexible posterior pelvic tilt suggests that he is able to be supported into a neutral or anterior pelvic tilt. Once he is supported into a neutral pelvic tilt, the thoracic kyphosis is minimized

and consequently realigns the cervical spine. Thus, from an anterior-to-posterior view, his weight can be more evenly distributed across his femurs. Remember, when one is in a posterior pelvic tilt, greater pressure is placed on the ischial tuberosities, thus increasing the risk of pressure injury development. Additionally, a posture of posterior pelvic tilt creates an overstretch to the latissimus dorsi, brings the arms into internal rotation, and limits the ability of the arms to reach above shoulder level.

The wheelchair has the following characteristics: mid-wheel drive, power mobility with power tilt, recline, and elevating leg rest. It is necessary that his wheelchair and seating system allow Terrence to be repositioned with power seat functions to prevent increased risk of orthopedic deformities and pressure injuries. Improving his posture would allow greater access to his environment by improving his ability to reach. He will have less difficulty drinking from a glass, combing his hair, and reaching in front of his body to retrieve items.

Also recommended is a swing away joystick mounted on the right. The occupational therapy practitioner recommended an air-filled pressure-distributing seat cushion that fits into the seat and a supportive back rest with lateral support built into the back rest. Additionally, a pelvic positioning belt was recommended to maintain his posture in the chair, a lap tray for improved weight bearing for his UEs, and a head rest for use while in a tilted or reclined position.

Chapter 6—Betty

Occupational Therapy Plan of Care

Betty was seen in occupational therapy seven times per week for the first 4 weeks and then five times per week for the following 2 weeks. Betty returned home after 6 weeks in the long-term care facility. Betty's discharge was determined by information provided by the rehabilitation team, her progress in therapy, her desire to return home, and family support to provide the assistance needed to return home. A summary of her goals and functional outcome follow.

Betty was discharged to home with orders for continued outpatient occupational therapy. It was recommended that she not drive until further occupational therapy or until cleared by her physician. Occupational therapy further recommends continued assistance as needed with simple IADLs to facilitate return to home. It was recommended that Betty did not need 24-hour assistance. Betty's family and friends coordinated assistance for simple IADL tasks and transportation needs. Her family installed grab bars in the bathroom to increase independence and safety with ADLs.

Occupational Therapy Outcomes

Short-Term Goals:

1. Client will be educated in and demonstrate independence with a home exercise program for increased left UE functional ability within 1 week. **Goal met**—Betty was trained in daily tasks she could perform to increase the use of her left UE.

2. Client will demonstrate supervision with stand pivot transfers using adaptive equipment appropriately by 2 weeks. **Goal met**—Betty demonstrated supervision with stand pivot transfers consistently by the end of 2 weeks.

3. Client will demonstrate supervision with standing balance to sweep floors by 2 weeks. **Goal met**—Betty demonstrated static standing ability by 2 weeks.

4. Client will demonstrate modified independence to supervision with all ADL tasks by 2 weeks. **Goal met**—Betty demonstrated independence with self-feeding, grooming, upper body dressing, and upper body bathing. Betty demonstrates supervision with lower body dressing, lower body bathing, and self-toileting due to concern for safety with standing balance.

Long-Term Goals:

1. Client will demonstrate modified independence with all functional stand pivot transfers by discharge. **Goal met**—Betty demonstrated modified independence with functional transfers due to the use of adaptive equipment (i.e., rolling walker and ankle-foot orthotic).

2. Client will demonstrate modified independence with self-care tasks using bilateral UEs by discharge. **Goal met**—Betty demonstrates the ability to complete ADL tasks using her bilateral UEs. Betty independently completes her upper body ADL tasks but requires modified independence with lower body ADL tasks due to adaptive equipment and methods for success. Examples include using grab bars for UE support during self-toileting when standing. She also uses a cane and rolling walker for UE support during standing for lower extremity (LE) dressing.

3. Client will demonstrate MMT and grip pinch strength within functional limits (WFL) in the left UE by discharge. **Goal not met**—Betty demonstrated significantly improved UE ability; however, she demonstrated and reported continued problems using her left UE as prior to onset. She stated at discharge, "I'm really disappointed that I can't move my left arm like I used to." Betty was able to demonstrate at discharge left UE active range of motion (AROM) at full available range of motion (ROM) with MMT left shoulder grossly 3+/5. Betty continues to demonstrate left UE impaired sequencing of muscle synergies and delayed initiation of muscle contractions. She displays no continued increased tone in the left UE.

4. Client will demonstrate modified independence with simple home management tasks by discharge. **Goal met**—Betty demonstrated safety and the ability to make simple meals, wash and fold clothes, and sweep the floor. Betty reported continued difficulty with vacuuming with supervision needed for dynamic standing balance safety. Betty did not demonstrate adequate driving ability to return to self-driving.

Occupational Therapy Services Provided

Betty's occupational therapy included the use of ADL and IADL retraining, therapeutic activities, therapeutic exercise, functional transfers, neuro re-education, caregiver and client education and training, and graded functional tasks. An occupational therapy assistant provided treatment for client education on adaptive methods to complete self-care tasks and to don and doff her ankle-foot orthotic. Education also included a home exercise program to improve left UE functional ability, safety, use of adaptive equipment, and functional transfer ability. Therapeutic exercise and therapeutic activities included AROM and passive range of motion (PROM), exercises, and physical agent modalities (PAMs) of electrical stimulation to enhance movement, decrease pain, and improve functional use. Neuro re-education in the form of neurodevelopmental treatment was provided to also improve left UE functional ability.

Occupation-based treatment approaches were also used. Betty completed ADL tasks using her affected left UE. She also completed functional transfers as needed to complete functional tasks, such as transferring into the wheelchair and onto the commode. Betty also performed simple IADL tasks to ensure ability upon return home. Overall, Betty demonstrated good progress toward occupational therapy goals.

Chapter 7—Linda

Occupational Therapy Plan of Care

Linda was seen in occupational therapy three times per week the first 3 weeks, two times per week for the following 3 weeks, and then one time per week for an additional 3 weeks. Linda was discharged to home with a home exercise program after a total of 9 weeks (18 sessions). Her discharge from occupational therapy was determined with input from Linda, the doctor, and recommendations from the occupational therapy practitioner based on her progress in therapy. The Medicare outpatient cap on occupational therapy services also influenced Linda's time in therapy. A summary of her goals and functional outcomes follows.

Occupational Therapy Outcomes

Short-Term Goals:

1. Client will be instructed in and comply with a home exercise program within 2 weeks. **Goal met**—Linda was instructed in a home exercise program within the first week of therapy consisting of daily tasks she could perform to increase use of her right UE. She demonstrated compliance by performing her home exercise program during the therapy session within 2 weeks.

2. Client will decrease pain from 3/10 to 0/10 at rest and will be able to sleep through the night within 4 weeks by sleeping on her left side or back and using a pillow under her right shoulder. **Goal met**—Linda reported she had no pain in her right shoulder at rest after 4 weeks of therapy. She demonstrated the use of postural changes at night and reported improved sleeping habits within 4 weeks.

3. Client will decrease pain from 8/10 to 4/10 at worst with transferring grandchildren out of car seats within 4 weeks by using modified lifting techniques. **Goal met**—Linda reported her pain had decreased with transferring her grandchildren out of car seats and changing her granddaughter's diapers to a 3/10 at worst after 4 weeks.

4. Client will increase AROM in all limited planes of right shoulder ROM by 10 degrees within 3 weeks. **Goal met**—Linda presented with increased right UE AROM within 3 weeks. Glenohumeral (GH) joint flexion was 100 degrees (an increase of 25 degrees); GH joint abduction was 75 degrees (an increase of 15 degrees); GH joint external rotation was 35 degrees (an increase of 10 degrees); and GH joint internal rotation was 45 degrees (an increase of 10 degrees).

5. Client will increase right grip strength by 5 pounds within 4 weeks. **Goal met**—Linda presented with an increase in her right grip to 50 pounds (an increase of 5 pounds) within 4 weeks.

6. Client will be able to perform donning/doffing of bra using right UE independently and with fewer complaints of pain within 4 weeks. **Goal met**—Linda demonstrated the ability to perform donning/doffing of bra using her right dominant UE independently with only minimal reports of discomfort within 4 weeks.

Long-Term Goals:

1. Client will demonstrate compliance and independence in home exercise program at discharge. **Goal met**—Linda demonstrated independence and compliance in a home exercise program that was modified to accommodate her progress. She was discharged with a structured, progressive home exercise program.

2. Client will be independent with use of right UE in self-care and occupational roles with only minimal complaints of discomfort within 3 months. **Goal met**—Linda demonstrated independent use of the right UE in domains of occupation at discharge. She reported only minimal discomfort when reaching overhead or placing her granddaughter in the car seat.

3. Client will demonstrate AROM in right shoulder and right grip strength to WFL within 3 months. **Goal met**—Linda demonstrated grip and AROM to WFL, even though she was slightly limited in all planes of right GH joint motion compared to her left shoulder.

Occupational Therapy Services Provided

Linda's occupational therapy included the use of ADL and IADL retraining, client education and training, therapeutic activities, therapeutic exercises, and graded functional tasks. An occupational therapy assistant with training and experience in the UE provided treatment for client education on adaptive methods to complete grooming, toileting, and donning and doffing her bra. Education consisted of a home exercise program and protection principles, which included sleeping postures and proper lifting and reaching techniques. The occupational therapy assistant also provided therapeutic exercise and therapeutic activities including AROM, active assist ROM, and PROM exercises. PAMs of electrical stimulation and ultrasound were implemented to decrease pain, stimulate tissue healing, and enhance movement for improved functional use. Graded functional tasks included upper body dressing, folding clothes, and reaching in a cabinet.

Linda demonstrated the use of occupation-based treatment approaches in therapy to ensure independent use of her right dominant UE upon discharge. She was able to perform all domains of occupation independently, including caring for her grandchildren after occupational therapy discharge. Overall, Linda demonstrated excellent progress toward her occupational therapy goals.

Chapter 8—David

Occupational Therapy Plan of Care

David was seen in occupational therapy three times per week for the first 3 weeks, two times per week for the following 3 weeks, and one time per week for an additional 6 weeks for a total of 12 weeks (21 treatment sessions). The number of visits and date of discharge were determined by several factors, including the doctor's orders, therapist's recommendations, and David's progress in therapy. His work schedule and insurance coverage also influenced his number of therapy visits. A summary of David's goals and functional outcomes follows.

Occupational Therapy Outcomes

Short-Term Goals:

1. Client will be instructed in and comply with a home exercise program within 2 weeks. **Goal met**—David demonstrated compliance and independence in a home exercise program within 2 weeks.

2. Client will present with decreased pain from 7/10 to 3/10 at worst during tool use and lifting tasks at work within 4 weeks by using modified lifting techniques, adapting tool handles, using cold modalities, and performing stretches. **Goal met**—David demonstrated less pain in the right elbow during tool use and lifting tasks at work using adaptive tools, protection principles, modalities, and stretches within 4 weeks. Pain during the resistive functional tasks was rated at a 3/10 at worst.

3. Client will increase right grip strength by 5 pounds with report of no greater pain within 4 weeks. **Goal met**—David demonstrated an increase in right grip strength to 100 pounds in the standard position and 85 pounds in the stressed position within 4 weeks with no increase in pain.

4. Client will be able to drive his truck and brush his teeth using his dominant hand with no complaints of pain in the right elbow within 3 weeks. **Goal not met**—David demonstrated the ability to brush his teeth without elbow pain but continued to report pain with driving tasks after 3 weeks.

5. Client will be able to work with a 20-pound lifting restriction on the right UE and fewer complaints of pain in the right elbow within 6 weeks. **Goal met**—David demonstrated the ability to return to his job at work with a 20-pound lifting restriction and only complained of 3/10 pain in the right elbow at the end of his workday within 6 weeks.

Long-Term Goals:

1. Client will demonstrate compliance and independence in a home exercise program at discharge. **Goal met**—David demonstrated compliance and independence in a structured and progressive home exercise program at discharge.

2. Client will be independent in self-care and occupational roles using the right UE with no complaints of pain and utilization of ergonomic considerations within 12 weeks. **Goal met**—David was able to perform ADL and IADL tasks independently and with no reports of pain in his right elbow. David was able to drive, work with no restrictions and practice baseball with his son using protection principles at discharge. He did choose to delay the remodeling project at home for 3 months to rest his injured right arm.

3. Client will demonstrate MMT and grip pinch strength WFL in the right UE within 12 weeks. **Goal met**—David presented with right wrist extensor strength grossly 5/5 with MMT. His right grip improved to 110 pounds in the standard position and 115 pounds in the stressed position. His right palmar pinch improved to 25 pounds.

4. Client will demonstrate the ability to fish without pain in his right UE at discharge. **Goal met**—David demonstrated the ability to participate in the leisure occupation of fishing independently with no pain at discharge.

Occupational Therapy Services Provided

David's occupational therapy included client education and instruction in adaptive equipment, protection principles, and ergonomic considerations. His occupational therapy treatment included therapeutic activities, therapeutic exercises, and graded functional tasks including work conditioning. An occupational therapy assistant experienced and trained in UE injuries provided treatment including tool adaptation and proper body mechanics during lifting and tool use. The occupational therapy assistant educated David in a structured home exercise program including friction massage, tennis elbow stretching, the use of cold, and bracing to decrease pain and inflammation and to increase healing. Therapeutic exercises and activities included ROM, strengthening, and PAMs of ultrasound and cold to decrease pain for improved functional use.

Occupation-based treatment included graded functional tasks during work conditioning of casting a fishing rod and using a hammer and power screwdriver.

At the time of discharge, David was able to participate in his occupational roles of father, carpenter, and fisherman independently and without pain. Overall, David demonstrated excellent progress, meeting all of his occupational therapy goals at discharge.

Chapter 9—Laura

Occupational Therapy Plan of Care

Laura was seen in occupational therapy three times per week for the first 4 weeks. Due to complications from her injury, there was an interruption in Laura's therapy for 3 weeks. After 4 weeks in occupational therapy and continued complaints of weakness, stiffness, and numbness in the median nerve distribution of her left hand, she received a nerve conduction study that revealed moderate carpal tunnel syndrome. Laura received surgical release of the carpal tunnel and resumed occupational therapy at 2 weeks after her surgery. She continued therapy three times per week for 3 weeks and then two times per week for the following 2 weeks. Laura completed a total of 25 therapy sessions, 12 before her carpal tunnel release and 13 after surgery. She was discharged at the 3-month mark from beginning occupational therapy, or 5.5 months after her fall resulting in a Colles fracture of the left wrist. Discharge was based on a team decision involving Laura, her doctor, and the occupational therapy practitioner. It was difficult for Laura to attend therapy the first 2 weeks because she was unable to drive and had to rely on family and friends for her transportation. A summary of Laura's goals and her functional outcomes follow.

Occupational Therapy Outcomes

Short-Term Goals:

1. Client will be instructed in and comply with a home exercise program within 2 weeks. **Goal met**—Laura demonstrated compliance and independence in a home exercise program given to her by the occupational therapy practitioner within 2 weeks by performing in-home therapy sessions.

2. Client will tolerate a formal evaluation of left grip and pinch strength when able and appropriate or within 4 weeks. **Goal met**—Laura demonstrated the ability to tolerate an assessment of her left grip and pinch strength within 4 weeks.

3. Client will demonstrate the ability to grade students' papers using the left, dominant hand and adaptive writing implements within 3 weeks. **Goal met**—Laura demonstrated the ability to return to her occupational role of teacher after 3 weeks. She was able to drive to work with a left wrist brace in place, and she was able to grade papers using a gel pen with an enlarged rubber grip.

4. Client will demonstrate self-feeding with the left hand and adaptive utensils within 2 weeks. **Goal met**—Laura demonstrated the ability to feed herself using her left dominant hand after using adaptive foam or pipe insulation to enlarge the handles of her fork and spoon.

5. Client will demonstrate decreased edema by 30 mL using edema control techniques of elevation, AROM, and wearing of an Isotoner glove within 3 weeks. **Goal met**—Laura demonstrated a 50 mL reduction in edema in the left hand and wrist within 3 weeks, which allowed her to make a straight fist, experience less pain, and drive to her teaching position.

6. Client will demonstrate an increase in AROM in all limited joints by 5 degrees each in 4 weeks. **Goal met**—Laura demonstrated an increase of more than 5 degrees in all limited joints of her forearm, wrist, thumb, and fingers by the end of 4 weeks.

Long-Term Goals:

1. Client will demonstrate compliance and independence in a home exercise program at discharge. **Goal met**—Laura demonstrated compliance and independence in a modified and progressive home exercise program at discharge.

2. Client will be independent in self-care and occupational roles using the left dominant hand and adaptive equipment within 3 months. **Goal met**—Laura demonstrated the ability to perform all occupational roles independently using her left dominant UE and adaptive equipment at discharge. She was able to perform grooming and household activities as well as drive to work and perform the duties of a teacher, including computer use and writing tasks, at discharge.

3. Client will demonstrate AROM to WFL in left forearm, wrist, and thumb and demonstrate a straight fist in left hand within 3 months. **Goal met**—Laura was able to perform all functional roles independently, showing gains in AROM to WFL in the left UE. However, she continued to show a limitation in AROM compared to her right UE, especially in forearm supination, wrist extension, ulnar deviation, and thumb flexion at discharge.

4. Client will demonstrate a decrease in edema by 50 mL in the left hand volumetrically in 3 months. **Goal met**—Laura's whole-hand edema had decreased by 75 mL when measured volumetrically at discharge.

5. Client will demonstrate functional ROM in left dominant hand by resuming her leisure activity of knitting in 3 months. **Goal met**—Laura demonstrated functional AROM in her left hand and wrist by discharge. She was enjoying knitting again and was making a scarf for her granddaughter at discharge.

Occupational Therapy Services Provided

Laura's occupational therapy included client education and instruction in adaptive equipment, therapeutic activities, therapeutic exercises, and graded functional tasks. An occupational therapy assistant trained and experienced in hand and wrist injuries provided treatment, including instruction in edema control techniques, compensatory techniques, and a home exercise program. Treatment in occupational therapy also included the use of adaptive equipment, therapeutic exercises and activities, AROM and PROM, and PAMs of electrical stimulation to decrease edema, enhance movement, and decrease pain for improved functional use.

Occupation-based treatment approaches were used. Laura completed tasks in therapy such as feeding, writing, and peeling vegetables to prepare for independent participation with occupational roles at home and work. Overall, Laura demonstrated excellent progress toward her occupational therapy goals.

Chapter 10—Sara

Occupational Therapy Plan of Care

Sara was seen in occupational therapy three times per week for 2 weeks, then two times per week for 4 weeks. Sara was discharged to a home exercise program after a total of 6 weeks (14 total sessions). The number of visits and date of discharge were determined by several factors, including the doctor's orders, recommendation from the occupational therapy practitioner, insurance coverage, and Sara's progress in therapy as well as her input. A summary of her goals and functional outcomes follows.

Occupational Therapy Outcomes

Short-Term Goals:
1. Client will be instructed in and comply with a home exercise program within 2 weeks. **Goal met**—Sara demonstrated compliance and independence in a home exercise program within 2 weeks.
2. Client will tolerate a formal evaluation of right grip and pinch strength when able and appropriate or within 3 weeks. **Goal met**—Sara demonstrated the ability to tolerate an assessment of her right grip and lateral three-jaw chuck and tip pinch strength within 3 weeks.
3. Client will be able to brush teeth with right hand using a toothbrush with an adapted handle within 2 weeks. **Goal met**—Sara demonstrated the ability to brush her teeth using her right hand and a power toothbrush with a wider handle within 2 weeks.
4. Client will demonstrate self-feeding with the right hand using adaptive utensils within 1 week. **Goal met**—Sara demonstrated the ability to feed herself using her right dominant hand after using adaptive foam or pipe insulation to enlarge the handles of her fork and spoon within 1 week.

5. Client will demonstrate decreased edema by 0.5 cm in right thumb to help with buttoning within 3 weeks. **Goal met**—Sara presented with decreased edema by 0.6 cm after being remeasured circumferentially at the right interphalangeal (IP) thumb joint and demonstrated the ability to button her shirt using both hands within 3 weeks.
6. Client will demonstrate an increase in AROM in right thumb by 5 degrees in metacarpophalangeal (MCP) and IP flexion and radial and palmar abduction. To be able to fully adduct thumb and to increase end stage opposition on the Kapandji scale from 3/10 to 6/10 to assist with dressing activities within 3 weeks. **Goal met**—Sara demonstrated more than a 5 degree increase in AROM of right thumb. She showed an increase in MCP flexion to 15 degrees, 30 degrees in IP flexion, 25 degrees in palmar abduction, and 37 degrees in radial abduction. She was able to fully adduct her thumb and oppose her thumb to the pad of her small finger. She was able to dress herself except for tying her tennis shoes within 3 weeks.

Long-Term Goals:
1. Client will demonstrate compliance and independence in a progressive home exercise program at discharge. **Goal met**—Sara demonstrated compliance and independence in a modified and progressive home exercise program at discharge.
2. Client will be independent in self-care tasks and occupational roles using right dominant hand and adaptive tools within 6 weeks. **Goal met**—Sara demonstrated the ability to perform all self-care tasks and occupational roles at home independently using her right hand and adaptive equipment at discharge. She was able to return to her job wearing a thumb brace and following lifting restrictions at discharge.
3. Client will demonstrate an increase in AROM in MCP and IP joint flexion by 30 degrees within 6 weeks to be independent in buttoning pants and tying shoes. **Goal met**—Sara demonstrated an increase in right thumb flexion by a total of 42 degrees and the ability to button her jeans and tie her shoes using her right hand as the dominant hand in bilateral activities at discharge.
4. Client will be able to return to work with 40-pound lifting restriction within 6 weeks. **Goal met**—Sara demonstrated the ability to perform her driving and food service duties at work requiring lifting up to 40 pounds at discharge.

5. Client will demonstrate the ability to knit and crochet for 30 minutes at a time with no pain within 6 weeks. **Goal met**—Sara demonstrated the ability to enjoy her leisure activity of knitting and crocheting for no more than 30 minutes at a time with no reported pain at discharge.

Occupational Therapy Services Provided

Sara's occupational therapy included client education and instruction in adaptive equipment, therapeutic activities, therapeutic exercises, and graded functional tasks. An occupational therapy assistant trained and experienced in hand injuries and diseases provided treatment, including instruction in edema and scar control techniques and a home exercise program. Treatment in occupational therapy also included the use of adaptive equipment, therapeutic exercises and activities, AROM and PROM, and PAMs of electrical stimulation and ultrasound to decrease edema and scar, to enhance movement and decrease pain for improved functional use. Occupational-based treatment approaches were used. Sara completed tasks in therapy such as feeding, writing, tying, buttoning, carrying trays, lifting boxes, and cooking to prepare for independent participation in occupational roles at home and work. Sara demonstrated excellent progress toward her occupational therapy goals and was able to return to work with a 40-pound lifting restriction after 6 weeks in therapy.

Chapter 12—Rachel

Occupational Therapy Plan of Care

Rachel was seen four times in 6 weeks for 1 hour each time. She was discharged with a home exercise program. Her discharge was determined with input from Rachel and recommendations from the occupational therapy practitioner based on her progress. A summary of her goals and functional outcomes follows.

Occupational Therapy Outcomes

Short-Term Goals:

1. Client will independently access a swimming pool via ladder, ramp, or stairs in 4 weeks to perform an exercise program. **Goal met**—Rachel independently accessed a pool via stairs with a railing.

2. Client will independently perform a home exercise program in the swimming pool in 4 weeks to increase LE strength. **Goal met**—Rachel demonstrated compliance and independence in a home exercise program at the pool within 4 weeks.

3. Client will demonstrate independence in three energy conservation techniques during an IADL task in 4 weeks. **Goal met**—Rachel demonstrated the ability to alternate heavy and light tasks throughout the day, prepare a weekly schedule for IADL tasks, and organize her workspace for ease of use.

4. Client will increase bilateral hip flexion strength to 3+/5 in 4 weeks to facilitate stepping up a curb. **Goal not met**—Rachel's LE strength did not improve after 4 weeks of participation in a home exercise program at the pool; however, she was compliant and motivated for the exercises so her strength may improve following discharge. At the time of discharge, Rachel was still unable to step up a curb independently.

Long-Term Goals:

1. Client will demonstrate increased occupational participation in valued leisure activities of yoga and swimming in 6 weeks. **Goal met**—Rachel participated in swimming four times over the course of 6 weeks as well as one yoga session. At discharge, Rachel's performance score on the Canadian Occupational Performance Measure improved from 3.8 to 5, and her satisfaction score changed from 2.4 to 4.6. An improvement of 2 or greater is considered clinically significant.

2. Client will be independent in home exercise program in 6 weeks. **Goal met**—Rachel was compliant with her home exercise program at the pool.

3. Client will be independent in energy conservation and work simplification techniques for all valued ADL, IADL, work, and leisure tasks in 6 weeks. **Goal met**—Rachel demonstrated the ability to adapt tasks and her routine to save energy and simplify tasks at both work and home.

4. Client will walk from her parking space to her office without falling or loss of balance in 6 weeks. **Goal not met**—Rachel continued to report loss of balance and inability to step up a curb when walking from parking space to office; however, she reported no falls in the 6-week period. At discharge, her Berg Balance score improved from 39/56 to 40/56, which continued to indicate medium fall risk.

Occupational Therapy Services Provided

Rachel's occupational therapy intervention included client education and instruction for fall prevention. An occupation-based treatment approach was used to focus on improving Rachel's occupational performance in her workplace and with IADLs in her home through energy conservation and work simplification techniques. She was instructed in an aquatic exercise program to increase LE strength and to encourage her return to her valued leisure activity of swimming. The occupational therapy practitioner also educated Rachel about the surgeries she had as a child and about health concerns such as fatigue, chronic pain, and joint deterioration that are common for adults with cerebral palsy (CP). Overall, Rachel demonstrated good progress toward her occupational therapy goals, meeting three out of four of her short-term goals and three out of four of her long-term goals. Due to her continued difficulty with LE pain, decreased LE strength, and declining gait, a referral was made to physical therapy. Additionally, due to her complaints of LE spasticity, a referral was made to a neurologist to consider Botox (botulinum toxin) injections for localized spasticity management.

Grip/Pinch and Testing Norms

Nine-Hole Peg Test Norm Scores

Table D-1 presents Nine-Hole Peg Test Average Male Participant Scores.
Table D-2 presents Nine-Hole Peg Test Average Female Participant Scores.

Box and Block Test Norm Scores

Table D-3 presents Box and Block Test Average Male Participant Scores.
Table D-4 presents Box and Block Test Average Female Participant Scores.

Grip And Pinch Norm Scores

Table D-5 presents Grip Strength Average Performance of Normal Subjects (ages 6-19).
Table D-6 presents Average Grip Strength Performance.
Table D-7 presents Average Tip Pinch Strength Performance.
Table D-8 presents Average Key Pinch Strength Performance.
Table D-9 presents Average Palmar Pinch Strength Performance.

Sain, S. J., & Roller, C. L. *Kinesiology for the Occupational Therapy Assistant: Essential Components of Function and Movement, Third Edition* (pp. 343-352). © 2024 Taylor & Francis Group.

TABLE D-1

Nine-Hole Peg Test Average and Standard Deviation of Male Participants' Scores (N = 314)

AGE	N	AVERAGE: RIGHT (seconds)	AVERAGE: LEFT (seconds)	STANDARD DEVIATION: RIGHT (seconds)	STANDARD DEVIATION: LEFT (seconds)
21 to 25	41	16.41	17.53	1.65	1.73
26 to 30	32	16.88	17.84	1.89	2.22
31 to 35	31	17.54	18.47	2.70	2.94
36 to 40	32	17.71	18.62	2.12	2.30
41 to 45	30	18.54	18.49	2.88	2.42
46 to 50	30	18.35	19.57	2.47	2.69
51 to 55	25	18.93	19.84	2.37	3.10
56 to 60	25	20.90	21.64	4.55	3.39
61 to 65	24	20.87	21.60	3.50	2.98
66 to 70	14	21.23	22.29	3.29	3.71
71+	25	25.79	25.95	5.60	4.54
All Male					
Subjects	314	18.99	19.79	3.91	3.66

Oxford, G. K., Vogel, K. A., Le, F., Mitchell, A., Muniz, S., & Vollmer, M. A. (2003). Brief report—Adult norms for a commercially available nine hole peg test for finger dexterity. *American Journal of Occupational Therapy, 57,* 570-573. Reproduced with permission from American Occupational Therapy Association in the format Textbook via Copyright Clearance Center.

TABLE D-2

Nine-Hole Peg Test Average and Standard Deviation of Female Participants' Scores (N = 389)

AGE	N	AVERAGE: RIGHT (seconds)	AVERAGE: LEFT (seconds)	STANDARD DEVIATION: RIGHT (seconds)	STANDARD DEVIATION: LEFT (seconds)
21 to 25	43	16.04	17.21	1.82	1.55
26 to 30	33	15.90	16.97	1.91	1.77
31 to 35	32	16.69	17.47	1.70	2.13
36 to 40	35	16.74	18.16	1.95	2.08
41 to 45	37	16.54	17.64	2.14	2.06
46 to 50	45	17.36	17.96	2.01	2.30
51 to 55	42	17.38	18.92	1.88	2.29
56 to 60	31	17.86	19.48	2.39	3.26
61 to 65	29	18.99	20.33	2.18	2.76
66 to 70	31	19.90	21.44	3.15	3.97
71+	31	22.49	24.11	6.02	5.66
All Female					
Subjects	389	17.67	18.91	3.17	3.44

TABLE D-3

Average Performance of Normal Males on the Box and Block Test (Number of Cubes Transferred in 1 Minute)

AGE	HAND	MEAN	SD	SE	LOW	HIGH
20 to 24	Right	88.2	8.8	1.6	70	105
	Left	86.4	8.5	1.6	70	102
25 to 29	Right	85.0	7.5	1.4	71	95
	Left	84.1	7.1	1.4	69	100
30 to 34	Right	81.9	9.0	1.7	68	96
	Left	81.3	8.1	1.6	69	99
35 to 39	Right	81.9	9.5	1.9	64	104
	Left	79.8	9.7	1.9	56	97
40 to 44	Right	83.0	8.1	1.6	69	101
	Left	80.0	8.8	1.7	59	93
45 to 49	Right	76.9	9.2	1.7	61	93
	Left	75.8	7.8	1.5	60	88
50 to 54	Right	79.0	9.7	1.9	62	106
	Left	77.0	9.2	1.8	60	97
55 to 59	Right	75.2	11.9	2.6	45	97
	Left	73.8	10.5	2.3	43	94
60 to 64	Right	71.3	8.8	1.8	52	84
	Left	70.5	8.1	1.6	47	82
65 to 69	Right	68.4	7.1	1.4	55	80
	Left	67.4	7.8	1.5	48	86
70 to 74	Right	66.3	9.2	1.8	50	86
	Left	64.3	9.8	1.9	45	84
75+	Right	63.0	7.1	1.4	47	75
	Left	61.3	8.4	1.7	46	74
All male subjects	Right	76.9	11.6	.66	45	106
	Left	75.4	11.4	.65	43	102

SD = standard deviation; SE = standard error.

Mathiowetz, V., Volland, G., Kashman, N., & Weber, K. (1985). Adult norms for the box and block test of manual dexterity. *American Journal of Occupational Therapy, 39* (6), 386-391. Reproduced with permission from American Occupational Therapy Association in the format Textbook via Copyright Clearance Center.

TABLE D-4

Average Performance of Normal Females on the Box and Block Test (Number of Cubes Transferred in 1 Minute)

AGE	HAND	MEAN	SD	SE	LOW	HIGH
20 to 24	Right	88.0	8.3	1.6	67	103
	Left	83.4	7.9	1.6	66	99
25 to 29	Right	86.0	7.4	1.4	63	96
	Left	80.9	6.4	1.2	63	93
30 to 34	Right	85.2	7.4	1.5	75	101
	Left	80.2	5.6	1.1	66	92
35 to 39	Right	84.8	6.1	1.2	71	95
	Left	83.5	6.1	1.2	72	97
40 to 44	Right	81.1	8.2	1.5	60	97
	Left	79.7	8.8	1.6	57	97
45 to 49	Right	82.1	7.5	1.5	68	99
	Left	78.3	7.6	1.5	59	91
50 to 54	Right	77.7	10.7	2.1	57	98
	Left	74.3	9.9	2.0	53	93
55 to 59	Right	74.7	8.9	1.8	56	94
	Left	73.6	7.8	1.6	54	85
60 to 64	Right	76.1	6.9	1.4	63	95
	Left	73.6	6.4	1.4	62	86
65 to 69	Right	72.0	6.2	1.2	60	82
	Left	71.3	7.7	1.4	61	89
70 to 74	Right	68.6	7.0	1.3	53	80
	Left	68.3	7.0	1.3	51	81
75+	Right	65.0	7.1	1.4	52	79
	Left	63.6	7.4	1.5	51	81
All female subjects	Right	78.4	10.4	.58	52	103
	Left	75.8	9.5	.53	51	99

SD = standard deviation; SE = standard error.

Mathiowetz, V., Volland, G., Kashman, N., & Weber, K. (1985). Adult norms for the box and block test of manual dexterity. *American Journal of Occupational Therapy, 39* (6), 386-391. Reproduced with permission from American Occupational Therapy Association in the format Textbook via Copyright Clearance Center.

TABLE D-5

Average Performance of Normal Subjects (Age 6-19) on Grip Strength (lbs)

AGE	HAND	MALES			FEMALES		
		Mean	*SD*	*Range*	*Mean*	*SD*	*Range*
6 to 7	Right	32.5	4.8	21 to 42	28.6	4.4	20 to 39
	Left	30.7	5.4	18 to 38	27.1	4.4	16 to 36
8 to 9	Right	41.9	7.4	27 to 61	35.3	8.3	18 to 55
	Left	39.0	9.3	19 to 63	33.0	6.9	16 to 49
10 to 11	Right	53.9	9.7	35 to 79	49.7	8.1	37 to 82
	Left	48.4	10.8	26 to 73	45.2	6.8	32 to 59
12 to 13	Right	58.7	15.5	33 to 98	56.8	10.6	39 to 79
	Left	55.4	16.9	22 to 107	50.9	11.9	25 to 76
14 to 15	Right	77.3	15.4	49 to 108	58.1	12.3	30 to 93
	Left	64.4	14.9	41 to 94	49.3	11.9	26 to 73
16 to 17	Right	94.0	19.4	64 to 149	67.3	16.5	23 to 126
	Left	78.5	19.1	41 to 123	56.9	14.0	23 to 87
18 to 19	Right	108.0	24.6	64 to 172	71.6	12.3	46 to 90
	Left	93.0	27.8	53 to 149	61.7	12.5	41 to 86

lbs = pounds; SD = standard deviation.

Mathiowetz, V., Wiemer, D., & Federman, S. (1986). Grip and pinch strength: Norms for 6- to 19-year-olds. *American Journal of Occupational Therapy, 40*(10), 705-711. Reproduced with permission from American Occupational Therapy Association in the format Textbook via Copyright Clearance Center.

TABLE D-6
Average Performance of All Subjects on Grip Strength (lbs)

AGE	HAND	MEN					WOMEN				
		Mean	SD	SE	Low	mm	Mean	SD	SE	Low	High
20 to 24	Right	121.0	20.6	3.8	91	167	70.4	14.5	2.8	46	95
	Left	104.5	21.8	4.0	71	150	61.0	13.1	2.6	33	88
25 to 29	Right	120.8	23.0	4.4	78	158	74.5	13.9	2.7	48	97
	Left	110.5	16.2	3.1	77	139	63.5	12.2	2.4	48	97
30 to 34	Right	121.8	22.4	4.3	70	170	78.7	19.2	3.8	46	137
	Left	110.4	21.7	4.2	64	145	68.0	17.7	3.5	36	115
35 to 39	Right	119.7	24.0	4.8	76	176	74.1	10.8	2.2	50	99
	Left	112.9	21.7	4.4	73	157	66.3	11.7	2.3	49	91
40 to 44	Right	116.8	20.7	4.1	84	165	70.4	13.5	2.4	38	103
	Left	112.8	18.7	3.7	73	157	62.3	13.8	2.5	35	94
45 to 49	Right	109.9	23.0	4.3	65	155	62.2	15.1	3.0	39	100
	Left	100.8	22.8	4.3	58	160	56.0	12.7	2.5	37	83
50 to 54	Right	121.0	20.6	3.8	91	167	70.4	14.5	2.8	46	95
	Left	101.9	17.0	3.4	70	143	57.3	10.7	2.1	35	76
55 to 59	Right	101.1	26.7	5.8	59	154	57.3	12.5	2.5	33	86
	Left	83.2	23.4	5.1	43	128	47.3	11.9	2.4	31	76
60 to 64	Right	89.7	20.4	4.2	51	137	55.1	10.1	2.0	37	77
	Left	76.8	20.3	4.1	27	116	45.7	10.1	2.0	29	66
65 to 69	Right	91.1	20.6	4.0	56	131	49.6	9.7	1.8	35	74
	Left	76.8	19.8	3.8	43	117	41.0	8.2	1.5	29	63
70 to 74	Right	75.3	21.5	4.2	32	108	49.6	11.7	2.2	33	78
	Left	64.8	18.1	3.7	32	93	41.5	10.2	1.9	23	67
75+	Right	65.7	21.0	4.2	40	135	42.6	11.0	2.2	25	65
	Left	55.0	17.0	3.4	31	119	37.6	8.9	1.7	24	61
All subjects	Right	104.3	28.3	1.6	32	176	62.8	17.0	0.96	25	137
	Left	93.1	27.6	1.6	27	160	53.9	15.7	.88	23	115

SD = standard deviation; SE = standard error.

This table was published in *Archives of Physical Medicine & Rehabilitation*, 66, Mathiowetz, V., Kashman, N., Volland, G., Weber, K., Dowe, M., & Rogers, S., "Grip and pinch strength: Normative data for adults." pp. 69-72, Copyright Elsevier (1985).

TABLE D-7
Average Performance of All Subjects on Tip Pinch (lbs)

AGE	HAND	MEN					WOMEN				
		Mean	SD	SE	Low	High	Mean	SD	SE	Low	High
20 to 24	Right	18.0	3.0	0.57	11	23	11.1	2.1	0.42	8	16
	Left	17.0	2.3	0.43	12	33	10.5	1.7	0.34	8	14
25 to 29	Right	18.3	4.4	0.84	10	34	11.9	1.8	0.35	8	16
	Left	17.5	5.2	0.99	12	36	11.3	1.8	0.35	9	18
30 to 34	Right	17.6	6.7	0.71	12	25	12.6	3.0	0.58	8	20
	Left	17.6	4.8	0.93	10	27	11.7	2.8	0.54	7	17
35 to 39	Right	18.0	3.6	0.73	12	27	11.6	2.5	0.50	8	19
	Left	17.7	3.8	0.76	10	24	11.9	2.4	0.47	8	16
40 to 44	Right	17.8	4.0	0.78	11	25	11.5	2.7	0.49	5	15
	Left	17.7	3.5	0.68	12	25	11.1	3.0	0.54	6	17
45 to 49	Right	18.7	4.9	0.92	12	30	13.2	3.0	0.60	9	19
	Left	17.6	4.1	0.77	12	28	12.1	2.7	0.55	7	18
50 to 54	Right	18.3	4.0	0.80	11	24	12.5	2.2	0.44	9	18
	Left	17.8	3.9	0.77	12	26	11.4	2.4	0.49	7	16
55 to 59	Right	15.0	3.7	0.81	10	26	10.4	1.4	0.29	8	13
	Left	16.6	3.3	0.73	11	24	11.7	1.7	0.34	9	16
60 to 64	Right	15.8	3.9	0.80	9	22	10.1	2.1	0.43	7	17
	Left	15.3	3.7	0.76	9	23	9.9	2.0	0.39	6	15
65 to 69	Right	17.0	4.2	0.81	11	27	10.6	2.0	0.39	7	15
	Left	15.4	2.9	0.55	10	21	10.5	2.4	0.45	7	17
70 to 74	Right	13.8	2.6	0.52	11	21	10.1	2.6	0.48	7	15
	Left	13.3	2.6	0.51	10	21	9.8	2.3	0.43	6	17
75+	Right	14.0	3.4	0.68	7	21	9.6	2.8	0.54	4	16
	Left	13.9	3.7	0.75	8	25	9.3	2.4	0.47	4	13
All subjects	Right	17.0	4.1	0.23	7	34	11.3	2.6	0.15	4	20
	Left	16.4	4.0	.023	8	36	10.8	2.4	0.14	4	18

SD = standard deviation; SE = standard error.

This table was published in *Archives of Physical Medicine & Rehabilitation*, 66, Mathiowetz, V., Kashman, N., Volland, G., Weber, K., Dowe, M., & Rogers, S., "Grip and pinch strength: Normative data for adults." pp. 69-72, Copyright Elsevier (1985).

TABLE D-8

Average Performance of All Subjects on Key Pinch (lbs)

AGE	HAND	MEN					WOMEN				
		Mean	*SD*	*SE*	*Low*	*High*	*Mean*	*SD*	*SE*	*Low*	*High*
20 to 24	Right	26.0	3.5	0.65	21	34	17.6	2.0	0.39	14	23
	Left	24.8	3.4	0.64	19	31	16.2	2.1	0.41	13	23
25 to 29	Right	26.7	4.9	0.94	19	41	17.7	2.1	0.41	14	22
	Left	25.0	4.4	0.85	19	39	16.6	2.1	0.41	13	22
30 to 34	Right	26.4	4.8	0.93	20	36	18.7	3.0	0.60	13	25
	Left	26.2	5.1	0.98	17	36	17.8	3.6	0.70	12	26
35 to 39	Right	26.1	3.2	0.65	21	32	16.6	2.0	0.40	12	21
	Left	25.6	3.9	0.77	18	32	16.0	2.7	0.53	12	22
40 to 44	Right	25.6	2.6	0.50	21	31	16.7	3.1	0.56	10	24
	Left	25.1	4.0	0.79	19	31	15.8	3.1	0.55	8	22
45 to 49	Right	25.8	3.9	0.73	19	35	17.6	3.2	0.65	13	24
	Left	24.8	4.4	0.84	18	42	16.6	2.9	0.58	12	24
50 to 54	Right	26.7	4.4	0.88	20	34	16.7	2.5	0.50	12	22
	Left	26.1	4.2	0.84	20	37	16.1	2.7	0.53	12	22
55 to 59	Right	24.2	4.2	0.92	18	34	15.7	2.5	0.50	11	21
	Left	23.0	4.7	1.02	13	31	14.7	2.2	0.44	12	19
60 to 64	Right	23.2	5.4	1.13	14	37	15.5	2.7	0.55	10	20
	Left	22.2	4.1	0.84	16	33	14.1	2.5	0.50	10	19
65 to 69	Right	23.4	3.9	0.75	17	32	15.0	2.6	0.49	10	21
	Left	22.0	3.6	0.70	17	28	14.3	2.8	0.53	10	20
70 to 74	Right	19.3	2.4	0.47	16	25	14.5	2.9	0.54	8	22
	Left	19.2	3.0	0.59	13	28	13.8	3.0	0.56	9	22
75+	Right	20.5	4.6	0.91	9	31	12.6	2.3	0.45	8	17
	Left	19.1	3.0	0.59	13	24	11.4	2.6	0.50	7	16
All subjects	Right	24.5	4.6	0.26	9	41	16.2	3.0	0.17	8	25
	Left	23.6	4.6	.026	11	42	15.3	3.1	0.18	7	26

SD = standard deviation; SE = standard error.

This table was published in *Archives of Physical Medicine & Rehabilitation*, 66, Mathiowetz, V., Kashman, N., Volland, G., Weber, K., Dowe, M., & Rogers, S., "Grip and pinch strength: Normative data for adults." pp. 69-72, Copyright Elsevier (1985).

TABLE D-9

Average Performance of All Subjects on Palmar Pinch (lbs)

AGE	HAND	MEN					WOMEN				
		Mean	*SD*	*SE*	*Low*	*High*	*Mean*	*SD*	*SE*	*Low*	*High*
20 to 24	Right	26.6	5.3	1.03	18	45	17.2	2.3	0.45	14	23
	Left	25.7	5.8	1.08	15	42	16.3	2.8	0.56	11	24
25 to 29	Right	26.0	4.3	0.84	19	35	17.7	3.2	0.62	13	29
	Left	25.1	4.2	0.82	19	36	17.0	3.0	0.58	13	26
30 to 34	Right	24.7	4.7	0.91	16	34	19.3	5.0	0.99	12	34
	Left	25.4	5.7	1.10	15	37	18.1	4.8	0.94	12	32
35 to 39	Right	26.2	4.1	0.83	19	36	17.5	4.2	0.85	13	29
	Left	25.9	5.4	1.17	14	40	17.1	3.4	0.69	12	24
40 to 44	Right	24.5	4.3	0.85	17	37	17.0	3.1	0.56	10	23
	Left	24.8	4.9	0.96	15	37	16.6	3.5	0.63	10	25
45 to 49	Right	24.0	3.3	0.63	19	33	17.9	3.0	0.60	12	27
	Left	23.7	3.8	0.71	18	33	17.5	2.8	0.57	12	24
50 to 54	Right	23.8	5.4	1.08	15	36	17.3	3.1	0.63	12	23
	Left	24.0	5.8	1.16	16	36	16.4	2.9	0.59	12	22
55 to 59	Right	23.7	4.8	1.06	16	34	16.0	3.1	0.63	11	26
	Left	21.3	4.5	0.99	12	8	15.4	3.0	0.61	11	21
60 to 64	Right	21.8	3.3	0.67	16	28	14.8	3.1	0.61	10	20
	Left	21.2	3.2	0.65	15	27	14.3	2.7	0.54	10	20
65 to 69	Right	21.4	3.0	0.58	15	25	14.2	3.1	0.59	8	20
	Left	21.2	4.1	0.80	14	30	13.7	3.4	0.64	8	22
70 to 74	Right	18.1	3.4	0.67	14	27	14.4	2.6	0.48	9	19
	Left	18.8	3.3	0.65	13	27	14.0	1.9	0.35	10	17
75+	Right	18.7	4.2	0.84	9	26	12.0	2.6	0.51	8	17
	Left	18.3	3.8	0.77	10	26	11.5	2.6	0.52	6	16
All subjects	Right	23.4	5.0	0.28	9	45	16.3	3.8	0.21	8	34
	Left	23.0	5.3	0.30	10	42	15.7	3.6	0.20	6	32

SD = standard deviation; SE = standard error.

This table was published in *Archives of Physical Medicine & Rehabilitation*, 66, Mathiowetz, V., Kashman, N., Volland, G., Weber, K., Dowe, M., & Rogers, S., "Grip and pinch strength: Normative data for adults," pp. 69-72, Copyright Elsevier (1985).

Financial Disclosures

Dr. Dana M. Howell reported no financial or proprietary interest in the materials presented herein.

Carolyn L. Roller reported no financial or proprietary interest in the materials presented herein.

Dr. Matthew J. Sabin reported no financial or proprietary interest in the materials presented herein.

Susan J. Sain reported no financial or proprietary interest in the materials presented herein.

Dr. Maribeth P. Vowell reported no financial or proprietary interest in the materials presented herein.

Index

abnormal atypical movement, 75

accessibility, 51

accessory motions, 25

active insufficiency, 51, 65-66

active range of motion, 75

activities, 1

activities of daily living, 1

activity demands, 15-16

activity limitations, 1, 267

adaptive motor behaviors, 75

afferent, 25

ambulation, 123

amphiarthrodial, 25

anatomical position, 25

anatomical snuff box, 203

antagonists, 149

anterior pelvic tilt, 97

anticipatory postural movements, 75, 83-84

areas of occupation, 1

arthrokinematic movement, 267

arthroplasty, 229

arthroscopy, 203

assessment, therapeutic exercise, healing, integration of, 280

assessment of body movement, 84-91

assistive technology, 283

atlas, 97

attrition rupture, 203

avascular necrosis, 203

avulsion fracture, 229

axis, 51, 97

backward pelvic rotation, 97

balance, 267

    therapeutic exercise, 278-279

balance/postural control, observation of, 103-105

base of support, 97

bed mobility, 283

beliefs, 1

    as client factor, 13-14

biaxial joint, 203

biomechanical model, 1

body functions, 1, 26-35, 75

    cardiovascular functions, 30-32

    movement-related functions, 27-30

    muscular functions, 32-34

    neuromuscular functions, 27-30

    respiratory system functions, 30-32

    skeletal functions, 34-35

body mechanics, 283

body movement, 75-96

    applications, 93

    assessment, 84-91

    gross manual muscle testing, 87-91

    gross range of motion, 85-87

    human movement for function, 76-84

        anticipatory postural movements, 83-84

        motor behavior, 78-80

        movement characteristics, 80-83

        Occupational Therapy Practice Framework: Domain and Process, Fourth Edition, 76-78

    measuring movement, 84-85

body structures, 1, 75, 107-116

    muscular system, 36-39

    nervous system, 35-36

    skeletal system, 39-43

boutonniere deformity, 229

Box and Block Test norm scores, 343

bridging, 283

buoyancy, 51

cardiovascular functions, 30-32

carpal tunnel syndrome, 229

carpometacarpal joint, 203

carrying angle, 179

center of gravity, 51, 97

central nervous system, 25

cerebrovascular accident, 135-136

cervical retraction, 97

cervical vertebrae, 108-109

characteristics of movement, 80-83

circumduction, 123, 203

client factors, 1, 13-14

    beliefs, 13-14

    spirituality, 13-14

    values, 13-14

close-pack position, 51, 67

closed environment, 283

closed kinematic chain, 51

coccygeal vertebrae, 109-111

Colles fracture, 203

community/home, mobility in, 287-292

    body mechanics, 290-292

    home vs. community environments, 288-290